Gastrointestinal Pathology

Editor

RONDELL P. GRAHAM

SURGICAL PATHOLOGY CLINICS

www.surgpath.theclinics.com

Consulting Editor
JASON L. HORNICK

December 2023 • Volume 16 • Number 4

ELSEVIER

1600 John F. Kennedy Boulevard • Suite 1800 • Philadelphia, Pennsylvania, 19103-2899

http://www.theclinics.com

SURGICAL PATHOLOGY CLINICS Volume 16, Number 4
December 2023 ISSN 1875-9181, ISBN-13: 978-0-443-18316-4

Editor: Taylor Hayes
Developmental Editor: Saswoti Nath

Surgical Pathology Clinics (ISSN 1875-9181) is published quarterly by Elsevier Inc., 360 Park Avenue South, New York, NY 10010. Months of issue are March, June, September, and December. Business and Editorial Office: Elsevier Inc., 1600 John F. Kennedy Blvd., Ste. 1800, Philadelphia, PA 19103-2899. Accounting and Circulation Offices: Elsevier Inc., 3251 Riverport Lane, Maryland Heights, MO 63043. Periodicals postage paid at New York, NY and at additional mailing offices. Subscription prices are $246.00 per year (US individuals), $354.00 per year (US institutions), $100.00 per year (US students/residents), $294.00 per year (Canadian individuals), $402.00 per year (Canadian Institutions), $295.00 per year (foreign individuals), $402.00 per year (foreign institutions), and $120.00 per year (international students/residents), $100.00 per year (Canadian students/residents). Foreign air speed delivery is included in all *Clinics'* subscription prices. All prices are subject to change without notice. **POSTMASTER:** Send address changes to *Surgical Pathology Clinics*, Elsevier, 3251 Riverport Lane, Maryland Heights, MO 63043. **Customer Service: 1-800-654-2452 (US). From outside the United States, call 1-314-447-8871. Fax: 1-314-447-8029. E-mail:** JournalsCustomerServiceusa@elsevier.com **(for print support)** and JournalsOnlineSupport-usa@elsevier.com **(for online support)**.

Reprints. For copies of 100 or more, of articles in this publication, please contact the Commercial Reprints Department, Elsevier Inc., 360 Park Avenue South, New York, NY 10010-1710. Tel. 212-633-3874; Fax: 212-633-3820; E-mail: reprints@elsevier.com.

Surgical Pathology Clinics of North America is covered in *MEDLINE/PubMed (Index Medicus)*.

Contributors

CONSULTING EDITOR

JASON L. HORNICK, MD, PhD
Director of Surgical Pathology and
Immunohistochemistry, Brigham and Women's
Hospital, Professor of Pathology, Harvard
Medical School, Boston, Massachusetts, USA

EDITOR

RONDELL P. GRAHAM, MBBS
Professor of Laboratory Medicine and
Pathology, Head of Section of GI/Liver
Pathology, Executive Vice Chair of Academics
and People, Division of Anatomic Pathology,
Consultant Lead for Lab Services and Partner
Development, Vice Chair of Test Development,
Department of Laboratory Medicine and
Pathology, Mayo Clinic, Rochester, Minnesota,
USA

AUTHORS

BENJAMIN MICHAEL ALLANSON, MBBS, FRCPA
Consultant Anatomical Pathologist,
Department of Anatomical Pathology,
PathWest, QEII Medical Centre, Nedlands,
Western Australia, Australia

ESTHER BARANOV, MD
Associate Pathologist, Brigham and Women's
Hospital, Instructor of Pathology, Harvard
Medical School, Boston, Massachusetts, USA

WON-TAK CHOI, MD, PhD
Associate Professor, Department of Pathology,
University of California, San Francisco, San
Francisco, California, USA

YURI FEDORIW, MD
Professor, Department of Pathology and
Laboratory Medicine, Lineberger
Comprehensive Cancer Center, University of
North Carolina School of Medicine, Chapel Hill,
North Carolina, USA

CYRIL FISHER, MD, DSc, FRCPath
Professor, Department of Pathology, University
Hospitals Birmingham NHS Foundation Trust,
Birmingham, United Kingdom; Division of
Molecular Pathology, The Institute of Cancer
Research, London, United Kingdom

CATHERINE E. HAGEN, MD
Assistant Professor, Department of Laboratory
Medicine and Pathology, Mayo Clinic,
Rochester, Minnesota, USA

DANIEL HOUGHTON, FRCPA, BMBS, PhD, BSc (Hons)
Consultant Anatomical Pathologist,
Department of Anatomical Pathology,
PathWest, QEII Medical Centre, Nedlands,
Western Australia, Australia

DIPTI M. KARAMCHANDANI, MD
Associate Professor, Department of Pathology,
The University of Texas Southwestern Medical
Center, Dallas, Texas, USA

MARIAN PRIYANTHI KUMARASINGHE, MBBS, MD, Dip Cytopath (RCPA), FRCPA
Consultant Pathologist, Clinical Professor,
Anatomical Pathology, PathWest, QEII
Medical Centre, School of Pathology and
Laboratory Medicine, UWA and Curtin
Medical School, Nedlands, Western Australia,
Australia

LAURA W. LAMPS, MD
Godfrey D. Stobbe Professor and Director of
Gastrointestinal Pathology, Department of
Pathology, University of Michigan, Ann Arbor,
Michigan, USA

KELSEY MCHUGH, MD
Assistant Professor, Department of
Pathology and Laboratory Medicine,
Mayo Clinic, Scottsdale, Arizona,
USA

JAMES MICHAEL MITCHELL, MD
Assistant Professor, Department of
Pathology, The University of Texas
Southwestern Medical Center, Dallas, Texas,
USA

JONATHAN A. NOWAK, MD, PhD
Associate Pathologist and Associate Director
of the Center for Advanced Molecular
Diagnostics, Brigham and Women's Hospital,
Assistant Professor of Pathology, Harvard
Medical School, Boston, Massachusetts,
USA

RISH K. PAI, MD, PhD
Professor, Department of Pathology and
Laboratory Medicine, Mayo Clinic, Scottsdale,
Arizona, USA

NICOLE C. PANARELLI, MD
Associate Professor of Pathology, Albert
Einstein College of Medicine, Bronx, New York,
USA

LIRON PANTANOWITZ, MD, MHA, PhD
Chair and Professor, Department of Pathology,
UPMC Shadyside Hospital, Pittsburgh,
Pennsylvania, USA

**TIMOTHY J. PRICE, MBBS, FRACP, DHlthSc
(Med)**
Professor, Department Medical Oncology, The
Queen Elizabeth Hospital and University of
Adelaide, Adelaide, South Australia, Australia

KHIN THWAY, MD, FRCPath
Sarcoma Unit, Royal Marsden Hospital,
Division of Molecular Pathology, The Institute
of Cancer Research, London, United Kingdom

LAURA M. WAKE, MD
Assistant Professor, Department of Pathology,
Johns Hopkins School of Medicine, Baltimore,
Maryland, USA

ALISHA D. WARE, MD
Assistant Professor, Department of Pathology
and Laboratory Medicine, University of North
Carolina School of Medicine, Chapel Hill, North
Carolina, USA

MUSTAFA YOUSIF, MD
Assistant Professor, Department of Pathology,
University of Michigan, Ann Arbor, Michigan,
USA

TAO ZHANG, MD
Surgical Pathology Fellow, Department of
Laboratory Medicine and Pathology, Mayo
Clinic, Rochester, Minnesota, USA

Contents

Preface: What's Coming Down the Tube: Current and Emerging Topics in Gastrointestinal Pathology
ix

Rondell P. Graham

Pathologic Evaluation of Therapeutic Biomarkers in Colorectal Adenocarcinoma
635

Esther Baranov and Jonathan A. Nowak

Molecular testing is an essential component of the pathologic evaluation of colorectal carcinoma providing diagnostic, prognostic, and predictive therapeutic information. Mismatch repair status evaluation is required for all tumors. Advanced and metastatic tumors also require determination of tumor mutational burden, *KRAS*, *NRAS*, and *BRAF* mutation status, *ERBB2* amplification status, and *NTRK* and *RET* gene rearrangement status to guide therapy. Multiple assays, including immunohistochemistry, microsatellite instability testing, *MLH1* promoter methylation, and next-generation sequencing, are typically needed. Pathologists must be aware of these requirements to optimally triage tissue. Advances in colorectal cancer molecular diagnostics will continue to drive refinements in colorectal cancer personalized therapy.

Deep Learning and Colon Cancer Interpretation: Rise of the Machine
651

Kelsey McHugh and Rish K. Pai

The rapidly evolving development of artificial intelligence (AI) has spurred the development of numerous algorithms that augment information obtained from routine pathologic review of hematoxylin and eosin-stained slides. AI tools that predict prognosis and underlying molecular alterations have been the focus of much of the research to date. The results of these studies highlight the tremendous potential of AI to enhance our pathology reports by providing rapid predictions of key features that influence therapy and outcomes.

What Therapeutic Biomarkers in Gastro-Esophageal Junction and Gastric Cancer Should a Pathologist Know About?
659

Marian Priyanthi Kumarasinghe, Daniel Houghton, Benjamin Michael Allanson, and Timothy J. Price

Malignancies of upper gastrointestinal tract are aggressive, and most locally advanced unresectable and metastatic cancers are managed by a combination of surgery and neoadjuvant/adjuvant chemotherapy and radiotherapy. Current therapeutic recommendations include targeted therapies based on biomarker expression of an individual tumor. All G/gastro-esophageal junction (GEJ) cancers should be tested for HER2 status as a reflex test at the time of diagnosis. Currently, testing for PDL 1 and mismatch repair protein status is optional. HER2 testing is restricted to adenocarcinomas only and endoscopic biopsies, resections, or cellblocks. Facilities should be available for performing validated immunohistochemical stains and in-situ hybridization techniques, and importantly, pathologists should be experienced with preanalytical and analytical issues and scoring criteria. Genomic profiling via next-generation sequencing (NGS) is another strategy that assess numerous mutations and other molecular events simultaneously, including HER2 amplification, MSS status, tumor mutation burden, and neurotrophic tropomyosin-receptor kinases gene fusions.

Artificial Intelligence-Enabled Gastric Cancer Interpretations: Are We There yet?   673

Mustafa Yousif and Liron Pantanowitz

The integration of digital pathology and artificial intelligence (AI) is revolutionizing pathology by providing pathologists with new tools to improve workflow, enhance diagnostic accuracy, and undertake novel discovery. The capability of AI to recognize patterns and features in digital images beyond human perception is particularly valuable, thereby providing additional information for prognostic and predictive purposes. AI-based tools diagnose gastric carcinoma in digital images, detect gastric carcinoma metastases in lymph nodes, automate Ki-67 scoring in gastric neuroendocrine tumors, and quantify tumor-infiltrating lymphocytes. This article provides an overview of all of these applications of AI pertaining to gastric cancer.

Characteristics, Reporting, and Potential Clinical Significance of Nonconventional Dysplasia in Inflammatory Bowel Disease   687

Won-Tak Choi

The term nonconventional dysplasia has been coined to describe several underrecognized morphologic patterns of epithelial dysplasia in inflammatory bowel disease (IBD), but to date, the full recognition of these newly characterized lesions by pathologists is uneven. The identification of nonconventional dysplastic subtypes is becoming increasingly important, as they often present as invisible/flat dysplasia and are more frequently associated with advanced neoplasia than conventional dysplasia on follow-up. This review describes the morphologic, clinicopathologic, and molecular characteristics of seven nonconventional subtypes known to date, as well as their potential significance in the clinical management of IBD patients.

Histopathologic Manifestations of Immune Checkpoint Inhibitor Therapy-Associated Gastrointestinal Tract Injury: A Practical Review   703

James Michael Mitchell and Dipti M. Karamchandani

Immune checkpoint inhibitors have revolutionized the management of many advanced cancers by producing robust remissions. They mostly target two immune regulatory pathways: cytotoxic T lymphocyte antigen-4 and programmed death-1 or its ligand. However, a flip side is the immune-related adverse events (irAEs) commonly affecting the gastrointestinal (GI) tract that can cause treatment interruptions or discontinuation. This practical review discusses the clinical and histopathologic findings of irAEs encountered in the luminal GI tract, along with histopathologic differentials that can mimic varied inflammatory, infectious, or other medication-associated etiologies and the importance of clinico-pathologic correlation for an accurate diagnosis.

Lymphomas and Amyloid in the Gastrointestinal Tract   719

Alisha D. Ware, Laura M. Wake, and Yuri Fedoriw

Lymphoproliferative disorders are a heterogeneous group of neoplasms with varying clinical, morphologic, immunophenotypic, and genetic characteristics. A subset of lymphomas have a proclivity for the gastrointestinal tract, although this region may also be involved by systemic lymphomas. In addition, a number of indolent lymphoproliferative disorders of the gastrointestinal tract have been defined over the past decade, and it is important to accurately differentiate these neoplasms to ensure that patients receive the proper management. Here, the authors review lymphoid neoplasms that show frequent gastrointestinal involvement and provide updates from the recent hematolymphoid neoplasm classification systems.

Gastrointestinal Biopsies in the Patient Post-Stem Cell Transplant: An Approach to
Diagnosis   745

Tao Zhang and Catherine E. Hagen

Graft-versus-host disease (GVHD) is a major complication of hematopoietic stem cell transplantation (SCT), leading to a significant morbidity and mortality. Histologically, gastrointestinal GVHD is characterized by crypt apoptosis and dropout. However, similar histologic features can also be seen in drug-induced injury and opportunistic infection. Knowledge of the timing of biopsy, patient medications, evidence of infection, and presence of GVHD at other organ sites can aid in the correct diagnosis and subsequent management of these patients. This review focuses on the pathologic differential diagnosis of apoptosis in gastrointestinal biopsies obtained from SCT patients.

Mast Cell Disorders of the Gastrointestinal Tract: Clarity out of Chaos   755

Nicole C. Panarelli

Pathologists are increasingly asked to evaluate mast cell infiltrates in the gastrointestinal tract when there is clinical concern for systemic mastocytosis or a variety of functional disorders, including irritable bowel syndrome and mast cell activation syndrome. Neoplastic mast cells have established quantitative, morphologic, and immunohistochemical features that facilitate their identification in gastrointestinal mucosal biopsies. Specific qualitative and quantitative findings are lacking for inflammatory mast cell–mediated disorders. This review covers histopathologic features of mast cell disorders that affect the gastrointestinal tract and offers practical guidance for their assessment in mucosal biopsies.

A Practical Approach to Small Round Cell Tumors Involving the Gastrointestinal Tract
and Abdomen   765

Khin Thway and Cyril Fisher

Small round cell neoplasms are diagnostically challenging owing to their clinical and pathologic overlap, necessitating use of large immunopanels and molecular analysis. Ewing sarcomas (ES) are the most common, but *EWSR1* is translocated in several diverse neoplasms, some with round cell morphology. Molecular advances enable classification of many tumors previously termed 'atypical ES'. The current WHO Classification includes two new undifferentiated round cell sarcomas (with *CIC* or *BCOR* alterations), and a group of sarcomas in which *EWSR1* partners with non-Ewing family transcription factor genes. This article reviews the spectrum of small round cell sarcomas within the gastrointestinal tract and abdomen.

Infectious Disease Pathology of the Gastrointestinal Tract: Diagnosing the Challenging
Cases   779

Laura W. Lamps

Infectious diseases of the GI tract mimic a variety of other GI diseases, including chronic idiopathic inflammatory bowel disease and ischemia. It can be challenging to identify pathogens in tissue sections as well, as many trainees are not exposed to infectious disease pathology other than in the context of microbiology. Our ability to diagnose infections in formalin fixed, paraffin embedded material has grown exponentially with the advent of new histochemical and immunohistochemical stains, as well as more options for molecular testing. Correlating these diagnostic techniques with morphology has led to increasing understanding of the histologic patterns that are associated with specific pathogens.

SURGICAL PATHOLOGY CLINICS

FORTHCOMING ISSUES

March 2024
Soft Tissue Pathology
Gregory W. Charville, *Editor*

June 2024
New Frontiers in Thoracic Pathology
Alain Borczuk, *Editor*

September 2024
The Current and Future Impact of Cytopathology on Patient Care
Christopher J. VandenBussche, *Editor*

RECENT ISSUES

September 2023
Liver Pathology: Diagnostic Challenges, Practical Considerations and Emerging Concepts
Lei Zhao, *Editor*

June 2023
Hematopathology
Aliyah R. Sohani, *Editor*

March 2023
Endocrine Pathology
Nicole A. Cipriani, *Editor*

SERIES OF RELATED INTEREST

Clinics in Laboratory Medicine
http://www.labmed.theclinics.com/
Medical Clinics
https://www.medical.theclinics.com/

THE CLINICS ARE AVAILABLE ONLINE!
Access your subscription at:
www.theclinics.com

Preface

What's Coming Down the Tube: Current and Emerging Topics in Gastrointestinal Pathology

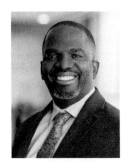

Rondell P. Graham, MBBS

Editor

To make this issue a high value to readers, I collaborated with an august group of expert pathologists to address timely current and emerging topics in gastrointestinal pathology. It was a great privilege to work with them, and they have my gratitude for well-written articles that address two categories of top-of-mind topics: select everyday issues and key emerging issues.

In the current issue, the authors provide practical approaches to handling current challenges related to diagnosing lymphoproliferative processes, the differential diagnoses in the post–stem cell transplant, interpreting small round blue cell tumors, along with best practices for diagnosing the gamut of infectious diseases that involve the tubal gut. Regarding emerging challenges, this issue includes articles wherein the increasing number of therapeutic biomarkers in gastric, gastroesophageal, and colorectal carcinoma, and the potential role of artificial intelligence in cancer interpretations are comprehensively discussed. Not all emerging issues are directly related to technology, and so, the hot topic of nonconventional dysplasia in inflammatory bowel disease and the vexing issue of mast cell activation syndrome are also presented.

Rondell P. Graham, MBBS
Division of Anatomic Pathology
Department of Laboratory Medicine and
Pathology
Mayo Clinic
200 First Street SW
Rochester, MN 55902, USA

E-mail address:
graham.rondell@mayo.edu

https://doi.org/10.1016/j.path.2023.05.001
1875-9181/23/© 2023 Published by Elsevier Inc.

Pathologic Evaluation of Therapeutic Biomarkers in Colorectal Adenocarcinoma

Esther Baranov, MD, Jonathan A. Nowak, MD, PhD*

KEYWORDS

- Colorectal adenocarcinoma • Mismatch repair • Microsatellite instability • Tumor mutational burden
- KRAS • NRAS • BRAF • ERBB2

Key points

- Molecular testing is an essential component of the pathologic evaluation of colorectal carcinoma that provides diagnostic, prognostic, and predictive information for therapeutic decisions.

- Evaluation of mismatch repair pathway status can efficiently screen patients for the presence of Lynch syndrome and can identify patients who are likely to benefit from immune checkpoint inhibition.

- Evaluation of RAS/MAPK driver status is required to identify patients eligible for EGFR, BRAF, and ERBB2 (HER2)-targeted therapy.

- Multiple assays, including immunohistochemistry, microsatellite instability testing, MLH1 promoter methylation testing, and next-generation sequencing, are typically needed to assess colorectal cancer biomarkers.

- Advances in colorectal cancer molecular diagnostics will likely drive refinements in colorectal cancer personalized therapy, including targeting KRAS-mutant colorectal cancers.

ABSTRACT

Molecular testing is an essential component of the pathologic evaluation of colorectal carcinoma providing diagnostic, prognostic, and predictive therapeutic information. Mismatch repair status evaluation is required for all tumors. Advanced and metastatic tumors also require determination of tumor mutational burden, KRAS, NRAS, and BRAF mutation status, ERBB2 amplification status, and NTRK and RET gene rearrangement status to guide therapy. Multiple assays, including immunohistochemistry, microsatellite instability testing, MLH1 promoter methylation, and next-generation sequencing, are typically needed. Pathologists must be aware of these requirements to optimally triage tissue. Advances in colorectal cancer molecular diagnostics will continue to drive refinements in colorectal cancer personalized therapy.

OVERVIEW

Colorectal carcinoma (CRC) is the third most-commonly diagnosed cancer worldwide and the second largest contributor to cancer-related death.[1,2] In addition, the incidence in individuals younger than 50 years of age (early-onset CRC) has increased steadily in recent years.[2] Since the original description of CRC pathogenesis as a stepwise series of linked molecular and morphologic events over 30 years ago, the burgeoning field of molecular biology and widely available clinical molecular diagnostics have defined molecularly distinct CRC subtypes with therapeutic relevance.[3–5] CRC pathogenesis is classically divided into 2 distinct, yet partially overlapping genetic pathways—the chromosomal instability ("CIN") pathway and microsatellite instability-high ("MSI-H") or mismatch repair (MMR) deficiency pathway. CIN pathway CRCs are characterized

---

Department of Pathology, Brigham & Women's Hospital, 75 Francis Street, Boston, MA 02115, USA
* Corresponding author.
E-mail address: janowak@bwh.harvard.edu

Surgical Pathology 16 (2023) 635–650
https://doi.org/10.1016/j.path.2023.05.002
1875-9181/23/© 2023 Elsevier Inc. All rights reserved.

by a high degree of chromosomal aneuploidy and frequent mutations in *APC*, *KRAS*, *SMAD4*, and *TP53*, whereas MMR-deficient CRCs are characterized by high numbers of mutations, a more stable copy number profile, and enrichment of some driver genes, such as *BRAF* and *RNF43*. Comprehensive molecular profiling of large numbers of CRCs in the past decade has refined these pathways and has transformed patient care by providing a clinically relevant molecular framework for CRC classification.

Evaluation of MMR status is required for all newly diagnosed colorectal cancers to screen patients for Lynch syndrome and to identify patients that are likely to benefit from immune checkpoint inhibitor therapy.[6–9] For patients with metastatic disease, testing for activating mutations in *KRAS*, *NRAS*, and *BRAF* is required to select therapies targeting *EGFR* and *BRAF*.[10–12] Evaluation of *ERBB2* (HER2) amplification status is also needed to appropriately select patients for anti-HER2 targeted therapy. In addition to the molecular testing required for these CRC-specific therapeutic indications, several therapies with pan-solid tumor approvals typically require molecular testing, including tumor mutational burden (TMB) and *NTRK1-3* and *RET* fusions. Given this array of testing indications, it is increasingly common for all patients with advanced-stage CRC to undergo molecular profiling by next-generation sequencing (NGS; **Fig. 1**). Herein, the authors review the molecular landscape of CRC with a focus on therapeutically relevant genes and methods for their assessment.

CAUSES OF MISMATCH REPAIR DEFICIENCY IN COLORECTAL CARCINOMA

Approximately 15% of all CRCs are hypermutated owing to MMR deficiency, also known as an MSI-H phenotype.[4,13] Roughly 12% of tumors develop sporadic or somatic-only MMR deficiency.[4,14] The remaining 3% to 4% of CRCs that are MMR deficient arise in the setting of Lynch syndrome owing to hereditary MMR gene defects.[4] Rates of MMR deficiency vary by anatomic location, with a 19%

rate of deficiency for colon carcinoma, and enrichment in the right side of the colon, as compared with a 3% rate of MMR deficiency in rectal carcinoma.[15,16] However, a greater relative percentage of MMR-deficient rectal adenocarcinomas is associated with Lynch syndrome.

The MMR system corrects mismatched bases as well as errors where one or several nucleotides have been inappropriately inserted or deleted during the process of DNA replication.[17] The key MMR proteins function in heterodimeric complexes with pairing between MLH1 and PMS2 and between MSH2 and MSH6. Typically, inactivating mutations in any MMR gene results in loss of expression of the corresponding protein. Furthermore, in the absence of MLH1 or MSH2 expression, expression of the corresponding partner protein PMS2 or MSH6 is also lost due to an inability to form a stabilizing heterodimeric complex. Somatic methylation of the *MLH1* promoter, in the context of a CpG island methylator phenotype, is the most common cause of MMR deficiency. However, inactivating mutations and copy number deletions can occur in all 4 MMR genes both in the context of Lynch syndrome and in sporadic tumors, leading to accumulation of missense and insertion/deletion mutations in tumors. Repetitive regions of the genome are particularly prone to accumulation of insertion and deletion errors during DNA replication. This phenomenon can be quantified by analyzing microsatellites, which are short stretches of DNA with 1 to 6 nucleotide repeat motifs. Alterations in the number of repeats in a microsatellite render the size of the microsatellite unstable within tumor cells and underlie MSI testing, the first molecular method developed to identify MMR deficiency.

Lynch syndrome, previously termed hereditary nonpolyposis colorectal cancer syndrome, is an autosomal dominant genetic cancer predisposition syndrome caused by genetic mutations any of the 4 core MMR genes or, more rarely, a germline deletion in the 3′ portion of *EPCAM* that leads to epigenetic silencing of *MSH2*.[18,19] Inactivation of the remaining nonmutated allele within tumor cells leads

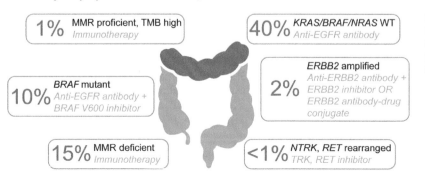

Fig. 1. Currently targetable molecular alterations in CRC and their prevalence across all stages of disease.

1% MMR proficient, TMB high *Immunotherapy*

40% *KRAS/BRAF/NRAS* WT *Anti-EGFR antibody*

10% *BRAF* mutant *Anti-EGFR antibody + BRAF V600 inhibitor*

2% ERBB2 amplified *Anti-ERBB2 antibody + ERBB2 inhibitor OR ERBB2 antibody-drug conjugate*

15% MMR deficient *Immunotherapy*

<1% *NTRK, RET* rearranged *TRK, RET inhibitor*

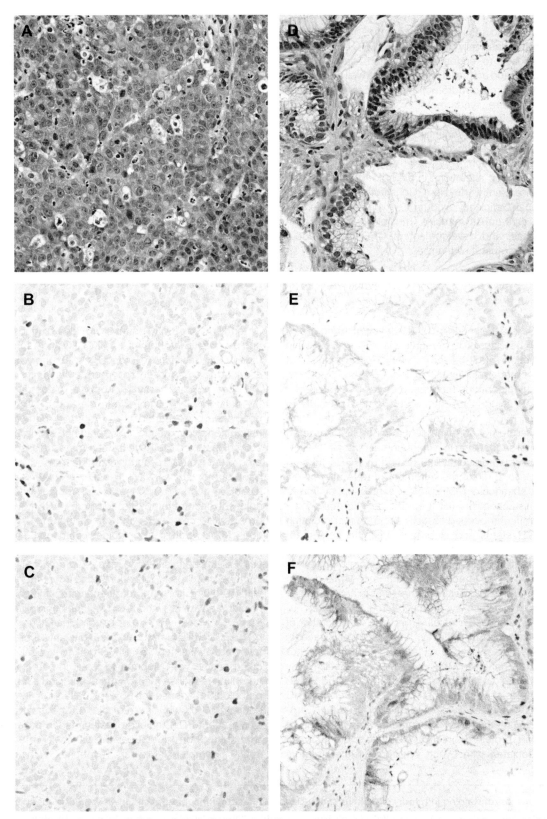

Fig. 2. **Mismatch repair–deficient (MMR-D) CRC.** Medullary morphology, strongly associated with MMR deficiency, characterized by solid/trabecular growth pattern of poorly differentiated cells with eosinophilic cytoplasm, prominent nucleoli, and increased intraepithelial lymphocytes (400x, *A*). IHC for MLH1 (*B*) and PMS2 (*C*)

to MSI and subsequent carcinogenesis. Lynch syndrome classically predisposes to CRC but also predisposes to endometrial, ovarian, gastric, small bowel, and urothelial carcinomas as well as glioblastoma (Turcot syndrome) and sebaceous neoplasia (Muir-Torre syndrome).[20–22] Identification of patients with Lynch syndrome is critical for enabling them to receive enhanced cancer screening and to evaluate their relatives who may also carry the same mutation. Very rarely, patients may inherit 2 pathogenic alterations in a single MMR gene and consequently develop Constitutional Mismatch Repair Deficiency syndrome, which is characterized by café-au-lait macules, multiple colorectal adenomas, and development of CRC in childhood, among other malignancies.[23,24]

DETECTION OF MISMATCH REPAIR DEFICIENCY

MSI is a hallmark of MMR-deficient tumors and can be classically detected via polymerase chain reaction (PCR)-based capillary electrophoresis at accepted microsatellite loci.[25] More recently, many algorithms have been developed to predict MMR using NGS data, and it is now possible to infer MMR status from both somatic-only and paired tumor:germline sequencing using targeted panel sequencing in a manner that matches or outperforms traditional MSI testing by PCR.[26–29]

Beyond direct measurement of DNA alterations, the absence of MMR protein expression by immunohistochemistry (IHC) on standard formalin-fixed paraffin-embedded tissue is accurate for predicting MMR status and is broadly used to screen for Lynch syndrome and to identify patients who may benefit from immune checkpoint inhibition (Fig. 2).[30–32] In addition, patterns of MMR protein loss can help predict whether tumors are likely sporadic or Lynch syndrome–related.[33,34] Intact nuclear expression of all 4 proteins is indicative of an intact MMR pathway, although rarely, patients may have missense mutations leading to a functionally inactive MMR protein that is still stably expressed.[35] Concurrent loss of MLH1 and PMS2 expression is the most common pattern of IHC loss and is usually caused by sporadic *MLH1* promoter methylation. In contrast, other patterns of MMR protein expression loss are more typically associated with Lynch syndrome–related tumors

and require germline sequencing and, potentially, somatic sequencing to identify the causative MMR gene mutation. IHC evaluation is typically straightforward, but may be subject to technical and interpretive pitfalls, such as suboptimal specimen processing or fixation, heterogeneous staining patterns or partial/subclonal loss of expression, and reduced expression of MMR proteins after chemoradiation.[36–39] Heterogenous or partial loss of MMR expression by IHC is a rare pattern associated with Lynch syndrome that is critical to recognize in practice (Fig. 2D–F, Fig. 3).[37] Finally, although MMR-deficient tumors often have characteristic histologic features (see Fig. 2) that can raise suspicion for MMR deficiency, none of these are sensitive enough to replace dedicated MMR testing.[40,41]

CLINICAL UTILITY OF MISMATCH REPAIR TESTING

Determination of MMR status provides diagnostic and prognostic information for all CRCs and informs therapeutic decisions for most CRCs. For more than a decade, it has been recognized that universal MMR testing for all newly diagnosed CRCs can identify patients with Lynch syndrome and provide a population-level morbidity and mortality benefit.[42] In addition to diagnostic utility for Lynch syndrome, staged-matched MMR-deficient tumors are associated with favorable prognosis and decreased likelihood of metastases.[43] MMR-deficient tumors also exhibit a worse response to fluorouracil-based adjuvant chemotherapy as compared with MMR-proficient tumors.[44] Beyond chemotherapy selection, MMR status also guides immunotherapy decisions, as MMR-deficient advanced or metastatic CRC has been shown to respond dramatically to immune checkpoint inhibition using monotherapy with PD-1 inhibitor pembrolizumab or PD-1 inhibitor nivolumab with or without CTLA-4 inhibitor ipilimumab.[6,7,45] More recently, use of combination nivolumab and ipilimumab as neoadjuvant therapy followed by surgery for MMR-deficient localized colon cancer was reported to result in pathologic complete response for 67% of patients and a major pathologic response for 95% of patients.[46] In the context of results from a trial of neoadjuvant single-agent PD-1 inhibitor dostarlimab in patients with stage II or II rectal cancer, which reported a 100% complete clinical response with no

shows loss of staining in tumor cells with intact nuclear staining in nonneoplastic cells. Invasive, mucinous adenocarcinoma (400x, *D*) in a patient with Lynch syndrome with a pathogenic *MSH2* germline variant. IHC shows loss of MSH2 (*E*) in tumor cells with intact nuclear staining in nonneoplastic cells and reduced nuclear staining of MSH6 with aberrant cytoplasmic staining (*F*).

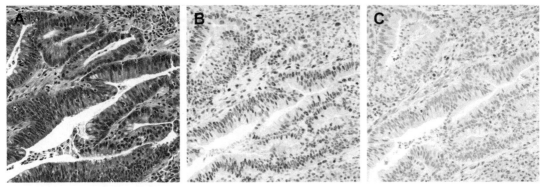

Fig. 3. **Partial loss pattern of MMR deficiency by IHC.** Moderately differentiated invasive colonic adenocarcinoma (400x, *A*). IHC for MLH1 shows intact nuclear staining in neoplastic and nonneoplastic cells (*B*). IHC for PMS2 reveals markedly reduced staining in tumor nuclei (partial loss pattern) with intact nuclear staining in adjacent nonneoplastic cells (*C*), an atypical MMR protein expression pattern that is important to recognize.

progression or recurrence over a median 1-year follow-up time, these results will likely result in neoadjuvant immunotherapy becoming standard of care for most MMR-deficient CRCs and raise the intriguing possibility of nonsurgical management of MMR-deficient localized colon cancer.[47]

TUMOR MUTATIONAL BURDEN AND ULTRAMUTATED *POLE/D1*-MUTATED COLORECTAL CARCINOMA

Although most CRCs with an elevated TMB are driven by MMR deficiency, mutations in several additional DNA repair pathways can lead to an elevated TMB. CRCs with missense mutations in the exonuclease domains of the *POLE* and *POLD1* genes, which encode the catalytic subunits of DNA polymerases Pol δ and Pol ε, respectively, typically acquire extremely high TMBs (>100 Mut/Mb) and are referred to as "ultramutated" owing to impaired proofreading activity of the mutant polymerases.[48–50] Such alterations occur in approximately 1% to 2% of CRCs.[4,48] Although rare, germline mutations in *POLE* and *POLD1* are highly penetrant and predispose to multiple or large adenomas and early-onset or multiple CRCs, with *POLD1* mutations also predisposing to endometrial carcinoma.[51]

POLE-mutated CRC is associated with younger average age at presentation, male predominance, early disease stage, and right-sided location.[48] These tumors also have a reduced risk of recurrence, improved disease-free survival in patients aged less than 80 years, and respond well to immune checkpoint inhibition.[48,52] *POLE/D1*-mutated CRC are typically *KRAS* and *BRAF* wild-type and MSS/MMR-proficient, although a subset of these tumors develop secondary MMR deficiency. Histologically, *POLE/D1*-mutated CRC can show a medullary or mucinous/signet-ring-cell phenotype classically associated with MMR-deficient CRC as well as a markedly increased density of tumor-infiltrating lymphocytes.[53,54] When present in MMR-proficient tumors, these histologic features should alert surgical pathologists to recommend NGS for evaluation of TMB and pathogenic *POLE/D1* mutations (**Fig. 4**).

Beyond MMR-deficient and *POLE/POLD1* mutant CRCs, tumors with biallelic pathogenic mutations in *MUTYH*, a component of the base excision repair pathway, have a moderately elevated mutational burden. *MUTYH*-mutant tumors often arise in the setting of *MUTYH*-associated polyposis, a hereditary polyposis and colorectal cancer predisposition syndrome.[55] Finally, a small number of CRCs harbor elevated TMBs without a clearly identifiable cause. Regardless of the underlying etiology, as part of the pan-solid tumor approval for pembrolizumab, unresectable or metastatic CRCs with a TMB $\geq$ 10 Mut/Mb are eligible for treatment with pembrolizumab after progression on prior treatment.[56,57]

RAS MUTATIONS IN COLORECTAL CARCINOMA

The RAS/MAPK signaling pathway and the related PI3K signaling pathway provide numerous therapeutic targets for CRC patients (**Fig. 5**). *KRAS* and *NRAS* are among the most commonly mutated genes in CRC, with activating *KRAS* mutations found in 40% to 45% of non-hypermutated CRC and activating *NRAS* mutations in 5% to 10%.[4,58] *KRAS* mutations are almost exclusively missense hot spot mutations, with 95% occurring in codons 12 and 13.[58] Of these, the most common protein changes are G12D, G12V, G13D, and G12C, in decreasing frequency.[59] *KRAS* and

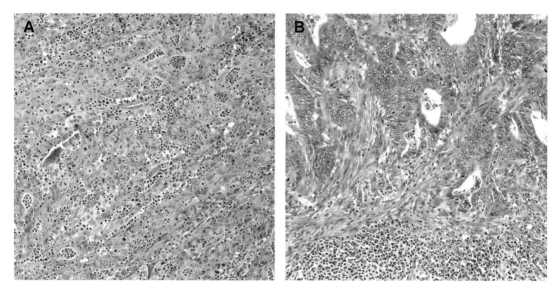

Fig. 4. **Histologic features of *POLE*-mutant ultramutated CRC.** Invasive, poorly differentiated carcinoma with medullary features and intact MMR protein IHC (200x, *A*). Invasive, moderately differentiated adenocarcinoma with classic intestinal-type morphology and an associated brisk Crohn-like lymphoid infiltrate (200x, *B*).

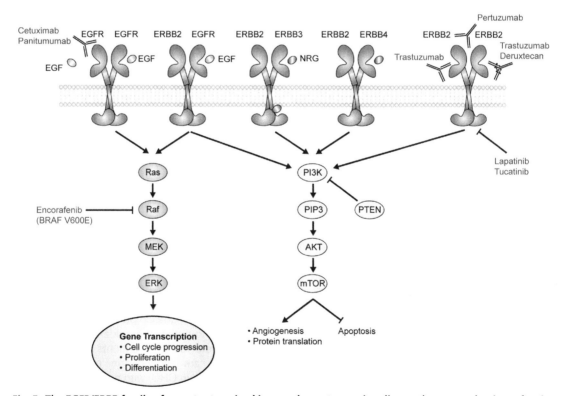

Fig. 5. **The EGFR/ERBB family of receptor tyrosine kinases, downstream signaling pathways, and points of action for targeted therapies.** Cetuximab and panitumumab are monoclonal antibodies directed against the extracellular domain of EGFR. Encorafenib is a small molecule kinase inhibitor with high selectivity for V600-mutant BRAF. Trastuzumab is a monoclonal antibody directed against the extracellular domain of ERBB2, whereas pertuzumab is an antibody that interferences with ERBB2 homodimerization. Tucatinib and lapatinib are small molecule tyrosine kinase inhibitors with high selectivity for ERBB2. Trastuzumab deruxtecan is an antibody-drug conjugate. (*Adapted from* Nowak 2020[76]; with permission.)

its homolog *NRAS* encode GTP-binding signal transducer proteins that respond to ligand-bound transphosphorylated receptor tyrosine kinases, like *EGFR*, and mediate downstream signaling in the *RAS/RAF/MEK/ERK* pathway.[60] *KRAS* and *NRAS* point mutations lead to constitutive activation of the downstream pathway, resulting in altered gene transcription, increased proliferation, and oncogenesis. *KRAS* mutations are independently associated with worse clinical outcomes, including shorter timer to recurrence, shorter survival after relapse, and worse overall survival.[61,62]

Until recently, it has proven challenging to develop targeted therapies for *KRAS* and *NRAS*-mutant CRC. Tumors in the left side of the colon that are *KRAS*, *NRAS*, and *BRAF*-wild-type benefit from addition of the EGFR inhibitors cetuximab or panitumumab to chemotherapy. However, tumors with activating mutations downstream of EGFR do not benefit from EGFR inhibition.[58,63] Consistent with this finding, tumors treated with EGFR inhibition often develop secondary, activating *KRAS* and *NRAS* mutations as resistance mechanisms that drive tumor progression.[11,64]

In the past 5 years, groundbreaking work has led to the development and approval of oral small molecule inhibitors that target G12C-mutant KRAS.[65,66] These inhibitors, adagrasib and sotorasib, covalently bind to the mutant cysteine residue, irreversibly locking G12C-mutant KRAS into an inactive state. Although only 3% to 4% of patients with metastatic CRC harbor *KRAS* p.G12C mutations, this approach represents a promising new class of therapies for CRC. When used as single agents, sotorasib and adagrasib have shown only modest activity in CRC, and various mechanisms of resistance have already been described.[67,68] However, simultaneous *EGFR* inhibition has been shown to prevent the development of resistance to KRAS G12C inhibitors in preclinical models.[69] In addition, heavily pretreated patients with *KRAS* G12C-mutated metastatic CRC have shown favorable response rates to treatment with adagrasib plus cetuximab.[70] These promising results pave the way for *KRAS*-targeted therapies, which have long been elusive. Many clinical trials are now underway testing *KRAS*-allele–specific inhibitors and pan-KRAS inhibitors alone and in combination with additional agents targeting the RAS/MAPK pathway.

BRAF V600E AND NON-V600 MUTATIONS IN COLORECTAL CARCINOMA

BRAF mutations, particularly *BRAF* p.V600E, are seen in 40% to 50% of MMR-deficient tumors and 3% to 5% of MMR-proficient tumors.[4,58,71]

Overall, *BRAF* V600E mutations are strongly associated with the so-called CpG island methylator phenotype, which is also characterized by somatic *MLH1* promoter methylation and, consequently, MMR deficiency.[72] *BRAF* V600E-mutated CRC shows higher rates of mucinous and signet-ring-cell histology and is associated with right-sided location, female predominance, and worse overall survival.[53,72,73] MMR-proficient *BRAF*-mutated CRC also shows increased rates of mucinous or signet-ring-cell morphology as well as increased rates of lymphatic invasion and lymph node metastases.[71,73] *BRAF* V600E mutations are associated with worse prognosis in both MMR-proficient and MMR-deficient tumors.[74] As with *KRAS* and *NRAS*, *BRAF* V600E mutations are associated with lack of response to EGFR inhibition.[58]

Despite notable success in targeting *BRAF* V600E mutations in other tumor types, identifying a treatment regimen active in CRC has proven challenging. However, results from the BEACON trial, which assessed the efficacy of BRAF-inhibitor encorafenib plus EGFR-inhibitor cetuximab, demonstrated increased overall survival and progression-free survival for treatment with dual-agent encorafenib and cetuximab in previously treated patients with *BRAF* V600E-mutated mCRC compared with standard chemotherapy.[12,75] Therefore, *BRAF* mutation testing is not only predictive of resistance to anti-EGFR targeted therapy, but also helps identify patients likely to benefit from BRAF V600E-directed therapy.

ERBB2 (HER2) AMPLIFICATION AND MUTATIONS

Alterations in *ERBB2* (alternatively referred to as *HER2*) are present in a small percentage of CRCs and are often mutually exclusive with other RAS/MAPK/PI3K pathway drivers (**Fig. 6**).[4,76] *ERBB2* encodes a member of the ERBB family of receptor tyrosine kinases, also including *ERBB1* (*EGFR*), *ERBB3* (*HER3*), and *ERBB4* (*HER4*). ERBB family receptors bind extracellular ligands, such as neuregulin and epidermal growth factor, inducing heterodimerization with each other and subsequent transphosphorylation that drives downstream signaling through the *RAS/MAPK* and *PI3K* signaling pathways.[77] Uniquely, ERBB2 does not bind ligands and heterodimerizes only with other family members under normal conditions. However, when overexpressed because of gene amplification, it homodimerizes and activates ligand-independent signaling. Activating

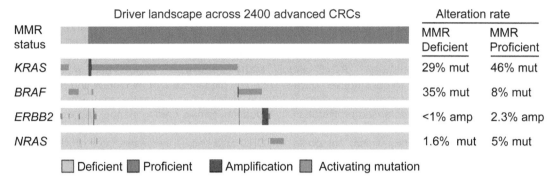

Fig. 6. **Landscape of therapeutically relevant RAS/MAPK/PI3K alterations in advanced CRC stratified by MMR status.** Oncogenic driver alterations in *KRAS*, *BRAF*, *NRAS*, and *ERBB2* are typically mutually exclusive, although a subset of tumors harbors co-occurring drivers. Activating *BRAF* mutations are more common in MMR-deficient tumors, whereas *KRAS* and *NRAS* mutations, along with *ERBB2* amplifications, are more common in MMR-proficient tumors. Activating *ERBB2* mutations are shown in addition to *ERBB2* amplification but are not currently used to guide therapy. Data represent 2423 consecutive colorectal cancers profiled using the OncoPanel platform at the Brigham and Women's Hospital and Dana-Farber Cancer Institute. amp, amplified; mut, mutant.

point mutations also occur in *ERBB2*, including several hotspot mutations within the extracellular domain (p.S310F/Y), juxtamembrane region (p. R678Q), and kinase domain (p.V777L/M and V842I), all of which are known to activate downstream signaling and promote oncogenesis in CRC.[78,79]

Oncogenic *ERBB2* alterations occur in approximately 5% of CRCs with amplification occurring in 3%, point mutations in 2%, and 0.5% of cases harboring both amplification and point mutations.[78,80,81] In some studies, higher rates of *ERBB2* amplification were reported in left-sided tumors; no other striking histologic or clinical correlates of *ERBB2*-altered tumors have been identified.[82] Although the prognostic utility of oncogenic *ERBB2* alterations is unclear, some studies report trends toward worse overall survival and shorter disease-free survival.[83] *KRAS* and *BRAF* are typically but not exclusively wild-type in *ERBB2*-altered CRC.[78]

Echoing the challenge, adopting BRAF-targeted therapy from other tumor types to CRC, single-agent targeting of *ERBB2* amplification in CRC has been unsuccessful. In conjunction with the development of new classes of ERBB2-targeted agents beyond the anti-ERBB2 antibody trastuzumab, clinical trials shifted to test multiagent regimens. The HERACLES, MyPathway phase 2, and MOUNTAINEER clinical trials revealed objective response rates (ORRs) of 30%, 32%, and 38% for trastuzumab combined with lapatinib, pertuzumab, or tucatinib, respectively. Lapatinib and tucatinib are both small molecular inhibitors of ERBB2 kinase activity, whereas pertuzumab is an antibody that interferes with ERBB2 homodimerization. These regimens are now approved

for advanced treatment-refractory, *ERBB2*-amplified, *RAS* and *BRAF*-wild-type CRC.[84–87] In addition, use of single-agent trastuzumab deruxtecan, an antibody-drug conjugate that uses trastuzumab to deliver deruxtecan, a topoisomerase I inhibitor, to ERBB2-overexpressing cells, showed a 45% ORR in *ERBB2*-amplified, *RAS* and *BRAF*-wild-type metastatic CRC, and is also now an approved therapy based on the DESTINY-CRC01 trial.[88]

In a companion study to the HERACLES trial, a CRC-specific approach for evaluating ERBB2 overexpression and amplification was described (**Fig. 7**).[89,90] Interestingly, CRC shows less intratumoral heterogeneity for ERBB2 overexpression than typically seen in esophagogastric carcinomas and more closely follows breast cancer in terms of ERBB2 expression pattern.[89] More recently, NGS has been shown to correlate very well with IHC and fluorescence *in situ* hybridization (FISH)-based identification of *ERBB2* amplification in CRC and may be a preferred screening modality given the relative rarity of *ERBB2* amplification.[91]

ONCOGENIC REARRANGEMENTS AS DRIVERS IN COLORECTAL CARCINOMA

Oncogenic chromosomal rearrangements that result in functional gene fusions are exceedingly rare in CRC. However, given the targetable nature of many of these fusions and the high overall prevalence of CRC, fusion testing should be standard of care for patients with metastatic CRC.[5,92,93] Although estimates of the overall prevalence of targetable oncogenic fusions in CRC vary based on methodology and cohort, most studies report

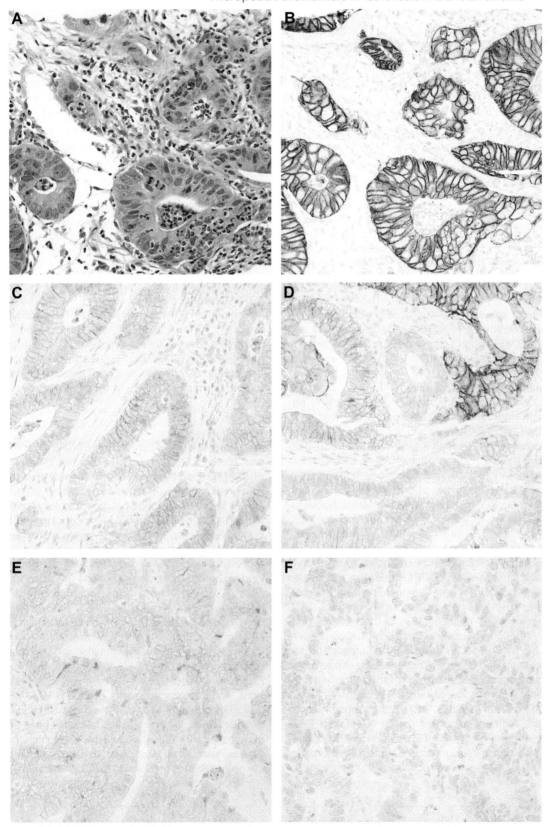

Fig. 7. **Evaluation of ERBB2 (HER2) protein expression by IHC in CRC.** Moderately differentiated CRC (400x, *A*) positive for ERBB2 IHC by HERACLES criteria, showing intense (3+) continuous membranous staining in ≥50% of cells (400x, *B*). CRC showing moderate (2+) membranous staining in ≥50% of cells (400x, *C*), which is considered equivocal and requires confirmation by FISH. CRC with heterogenous patterns of ERBB2 membranous

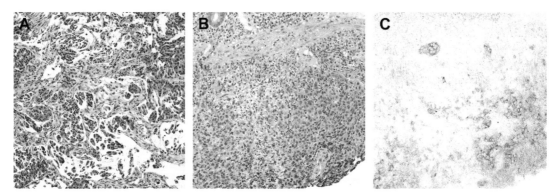

Fig. 8. NTRK-rearranged CRC. Moderately differentiated MLH1/PMS2-deficient CRC with mucinous features found to have a *TPR::NTRK1* fusion by molecular testing (200x, *A*). Poorly differentiated MLH1/PMS2-deficient medullary carcinoma also found to have a *TPR::NTRK1* fusion (200x, *B*), with concurrent pan-TRK IHC (200x, *C*) highlighting positive tumor cells with strong membranous and cytoplasmic staining.

rates of 1% to 2% or less.[92–94] These fusions are spread across numerous genes, including *BRAF*, *ALK*, *RET*, *ROS1*, *NTRK1*, *NTRK3*, *FGFR1*, and *ERBB2*, although fusion rates for any single gene are significantly less than 1%.[92–95] For example, *NTRK1-3*–rearranged CRC makes up less than half a percent of CRC in large studies.[96]

Oncogenic fusions are enriched in elderly patients with right-sided, *RAS* and *BRAF*-wild type, MMR-deficient tumors and are associated with a poorer prognosis than fusion-negative MMR-deficient tumors.[94,95,97,98] Histologically, these tumors are morphologically heterogeneous, although they typically exhibit the poorly differentiated and lymphocyte-rich appearance of MMR-deficient tumors (**Figs. 8** and **9**).[98] Although IHC for ALK, ROS1, and TRK proteins has been used routinely in other tumors for detection of actionable fusions, and pan-TRK IHC has been shown to accurately detect CRCs with *NTRK* fusions, the low overall frequency of any one fusion effectively necessitates the use of DNA or RNA-based NGS methods.[96,99]

Although the overall rarity of fusion-positive CRC has made it challenging to understand the best targeted treatment options for these patients, data from phase I and II basket trials, drawing from clinical knowledge gained by treating numerous different tumor types, have led to recommendations for targeted agent use in *NTRK* and *RET*-rearranged metastatic CRC. Currently, for locally advanced or metastatic CRC, the TRK inhibitors larotrectinib and entrectinib are approved for

NTRK-rearranged tumors, whereas the RET inhibitor selpercatinib is approved for *RET*-rearranged tumors.[5,100–102] Additional trials are needed to determine the optimal treatment strategy for fusion-positive *NTRK* and *RET*-rearranged tumors that are also MMR-deficient and therefore eligible for both immunotherapy and targeted therapy.

SUMMARY

Routine molecular classification of CRC over the past 25 years has focused on evaluating the status of the MMR system primarily to identify patients with Lynch syndrome. More recently, *KRAS*, *BRAF*, and *NRAS* testing became routine in order to guide the use of anti-EGFR monoclonal antibodies. However, in the past 6 years, numerous additional molecularly targeted therapies and immunotherapies have significantly expanded the landscape of targetable alterations in CRC. Success in using immunotherapy for treating MMR-deficient and hypermutated CRCs has resulted from several decades of studies focused on unraveling how mutations can elicit an antitumor immune response. Similarly, multiagent therapies now approved for *BRAF* V600E-mutated and *ERBB2*-amplified tumors have benefited not only from deep characterization of the RAS/MAPK and PI3K signaling pathways in preclinical models but also, crucially, from clinical trials that have uncovered tumor-type–specific effects for inhibitors of these pathways. In addition, treatment of multiple targetable alterations in CRC has benefited

staining, predominantly 1$^+$ to 2$^+$ with a focus of 3$^+$ staining (400x, *D*). A faint blush of cytoplasmic staining is interpreted as negative (1$^+$) (400x, *E*). Negative (0) staining for ERBB2 with no nuclear, membranous, or cytoplasmic expression (400x, *F*).

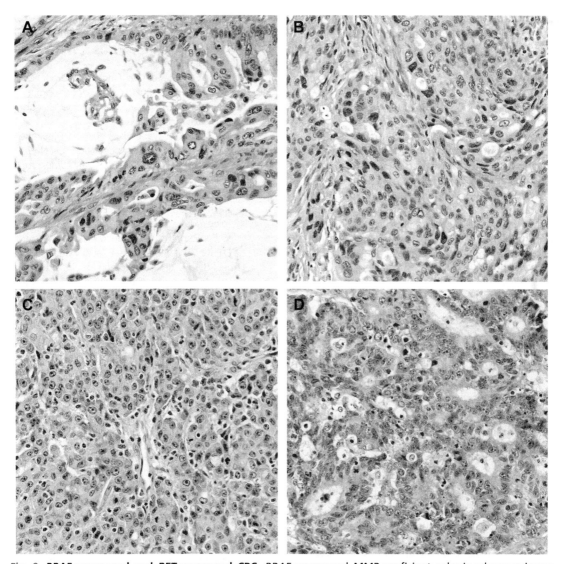

Fig. 9. **BRAF-rearranged and RET-rearranged CRC.** *BRAF*-rearranged MMR-proficient colonic adenocarcinoma with mucinous features (400x, *A*) and other areas showing squamoid morphology (400x, *B*). Molecular testing revealed a *BAIAP2L1::BRAF* rearrangement and no other RAS/RAF driver alteration. *RET*-rearranged, MLH1/PMS2-deficient medullary carcinoma with a trabecular growth pattern, amphophilic cytoplasm, and brisk eosinophilic and lymphocytic infiltrate (400x, *C*). Molecular testing revealed a *CCDC6::RET* rearrangement. Another *RET*-rearranged, MLH1/PMS2-deficient colonic adenocarcinoma with prominent cribriform morphology (400x, *D*) and IHC showing patchy, partial loss of staining of MSH6 expression. Molecular testing revealed a *CCDC6::RET* rearrangement, *MLH1* promoter methylation, and 2 subclonal *MSH6* frameshift mutations.

from the recognition that some biomarkers, such as MMR status, TMB, and gene fusions, maintain their predictive power across many solid tumors and can therefore function as cancer-type–agnostic biomarkers.

Moving forward, it is likely that KRAS inhibitors will be the next addition to the roster of targeted molecular agents approved for CRC. With the increasing use of agents targeting multiple proteins in the RAS/MAPK and PI3K pathways, it will be increasingly important to identify the secondary resistance mechanisms that will inevitably occur in patients treated with targeted therapy. Fortunately, the increasing number of agents approved for targeting these pathways may also make treatment of secondary resistance mechanisms more tractable. Routine evaluation of cell-free tumor DNA may provide a noninvasive method of monitoring disease recurrence and the development of resistance to therapy. It is also possible that advances in immunotherapy may identify targetable subsets of patients with non-hypermutated

MMR-proficient CRC. In the more distant future, evaluation of a patient's tumor-associated intestinal microbiome may provide insight into the tumor microenvironment and metabolic state. Regardless of which new biomarkers prove to have clinical utility, it is increasingly clear that the molecular alterations in CRC will need to be evaluated in the larger context of the patient's environmental, lifestyle, and genetic factors, as evidenced by the recent, yet largely unexplained increase in early-onset CRC. Dissecting these complex interrelationships will likely increase the value of classically recognized genotype-phenotype molecular alterations in CRC and may drive development of future therapies, much like the discovery of Lynch syndrome in the 1990s led to the success of immunotherapy for MMR-deficient tumors nearly 25 years later.

CLINICS CARE POINTS

- MMR testing should be performed for all newly diagnosed CRCs and the cause of MMR deficiency, if identified, should be determined.

- MMR protein IHC patterns should correlate with molecular results. If findings are discrepant, suspect an assay failure or misinterpreted IHC result.

- An elevated TMB in CRC is nearly always due to MMR deficiency or POLE/POLED1 mutations.

- Most CRCs have a driver gene alteration in the RAS/MAPK pathway. These are typically mutually exclusive and should be tested, typically by NGS, in all advanced and metastatic tumors.

- ERBB2 (HER2) protein expression in CRC should be reported using the CRC-specific HERACLES trial criteria.

REFERENCES

1. Sung H, Ferlay J, Siegel RL, et al. Global Cancer Statistics 2020: GLOBOCAN Estimates of Incidence and Mortality Worldwide for 36 Cancers in 185 Countries. CA Cancer J Clin 2021;71(3): 209–49. https://doi.org/10.3322/caac.21660.

2. Siegel RL, Miller KD, Goding Sauer A, et al. Colorectal cancer statistics, 2020. CA Cancer J Clin 2020;70(3): 145–64. https://doi.org/10.3322/caac.21601.

3. Fearon ER, Vogelstein B. A genetic model for colorectal tumorigenesis. Cell 1990;61(5):759–67. https://doi.org/10.1016/0092-8674(90)90186-i.

4. Cancer Genome Atlas N. Comprehensive molecular characterization of human colon and rectal cancer. Nature 2012;487(7407):330–7. https://doi.org/10.1038/nature11252.

5. National Comprehensive Cancer Network. Colon Cancer (Version 3.2022). Accessed February 1, 2023. https://www.nccn.org/professionals/physician_gls/pdf/colon.pdf.

6. Le DT, Uram JN, Wang H, et al. PD-1 Blockade in Tumors with Mismatch-Repair Deficiency. N Engl J Med 2015;372(26):2509–20. https://doi.org/10.1056/NEJMoa1500596.

7. Le DT, Durham JN, Smith KN, et al. Mismatch repair deficiency predicts response of solid tumors to PD-1 blockade. Science 2017;357(6349):409–13. https://doi.org/10.1126/science.aan6733.

8. Le DT, Kim TW, Van Cutsem E, et al. Phase II Open-Label Study of Pembrolizumab in Treatment-Refractory, Microsatellite Instability-High/Mismatch Repair-Deficient Metastatic Colorectal Cancer: KEYNOTE-164. J Clin Oncol 2020;38(1):11–9. https://doi.org/10.1200/JCO.19.02107.

9. Diaz LA Jr, Shiu KK, Kim TW, et al. Pembrolizumab versus chemotherapy for microsatellite instability-high or mismatch repair-deficient metastatic colorectal cancer (KEYNOTE-177): final analysis of a randomised, open-label, phase 3 study. Lancet Oncol 2022;23(5):659–70. https://doi.org/10.1016/S1470-2045(22)00197-8.

10. Benvenuti S, Sartore-Bianchi A, Di Nicolantonio F, et al. Oncogenic activation of the RAS/RAF signaling pathway impairs the response of metastatic colorectal cancers to anti-epidermal growth factor receptor antibody therapies. Cancer Res 2007;67(6):2643–8. https://doi.org/10.1158/0008-5472.CAN-06-4158.

11. Bertotti A, Papp E, Jones S, et al. The genomic landscape of response to EGFR blockade in colorectal cancer. Nature 2015;526(7572):263–7. https://doi.org/10.1038/nature14969.

12. Tabernero J, Grothey A, Van Cutsem E, et al. Encorafenib Plus Cetuximab as a New Standard of Care for Previously Treated BRAF V600E-Mutant Metastatic Colorectal Cancer: Updated Survival Results and Subgroup Analyses from the BEACON Study. J Clin Oncol 2021;39(4):273–84. https://doi.org/10.1200/JCO.20.02088.

13. Guinney J, Dienstmann R, Wang X, et al. The consensus molecular subtypes of colorectal cancer. Nat Med 2015;21(11):1350–6. https://doi.org/10.1038/nm.3967.

14. Weisenberger DJ, Siegmund KD, Campan M, et al. CpG island methylator phenotype underlies sporadic microsatellite instability and is tightly associated with BRAF mutation in colorectal cancer. Nat Genet 2006;38(7):787–93. https://doi.org/10.1038/ng1834.

15. Hause RJ, Pritchard CC, Shendure J, et al. Classification and characterization of microsatellite instability across 18 cancer types. Nat Med 2016; 22(11):1342–50. https://doi.org/10.1038/nm.4191.

16. Papke DJ Jr, Yurgelun MB, Noffsinger AE, et al. Prevalence of Mismatch-Repair Deficiency in Rectal Adenocarcinomas. N Engl J Med 2022;387(18): 1714–6. https://doi.org/10.1056/NEJMc2210175.

17. Jiricny J. The multifaceted mismatch-repair system. Nat Rev Mol Cell Biol 2006;7(5):335–46. https://doi.org/10.1038/nrm1907.

18. Woods MO, Williams P, Careen A, et al. A new variant database for mismatch repair genes associated with Lynch syndrome. Hum Mutat 2007;28(7): 669–73. https://doi.org/10.1002/humu.20502.

19. Ligtenberg MJ, Kuiper RP, Chan TL, et al. Heritable somatic methylation and inactivation of MSH2 in families with Lynch syndrome due to deletion of the 3' exons of TACSTD1. Nat Genet 2009;41(1): 112–7. https://doi.org/10.1038/ng.283.

20. Bonadona V, Bonaiti B, Olschwang S, et al. Cancer risks associated with germline mutations in MLH1, MSH2, and MSH6 genes in Lynch syndrome. JAMA 2011;305(22):2304–10. https://doi.org/10.1001/jama.2011.743.

21. Barrow E, Hill J, Evans DG. Cancer risk in Lynch Syndrome. Fam Cancer 2013;12(2):229–40. https://doi.org/10.1007/s10689-013-9615-1.

22. Ponti G, Ponz de Leon M. Muir-Torre syndrome. Lancet Oncol 2005;6(12):980–7. https://doi.org/10.1016/S1470-2045(05)70465-4.

23. Durno CA, Holter S, Sherman PM, et al. The gastrointestinal phenotype of germline biallelic mismatch repair gene mutations. Am J Gastroenterol 2010; 105(11):2449–56. https://doi.org/10.1038/ajg.2010.215.

24. Aronson M, Colas C, Shuen A, et al. Diagnostic criteria for constitutional mismatch repair deficiency (CMMRD): recommendations from the international consensus working group. J Med Genet 2022;59(4):318–27. https://doi.org/10.1136/jmedgenet-2020-107627.

25. Cicek MS, Lindor NM, Gallinger S, et al. Quality assessment and correlation of microsatellite instability and immunohistochemical markers among population- and clinic-based colorectal tumors results from the Colon Cancer Family Registry. J Mol Diagn 2011;13(3):271–81. https://doi.org/10.1016/j.jmoldx.2010.12.004.

26. Nowak JA, Yurgelun MB, Bruce JL, et al. Detection of Mismatch Repair Deficiency and Microsatellite Instability in Colorectal Adenocarcinoma by Targeted Next-Generation Sequencing. J Mol Diagn 2017;19(1):84–91. https://doi.org/10.1016/j.jmoldx.2016.07.010.

27. Salipante SJ, Scroggins SM, Hampel HL, et al. Microsatellite instability detection by next generation sequencing. Clin Chem 2014;60(9):1192–9. https://doi.org/10.1373/clinchem.2014.223677.

28. Ratovomanana T, Cohen R, Svrcek M, et al. Performance of Next-Generation Sequencing for the Detection of Microsatellite Instability in Colorectal Cancer With Deficient DNA Mismatch Repair. Gastroenterology 2021;161(3):814–826 e7. https://doi.org/10.1053/j.gastro.2021.05.007.

29. Middha S, Zhang L, Nafa K, et al. Reliable Pan-Cancer Microsatellite Instability Assessment by Using Targeted Next-Generation Sequencing Data. JCO Precis Oncol 2017. https://doi.org/10.1200/PO.17.00084.

30. Zhu L, Huang Y, Fang X, et al. A Novel and Reliable Method to Detect Microsatellite Instability in Colorectal Cancer by Next-Generation Sequencing. J Mol Diagn 2018;20(2):225–31. https://doi.org/10.1016/j.jmoldx.2017.11.007.

31. Lindor NM, Burgart LJ, Leontovich O, et al. Immunohistochemistry versus microsatellite instability testing in phenotyping colorectal tumors. J Clin Oncol 2002;20(4):1043–8. https://doi.org/10.1200/JCO.2002.20.4.1043.

32. Hissong E, Crowe EP, Yantiss RK, et al. Assessing colorectal cancer mismatch repair status in the modern era: a survey of current practices and re-evaluation of the role of microsatellite instability testing. Mod Pathol 2018;31(11):1756–66. https://doi.org/10.1038/s41379-018-0094-7.

33. Pearlman R, Markow M, Knight D, et al. Two-stain immunohistochemical screening for Lynch syndrome in colorectal cancer may fail to detect mismatch repair deficiency. Mod Pathol 2018;31(12):1891–900. https://doi.org/10.1038/s41379-018-0058-y.

34. Jaffrelot M, Fares N, Brunac AC, et al. An unusual phenotype occurs in 15% of mismatch repair-deficient tumors and is associated with non-colorectal cancers and genetic syndromes. Mod Pathol 2022;35(3):427–37. https://doi.org/10.1038/s41379-021-00918-3.

35. Chen W, Hampel H, Pearlman R, et al. Unexpected expression of mismatch repair protein is more commonly seen with pathogenic missense than with other mutations in Lynch syndrome. Hum Pathol 2020;103:34–41. https://doi.org/10.1016/j.humpath.2020.07.001.

36. Graham RP, Kerr SE, Butz ML, et al. Heterogenous MSH6 loss is a result of microsatellite instability within MSH6 and occurs in sporadic and hereditary colorectal and endometrial carcinomas. Am J Surg Pathol 2015;39(10):1370–6. https://doi.org/10.1097/PAS.0000000000000459.

37. Watson N, Grieu F, Morris M, et al. Heterogeneous staining for mismatch repair proteins during population-based prescreening for hereditary nonpolyposis colorectal cancer. J Mol Diagn 2007;9(4): 472–8. https://doi.org/10.2353/jmoldx.2007.060162.

38. McCarthy AJ, Capo-Chichi JM, Spence T, et al. Heterogenous loss of mismatch repair (MMR) protein expression: a challenge for immunohistochemical interpretation and microsatellite instability (MSI) evaluation. J Pathol Clin Res 2019;5(2): 115–29. https://doi.org/10.1002/cjp2.120.

39. Kuan SF, Ren B, Brand R, et al. Neoadjuvant therapy in microsatellite-stable colorectal carcinoma induces concomitant loss of MSH6 and Ki-67 expression. Hum Pathol 2017;63:33–9. https://doi.org/10.1016/j.humpath.2017.02.003.

40. Shia J, Ellis NA, Paty PB, et al. Value of histopathology in predicting microsatellite instability in hereditary nonpolyposis colorectal cancer and sporadic colorectal cancer. Am J Surg Pathol 2003;27(11): 1407–17. https://doi.org/10.1097/00000478-200311000-00002.

41. Alexander J, Watanabe T, Wu TT, et al. Histopathological identification of colon cancer with microsatellite instability. Am J Pathol 2001;158(2):527–35. https://doi.org/10.1016/S0002-9440(10)63994-6.

42. Evaluation of Genomic Applications in P, Prevention Working G. Recommendations from the EGAPP Working Group: genetic testing strategies in newly diagnosed individuals with colorectal cancer aimed at reducing morbidity and mortality from Lynch syndrome in relatives. Genet Med 2009;11(1):35–41. https://doi.org/10.1097/GIM.0b013e31818fa2ff.

43. Sinicrope FA, Rego RL, Halling KC, et al. Prognostic impact of microsatellite instability and DNA ploidy in human colon carcinoma patients. Gastroenterology 2006;131(3):729–37. https://doi.org/10.1053/j.gastro.2006.06.005.

44. Ribic CM, Sargent DJ, Moore MJ, et al. Tumor microsatellite-instability status as a predictor of benefit from fluorouracil-based adjuvant chemotherapy for colon cancer. N Engl J Med 2003; 349(3):247–57. https://doi.org/10.1056/NEJMoa022289.

45. Andre T, Shiu KK, Kim TW, et al. Pembrolizumab in Microsatellite-Instability-High Advanced Colorectal Cancer. N Engl J Med 2020;383(23):2207–18. https://doi.org/10.1056/NEJMoa2017699.

46. Chalabi M, Verschoor YL, van den Berg J, et al. LBA7 Neoadjuvant immune checkpoint inhibition in locally advanced MMR-deficient colon cancer: The NICHE-2 study. Ann Oncol 2022;33:S1389. https://doi.org/10.1016/j.annonc.2022.08.016.

47. Cercek A, Lumish M, Sinopoli J, et al. PD-1 Blockade in Mismatch Repair-Deficient, Locally Advanced Rectal Cancer. N Engl J Med 2022;386(25): 2363–76. https://doi.org/10.1056/NEJMoa2201445.

48. Domingo E, Freeman-Mills L, Rayner E, et al. Somatic POLE proofreading domain mutation, immune response, and prognosis in colorectal cancer: a retrospective, pooled biomarker study.

Lancet Gastroenterol Hepatol 2016;1(3):207–16. https://doi.org/10.1016/S2468-1253(16)30014-0.

49. Campbell BB, Light N, Fabrizio D, et al. Comprehensive Analysis of Hypermutation in Human Cancer. Cell 2017;171(5):1042–56. https://doi.org/10.1016/j.cell.2017.09.048, e10.

50. Rayner E, van Gool IC, Palles C, et al. A panoply of errors: polymerase proofreading domain mutations in cancer. Nat Rev Cancer 2016;16(2):71–81. https://doi.org/10.1038/nrc.2015.12.

51. Palles C, Cazier JB, Howarth KM, et al. Germline mutations affecting the proofreading domains of POLE and POLD1 predispose to colorectal adenomas and carcinomas. Nat Genet 2013;45(2): 136–44. https://doi.org/10.1038/ng.2503.

52. Silberman R, FS D, Lo AA, et al. Complete and Prolonged Response to Immune Checkpoint Blockade in POLE-Mutated Colorectal Cancer. JCO Precis Oncol 2019;3:1–5. https://doi.org/10.1200/PO.18.00214.

53. Shia J, Schultz N, Kuk D, et al. Morphological characterization of colorectal cancers in The Cancer Genome Atlas reveals distinct morphology-molecular associations: clinical and biological implications. Mod Pathol 2017;30(4):599–609. https://doi.org/10.1038/modpathol.2016.198.

54. Forgo E, Gomez AJ, Steiner D, et al. Morphological, immunophenotypical and molecular features of hypermutation in colorectal carcinomas with mutations in DNA polymerase epsilon (POLE). Histopathology 2020;76(3):366–74. https://doi.org/10.1111/his.13984.

55. Georgeson P, Harrison TA, Pope BJ, et al. Identifying colorectal cancer caused by biallelic MUTYH pathogenic variants using tumor mutational signatures. Nat Commun 2022;13(1):3254. https://doi.org/10.1038/s41467-022-30916-1.

56. Marabelle A, Fakih M, Lopez J, et al. Association of tumour mutational burden with outcomes in patients with advanced solid tumours treated with pembrolizumab: prospective biomarker analysis of the multicohort, open-label, phase 2 KEYNOTE-158 study. Lancet Oncol 2020;21(10):1353–65. https://doi.org/10.1016/S1470-2045(20)30445-9.

57. Strickler JH, Hanks BA, Khasraw M. Tumor Mutational Burden as a Predictor of Immunotherapy Response: Is More Always Better? Clin Cancer Res 2021;27(5):1236–41. https://doi.org/10.1158/1078-0432.CCR-20-3054.

58. De Roock W, Claes B, Bernasconi D, et al. Effects of KRAS, BRAF, NRAS, and PIK3CA mutations on the efficacy of cetuximab plus chemotherapy in chemotherapy-refractory metastatic colorectal cancer: a retrospective consortium analysis. Lancet Oncol 2010;11(8):753–62. https://doi.org/10.1016/S1470-2045(10)70130-3.

59. Patelli G, Tosi F, Amatu A, et al. Strategies to tackle RAS-mutated metastatic colorectal cancer. ESMO Open 2021;6(3):100156. https://doi.org/10.1016/j.esmoop.2021.100156.

60. Malumbres M, Barbacid M. RAS oncogenes: the first 30 years. Nat Rev Cancer 2003;3(6):459–65. https://doi.org/10.1038/nrc1097.

61. Taieb J, Le Malicot K, Shi Q, et al. Prognostic Value of BRAF and KRAS Mutations in MSI and MSS Stage III Colon Cancer. J Natl Cancer Inst 2017;109(5). https://doi.org/10.1093/jnci/djw272.

62. Taieb J, Zaanan A, Le Malicot K, et al. Prognostic Effect of BRAF and KRAS Mutations in Patients With Stage III Colon Cancer Treated With Leucovorin, Fluorouracil, and Oxaliplatin With or Without Cetuximab: A Post Hoc Analysis of the PETACC-8 Trial. JAMA Oncol 2016;2(5):643–53. https://doi.org/10.1001/jamaoncol.2015.5225.

63. Amado RG, Wolf M, Peeters M, et al. Wild-type KRAS is required for panitumumab efficacy in patients with metastatic colorectal cancer. J Clin Oncol 2008;26(10):1626–34. https://doi.org/10.1200/JCO.2007.14.7116.

64. Diaz LA Jr, Williams RT, Wu J, et al. The molecular evolution of acquired resistance to targeted EGFR blockade in colorectal cancers. Nature 2012;486(7404):537–40. https://doi.org/10.1038/nature11219.

65. Canon J, Rex K, Saiki AY, et al. The clinical KRAS(G12C) inhibitor AMG 510 drives antitumour immunity. Nature 2019;575(7781):217–23. https://doi.org/10.1038/s41586-019-1694-1.

66. Hallin J, Engstrom LD, Hargis L, et al. The KRAS(G12C) Inhibitor MRTX849 Provides Insight toward Therapeutic Susceptibility of KRAS-Mutant Cancers in Mouse Models and Patients. Cancer Discov 2020;10(1):54–71. https://doi.org/10.1158/2159-8290.CD-19-1167.

67. Fakih MG, Kopetz S, Kuboki Y, et al. Sotorasib for previously treated colorectal cancers with KRAS(G12C) mutation (CodeBreaK100): a prespecified analysis of a single-arm, phase 2 trial. Lancet Oncol 2022;23(1):115–24. https://doi.org/10.1016/S1470-2045(21)00605-7.

68. Awad MM, Liu S, Rybkin II, et al. Acquired Resistance to KRAS(G12C) Inhibition in Cancer. N Engl J Med 2021;384(25):2382–93. https://doi.org/10.1056/NEJMoa2105281.

69. Amodio V, Yaeger R, Arcella P, et al. EGFR Blockade Reverts Resistance to KRAS(G12C) Inhibition in Colorectal Cancer. Cancer Discov 2020;10(8):1129–39. https://doi.org/10.1158/2159-8290.CD-20-0187.

70. Yaeger R, Weiss J, Pelster MS, et al. Adagrasib with or without Cetuximab in Colorectal Cancer with Mutated KRAS G12C. N Engl J Med 2023;388(1):44–54. https://doi.org/10.1056/NEJMoa2212419.

71. Samowitz WS, Sweeney C, Herrick J, et al. Poor survival associated with the BRAF V600E mutation in microsatellite-stable colon cancers. Cancer Res 2005;65(14):6063–9. https://doi.org/10.1158/0008-5472.CAN-05-0404.

72. Ogino S, Nosho K, Kirkner GJ, et al. CpG island methylator phenotype, microsatellite instability, BRAF mutation and clinical outcome in colon cancer. Gut 2009;58(1):90–6. https://doi.org/10.1136/gut.2008.155473.

73. Pai RK, Jayachandran P, Koong AC, et al. BRAF-mutated, microsatellite-stable adenocarcinoma of the proximal colon: an aggressive adenocarcinoma with poor survival, mucinous differentiation, and adverse morphologic features. Am J Surg Pathol 2012;36(5):744–52. https://doi.org/10.1097/PAS.0b013e31824430d7.

74. Goldstein J, Tran B, Ensor J, et al. Multicenter retrospective analysis of metastatic colorectal cancer (CRC) with high-level microsatellite instability (MSI-H). Ann Oncol 2014;25(5):1032–8. https://doi.org/10.1093/annonc/mdu100.

75. Kopetz S, Grothey A, Yaeger R, et al. Encorafenib, Binimetinib, and Cetuximab in BRAF V600E-Mutated Colorectal Cancer. N Engl J Med 2019;381(17):1632–43. https://doi.org/10.1056/NEJMoa1908075.

76. Nowak JA. HER2 in Colorectal Carcinoma: Are We There yet? Surg Pathol Clin 2020;13(3):485–502. https://doi.org/10.1016/j.path.2020.05.007.

77. Arteaga CL, Engelman JA. ERBB receptors: from oncogene discovery to basic science to mechanism-based cancer therapeutics. Cancer Cell 2014;25(3):282–303. https://doi.org/10.1016/j.ccr.2014.02.025.

78. Ross JS, Fakih M, Ali SM, et al. Targeting HER2 in colorectal cancer: The landscape of amplification and short variant mutations in ERBB2 and ERBB3. Cancer 2018;124(7):1358–73. https://doi.org/10.1002/cncr.31125.

79. Pahuja KB, Nguyen TT, Jaiswal BS, et al. Actionable Activating Oncogenic ERBB2/HER2 Transmembrane and Juxtamembrane Domain Mutations. Cancer Cell 2018;34(5):792–806 e5. https://doi.org/10.1016/j.ccell.2018.09.010.

80. Ali SM, Sanford EM, Klempner SJ, et al. Prospective comprehensive genomic profiling of advanced gastric carcinoma cases reveals frequent clinically relevant genomic alterations and new routes for targeted therapies. Oncol 2015;20(5):499–507. https://doi.org/10.1634/theoncologist.2014-0378.

81. Bang YJ, Van Cutsem E, Feyereislova A, et al. Trastuzumab in combination with chemotherapy versus chemotherapy alone for treatment of HER2-positive advanced gastric or gastro-oesophageal junction

cancer (ToGA): a phase 3, open-label, randomised controlled trial. Lancet 2010;376(9742):687–97. https://doi.org/10.1016/S0140-6736(10)61121-X.

82. Corrections to "Distal and proximal colon cancers differ in terms of molecular, pathological, and clinical features". Ann Oncol 2015;26(2):445. https://doi.org/10.1093/annonc/mdu548.

83. Ingold Heppner B, Behrens HM, Balschun K, et al. HER2/neu testing in primary colorectal carcinoma. Br J Cancer 2014;111(10):1977–84. https://doi.org/10.1038/bjc.2014.483.

84. Sartore-Bianchi A, Trusolino L, Martino C, et al. Dual-targeted therapy with trastuzumab and lapatinib in treatment-refractory, KRAS codon 12/13 wild-type, HER2-positive metastatic colorectal cancer (HERACLES): a proof-of-concept, multicentre, open-label, phase 2 trial. Lancet Oncol 2016; 17(6):738–46. https://doi.org/10.1016/S1470-2045(16)00150-9.

85. Meric-Bernstam F, Hurwitz H, Raghav KPS, et al. Pertuzumab plus trastuzumab for HER2-amplified metastatic colorectal cancer (MyPathway): an updated report from a multicentre, open-label, phase 2a, multiple basket study. Lancet Oncol 2019; 20(4):518–30. https://doi.org/10.1016/S1470-2045(18)30904-5.

86. Biller LH, Schrag D. Diagnosis and Treatment of Metastatic Colorectal Cancer: A Review. JAMA 2021;325(7):669–85. https://doi.org/10.1001/jama.2021.0106.

87. Siena S, Elez E, Peeters M, et al. PD-1 MOUNTAINEER: Open-label, phase 2 study of tucatinib combined with trastuzumab for HER2-positive metastatic colorectal cancer (SGNTUC-017, trial in progress). Ann Oncol 2021;32:S199. https://doi.org/10.1016/j.annonc.2021.05.019.

88. Siena S, Di Bartolomeo M, Raghav K, et al. Trastuzumab deruxtecan (DS-8201) in patients with HER2-expressing metastatic colorectal cancer (DESTINY-CRC01): a multicentre, open-label, phase 2 trial. Lancet Oncol 2021;22(6):779–89. https://doi.org/10.1016/S1470-2045(21)00086-3.

89. Valtorta E, Martino C, Sartore-Bianchi A, et al. Assessment of a HER2 scoring system for colorectal cancer: results from a validation study. Mod Pathol 2015;28(11):1481–91. https://doi.org/10.1038/modpathol.2015.98.

90. Correction to Lancet Oncol 2016; 17: 738. Lancet Oncol 2016;17(10):e420. https://doi.org/10.1016/S1470-2045(16)30463-6.

91. Cenaj O, Ligon AH, Hornick JL, et al. Detection of ERBB2 Amplification by Next-Generation Sequencing Predicts HER2 Expression in Colorectal Carcinoma. Am J Clin Pathol 2019;152(1):97–108. https://doi.org/10.1093/ajcp/aqz031.

92. Zehir A, Benayed R, Shah RH, et al. Mutational landscape of metastatic cancer revealed from prospective clinical sequencing of 10,000 patients. Nat Med 2017;23(6):703–13. https://doi.org/10.1038/nm.4333.

93. Stransky N, Cerami E, Schalm S, et al. The landscape of kinase fusions in cancer. Nat Commun 2014;5:4846. https://doi.org/10.1038/ncomms5846.

94. Kloosterman WP, Coebergh van den Braak RRJ, Pieterse M, et al. A Systematic Analysis of Oncogenic Gene Fusions in Primary Colon Cancer. Cancer Res 2017;77(14):3814–22. https://doi.org/10.1158/0008-5472.CAN-16-3563.

95. Pietrantonio F, Di Nicolantonio F, Schrock AB, et al. ALK, ROS1, and NTRK Rearrangements in Metastatic Colorectal Cancer. J Natl Cancer Inst 2017; 109(12). https://doi.org/10.1093/jnci/djx089.

96. Solomon JP, Linkov I, Rosado A, et al. NTRK fusion detection across multiple assays and 33,997 cases: diagnostic implications and pitfalls. Mod Pathol 2020;33(1):38–46. https://doi.org/10.1038/s41379-019-0324-7.

97. Santos C, Sanz-Pamplona R, Salazar R. RET-fusions: a novel paradigm in colorectal cancer. Ann Oncol 2018;29(6):1340–3. https://doi.org/10.1093/annonc/mdy132.

98. Lasota J, Chlopek M, Lamoureux J, et al. Colonic Adenocarcinomas Harboring NTRK Fusion Genes: A Clinicopathologic and Molecular Genetic Study of 16 Cases and Review of the Literature. Am J Surg Pathol 2020;44(2):162–73. https://doi.org/10.1097/PAS.0000000000001377.

99. Sholl LM, Zheng M, Nardi V, et al. Predictive 'biomarker piggybacking': an examination of reflexive pan-cancer screening with pan-TRK immunohistochemistry. Histopathology 2021;79(2):260–4. https://doi.org/10.1111/his.14351.

100. Doebele RC, Drilon A, Paz-Ares L, et al. Entrectinib in patients with advanced or metastatic NTRK fusion-positive solid tumours: integrated analysis of three phase 1-2 trials. Lancet Oncol 2020; 21(2):271–82. https://doi.org/10.1016/S1470-2045(19)30691-6.

101. Hong DS, DuBois SG, Kummar S, et al. Larotrectinib in patients with TRK fusion-positive solid tumours: a pooled analysis of three phase 1/2 clinical trials. Lancet Oncol 2020;21(4):531–40. https://doi.org/10.1016/S1470-2045(19)30856-3.

102. Subbiah V, Wolf J, Konda B, et al. Tumour-agnostic efficacy and safety of selpercatinib in patients with RET fusion-positive solid tumours other than lung or thyroid tumours (LIBRETTO-001): a phase 1/2, open-label, basket trial. Lancet Oncol 2022; 23(10):1261–73. https://doi.org/10.1016/S1470-2045(22)00541-1.

Deep Learning and Colon Cancer Interpretation
Rise of the Machine

Kelsey McHugh, MD, Rish K. Pai, MD, PhD*

KEYWORDS

- Digital pathology • Artificial intelligence • Colorectal cancer • Whole-slide imaging

Key points

- Machine learning tools for colorectal cancer have focused on predicting outcomes as well as underlying molecular alterations such as microsatellite instability status.
- AI tools for colorectal cancer have the potential to augment current pathologic reporting and provide valuable information to clinicians and pathologists using hematoxylin and eosin-stained slides.
- Many barriers to implementation exist including costs for slide digitization, algorithm development, and algorithm deployment.

ABSTRACT

The rapidly evolving development of artificial intelligence (AI) has spurred the development of numerous algorithms that augment information obtained from routine pathologic review of hematoxylin and eosin-stained slides. AI tools that predict prognosis and underlying molecular alterations have been the focus of much of the research to date. The results of these studies highlight the tremendous potential of AI to enhance our pathology reports by providing rapid predictions of key features that influence therapy and outcomes.

OVERVIEW

Colorectal carcinoma (CRC) is the second leading cause of cancer deaths in the United States.[1] Treatment and prognosis of CRC are determined, in part, by histologic features, tumor, node, metastasis (TNM) staging, and underlying molecular alterations.[2] CRC is histologically and molecularly heterogeneous, and the current pathologic assessment does not capture this variability in a useful manner. The heterogeneity can help predict underlying molecular alterations as well as identify tumors with a distinct clinical behavior. For example, pathologists have long been aware of the associations between mismatch repair (MMR) deficiency and tumor grade, mucinous differentiation, and immune cell infiltration.[3–7] More recently, the presence of tumor budding (TB) and poorly differentiated clusters (PDCs) have been shown to provide important prognostic information and are thought to be the histologic representation of epithelial-mesenchymal transition.[6,8–11] Lastly, stroma-rich tumors and tumors with immature desmoplastic stroma are associated with worse outcomes.[12–15] Given the increasing number of proposed prognostic and predictive features, it can be challenging for pathologists to determine what to report in CRC and for oncologists to decipher the meaning of each feature. In addition, there is suboptimal interobserver agreement among pathologists, and differences in reporting exist between community and subspecialized gastrointestinal pathologists.[16–20] Given recent advances in deep learning and computer vision, there is an opportunity to develop algorithms that reliably predict prognosis, response to therapy, and specific molecular alterations. Such tools could help standardize reporting of CRC and reduce interobserver

Department of Pathology and Laboratory Medicine, Mayo Clinic Arizona, 13400 East Shea Boulevard, Scottsdale, AZ 85253, USA

* Corresponding author.

E-mail address: pai.rish@mayo.edu

Surgical Pathology 16 (2023) 651–658
https://doi.org/10.1016/j.path.2023.05.003
1875-9181/23/© 2023 Elsevier Inc. All rights reserved.

Table 1
Selected articles employing deep learning in colorectal cancer

Article	Goal	Method Used	Number of Cases Analyzed	Performance Metrics
Wei et al,[22] 2020	Develop a model to classify colonic polyps	High supervised learning with manual annotations	2704 cropped images from 458 WSI	Overall 87.6% accuracy
Echle et al,[26] 2020	Develop a model to predict MSI in CRC	High supervised learning with manual annotations	6406 WSI for model training 771 WSI for model validation	AUC of 0.95 in the external validation cohort
Sirinukunwattana et al,[27] 2021	Develop a model to predict CRC CMS	High supervised learning with manual annotations	506 WSI for model training 696 WSI for model validation	AUCs of 0.84 and 0.85 in the resection and biopsy external validation cohorts, respectively
Bilal et al,[29] 2021	Develop a model to predict key molecular alterations in CRC	Weakly supervised learning with the development of multiple models pipeline to arrive at final prediction	502 WSI for model training 47 slides for model validation of MSI prediction results	Mean AUCs for the following predictions: hypermutation 0.81, MSI 0.86, CIN 0.83, $BRAF^{mut}$ 0.79, $TP53^{mut}$ 0.73
Skrede et al,[32] 2020	Develop a prognostic digital biomarker	Weakly supervised learning with development of multiple models to arrive at a final prediction	828 for model development 1122 validation of prognostic model	c-index of 0.674 in the external validation cohort
Pai et al,[35] 2021	Develop a prognostic digital biomarker	High supervised learning with manual annotations	559 for model development 2411 training prognostic of model 938 validation of prognostic model	c-index of 0.744 in an external validation cohort

Abbreviations: CIN, chromosomal instability; CMS, consensus molecular subtypes; CRC, colorectal carcinoma; MSI, microsatellite instability; mut, mutation; WSI, whole slide images.

variability. In this review, we summarize recent developments in applying artificial intelligence (AI) tools to CRC (**Table 1**).

BASIC MACHINE LEARNING FOR SURGICAL PATHOLOGISTS

AI was a term first coined by McCarthy in 1956 to describe the use of computational methods to make a prediction. Machine learning is a form of AI and involves training a machine to learn from curated data to make subsequent predictions on new data. Since the advent of whole slide scanners, machine learning has been used to perform various tasks in pathology, most commonly image analysis. This type of machine learning is often regarded as traditional machine learning to separate this from new methods such as deep learning. Traditional machine learning uses predefined features (eg, pixel intensity, nuclear size, and so on) to set thresholds, which are then applied to an image. Such hand-crafted techniques are routinely employed to perform quantitative analysis of immunohistochemistry. Deep learning is a much more powerful type of machine learning that employs

convolutional neural networks (CNNs) to learn how to perform a task. A CNN is a multilayered network of millions of artificial neurons that can learn from complex data similar to a human brain. Because CNNs are not reliant on predetermined features, deep learning models vastly outperform traditional machine learning techniques.

It is beyond the scope of this review to discuss in detail different deep learning methods, but surgical pathologists should have a broad understanding of how deep learning methods are employed in pathology. Supervised deep learning is the most common type of deep learning used in pathology and can be performed using two broad methods (**Fig. 1**). Pathologists are most familiar with highly supervised deep learning wherein pathologists annotate regions on a slide, and the image data are extracted from the annotated regions and used to train a CNN to detect that feature of interest. Such methodology is very powerful but requires manual annotations by pathologists, which is time-consuming and costly. Features that have high interobserver variability will also require numerous annotations to train a reasonably performing CNN. While being more labor-intensive, such methods have the advantage of being

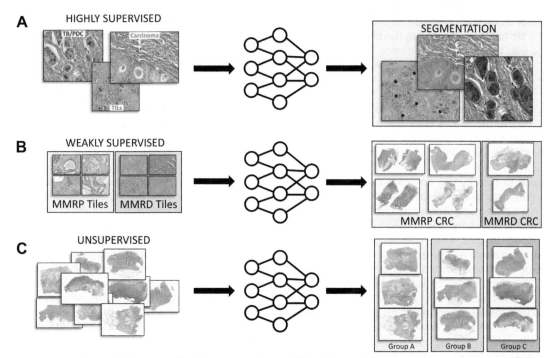

Fig. 1. Types of deep learning in pathology. (*A*) Highly supervised learning takes advantage of pathologist annotations of individual features. The annotated areas are extracted, and a convolutional neural network can be trained to identify these features. (*B*) Weakly supervised learning is a powerful alternative to time-consuming manual annotations. In this method, image tiles are labeled with a feature of interest, and the entire tile is fed into a neural network. This process does not require knowledge of features associated with the outcome of interest and can be used to identify novel histologic features. (*C*) In unsupervised learning, there is no labeling of the image tiles. This method could be used to identify novel associations between image data.

explainable as the feature is often well-defined and easily recognized by a pathologist. The advantage of highly supervised deep learning is not in the discovery of new findings but rather improved quantification and identification of specific features, which would be impossible for a pathologist to manually determine.

Another commonly used deep learning method employs the use of image tiles that are labeled with a specific feature, outcome, or molecular alteration. Often all the tiles in a whole slide image are given the same label even though some tiles will be noninformative. Features are extracted from these tiles and fed into a CNN to learn which tiles correspond to the specific outcome of interest. Tiles can be from the entire whole slide image or a specific portion of the image, such as tumor regions only. This weakly supervised methodology does not lend itself to easy explainability but can be useful to discover novel features. Additional techniques such as multiple-instance learning with or without attention have been used to improve model performance. Multiple-instance learning recognizes that not all tiles within an image reflect the underlying label, and combined with attention, each tile is weighted based on how much it contributes to the classification. The output from such a model is often represented as a tile heatmap identifying the tiles within an image with the strongest prediction for that feature.

DEEP LEARNING AS A DIAGNOSTIC AID

In contrast to other fields of pathology where training AI models to diagnose cancer has been the focus of most research, there are only very few studies using AI to diagnose CRC or precursor lesions. Korbar and colleagues developed an AI model to classify five common colorectal polyps (hyperplastic polyp, sessile serrated lesion, traditional serrated adenoma, tubular adenoma, and tubulovillous/villous adenoma).[21] They used 2704 cropped images from 458 whole-slide images that were annotated by expert gastrointestinal pathologists to train the model and tested the model on 239 whole-slide images. A variety of neural architectures were tested, and the best performing model (ResNet-D) achieved an overall accuracy of 93.0%, with the lowest accuracy for hyperplastic polyps (89.8%) and sessile serrated lesions (89.5%). In a follow-up study, the authors obtained an external data set of 238 slides from 179 patients to test their model using only 4 classes (excluding traditional serrated adenoma).[22] Five gastrointestinal pathologists reviewed these slides, and a consensus diagnosis was recorded. Using their model, an accuracy of 87.0% was obtained

when compared to the consensus diagnosis which compared favorably with the local pathologist's accuracy of 86.6%. Overall, these data suggest that such models may serve as a useful screen for pathologists by identifying areas of interest to improve efficiency and accuracy. However, more work is needed to determine the operating properties of such a model in a busy clinical practice.

DEEP LEARNING AS A PREDICTIVE BIOMARKER

Utilizing deep learning-based algorithms as surrogate markers for various genetic alterations in CRC holds great promise in gleaning significant prognostic and targeted therapeutic information from hematoxylin and eosin (H&E)-stained whole-slide images. Authors across the globe have demonstrated the utility of deep learning algorithms as powerful tools in predicting tumor mutation status, with sensitivities for microsatellite instability (MSI) detection that rival those of current standards of practice such as MMR protein immunohistochemistry.

In 2019, Kather and colleagues tested five CNNs and trained the best-performing model (Resnet18) to classify CRC with MSI versus microsatellite stable (MSS) tumors on two cohorts of whole-slide images which included 360 formalin-fixed paraffin-embedded (FFPE) samples and 378 snap-frozen samples.[23] They achieved an area under the curve (AUC) for MSI detection of 0.84 and 0.77 in their FFPE and snap-frozen cohorts, respectively. Upon application of their trained neural network to an external validation set of 378 patients, the model yielded an AUC of 0.84.[23] This AUC for MSI detection is similar to those generated by other authors including Cao and colleagues whose model, trained on 429 CRC cases from the Cancer Genome Atlas (AUC of 0.88), achieved an AUC of 0.85 in an external validation set of 785 CRC from an Asian CRC cohort.[24] Similarly, the MSINet model generated by Yamashita and colleagues, trained on only 100 whole-slide images equally divided between MSS and MSI tumors, achieved an AUC of 0.865 on an external data set of 40 cases equally divided between MSS and MSI tumors.[25] These authors did demonstrate superiority of their deep learning model in MSI detection when compared to five experienced gastrointestinal pathologists, who achieved a mean AUC of 0.605 for MSI detection on the external data set.[25] The largest effort to date in training and validating a deep learning system for MSI detection in CRC comes from a consortium of authors from institutions in Germany, the Netherlands, the United Kingdom, and the United States. Echle and colleagues utilized whole-slide images paired with molecular data from more than 8000 patients in their endeavor, achieving an AUC of 0.92 for MSI detection in their international training cohort.[26] External validation of the model on 771 whole-slide images from a population-based cohort generated an AUC of 0.95 for MSI detection.[26] Noteworthy take-aways from this international effort include data demonstrating the susceptibility of deep learning systems to "overfit" the cohorts they are trained on, compromising the applicability of models to other or more generalized cohorts. Echle and colleagues also nicely demonstrated a "learning curve" in which the AUC for MSI detection continued to increase as more patients were used to train the deep learning model until an AUC plateau (AUC of 0.92) was reached at approximately 5000 patients.[26] These data show that approximately 5000 patients are necessary and sufficient to train deep learning detectors of MSI.[26]

Beyond MSI, deep learning models have also been successfully trained to detect an array of other clinically and therapeutically significant molecular alterations commonly identified in CRC. Sirinukunwattana and colleagues trained inception V3 deep neural networks to predict CRC consensus molecular subtypes (CMS), initially set forth by Guinney and colleagues based on gene expression profiling data, through image analysis of 1540 slides from three independent data sets including 1134 resection samples and 406 biopsy samples.[27,28] Overall classification accuracies into one of four CRC CMSs were an AUC of 0.84 and an AUC of 0.85 for external validation cohorts of resection and biopsy specimens, respectively.[27] Authors from the United Kingdom had similar success in training a deep learning framework that involved three separate CNN models to predict the presence of hypermutation, MSI, chromosomal instability, CpG island methylator phenotype (CIMP)-high, BRAF mutation, TP53 mutation, and KRAS mutation in CRC. The deep learning method of those authors, Bilal and colleagues, yielded mean AUCs for the following predictions: 0.81 for hypermutation, 0.86 for MSI, 0.83 for chromosomal instability, 0.79 for BRAF mutation, 0.73 for TP53 mutation, 0.60 for KRAS mutation, and 0.79 for CIMP-high status.[29]

In summary, the aforementioned studies nicely demonstrate the utility of AI and deep learning-based algorithms as predictive biomarkers in CRC. At a minimum, these algorithms hold promise as high-sensitivity prescreening methodologies that would allow for reflexive molecular testing as the gold standard when warranted.

DEEP LEARNING AS A PROGNOSTIC BIOMARKER

Using deep learning to prognosticate has been an area of active research in CRC with the development of several digital biomarkers of prognosis. In an early study, Kather and colleagues trained a CNN to perform a simple segmentation to identify fat, debris, lymphoid aggregates, mucin, smooth muscle, normal colonic mucosa, tumor stroma, and tumor epithelium using annotations on 86 H&Es of CRCs.[30] A stroma score was derived from this algorithm and was shown to have prognostic value in an independent cohort of 409 stage I-IV CRCs. Subsequently, Wulczyn and colleagues developed a deep learning system to predict disease-specific survival for stage II and III CRCs using image tiles from tumor regions and achieved an AUC of 0.70 in predicting 5-year survival in a validation cohort.[31] In this study, human-interpretable features to explain the variance in survival was attempted by manual review of image tiles that strongly contributed to the model. The presence of PDCs adjacent to adipose tissue was identified as a possible predictor of poor survival. These early studies highlighted the potential of deep learning in predicting prognosis in CRC.

More recently, in *The Lancet*, Srkede and colleagues used image tiles from 828 patients to predict prognosis (DoMore-v1-CRC).[32] For the ground truth, patients were assigned to the good prognosis group if younger than 85 years and had greater than 6 years in follow-up without recurrence or cancer-specific death. Poor prognosis was defined as age less than 85 years with cancer-specific deaths occurring between 100 days and 2.5 years after surgery. All other patients were considered to have a nondistinct outcome and were used to tune the models. A total of 10 models were trained, 5 using image tiles with 10x resolution and 5 using image tiles with 40x resolution. The models were trained on the collection of tiles from a single whole-slide image labeled with the specific outcome. The networks were trained end-to-end from the image to the patient outcome. The prediction from the 10x and 40x resolution models was used to assign the final prediction as good, poor, or uncertain. The model was validated in an external cohort of 1122 stage III and high-risk stage II tumors from the QUASAR 2 clinical trial evaluating capecitabine plus bevacizumab or capecitabine alone.[33] The DoMore-v1-CRC provided a concordance (c) index of 0.674 (95% CI 0.624–0.719) in the validation cohort. The c-index reflects a measure of how well a model predicts the ordering of patient's time to recurrence. A c-index of 0.5 indicates a random model, whereas a c-index of 1 is a perfect ranking of time to recurrence. The DoMore-v1-CRC resulted in a hazard ratio of 2.71 (95% CI 1.25–5.86, $P = .011$) for poor prognosis stage II tumors and a cancer-specific survival hazard ratio of 2.95 (95% CI 1.81–4.82, $P < .0001$) for poor prognosis stage III tumors in the validation cohort. There was a strong association between the DoMore-v1-CRC classification and pT stage, pN stage, histological grade, and location. Subsequently, the same group combined DoMore-v1-CRC with other risk factors to generate a clinical decision-support tool to provide robust risk stratification for stage II and III CRCs.[34] This model incorporates pN stage, pT stage, and number of lymph nodes sampled with the DoMore-v1-CRC prognostic groups. The QUASAR 2 trial served as the validation cohort for this integrated scheme. The integrated scheme provided robust stratification for stage III tumors with a cancer-specific survival hazard ratio of 10.44 (95% CI 5.11–20.03, $P < .0001$) for high-risk tumors and outperformed standard risk stratification schemes. The DoMore-v1-CRC integrated risk stratification for stage II tumors was less robust with a log-rank P value of 0.035 in Kaplan-Meier analysis. Overall, these results highlighted the potential of AI to provide a robust risk-stratification scheme for CRC.

Recently, our group has developed a digital biomarker of recurrence for stage I-III CRC that utilizes highly supervised deep learning methods. First, a deep learning segmentation model (QuantCRC) was trained using 24,157 annotations on 559 images of CRC.[35] This model uses CNNs to quantify the amount of stroma and stromal subtypes (immature, inflammatory, and mature); tumor and tumor grade; signet ring cells; tumor infiltrating lymphocytes; TB and PDCs (as one combined feature); necrosis; and mucin. QuantCRC was validated against annotations made by expert gastrointestinal pathologists. We hypothesized that better quantification of known histological features associated with clinical outcomes would be able to provide a robust prediction of recurrence-free survival (RFS). To test this hypothesis, QuantCRC was applied to 2441 stage I-III CRCs with recurrence data from the well-established Colon Cancer Family Registry Cohort.[36] A multivariable Cox model incorporating 15 QuantCRC features, MMR status, and overall stage was trained on 80% of this cohort and tested on the remaining 20%. Based on the 33rd and 66th percentiles for predicted 36-month RFS, low-risk, intermediate-risk, and high-risk prognostic groups for each stage were identified and validated in a separate cohort of 938 CRCs. The c-index for

this model in the validation cohort was 0.744 (95% CI 0.741–754). For stage III CRCs, the high-risk group resulted in a univariate hazard ratio for RFS of 2.72 (95% CI 1.62–4.89, $P < .001$). For stage II CRCs, the high-risk group resulted in a hazard ratio of 3.18 (95% CI 1.51–6.73, $P = .002$). The prognostic groups were independent predictors of RFS after adjusting for established risk factors for stage III and II CRCs. Additional studies are needed to validate this finding and to integrate these prognostic risk groups into current risk-stratification schemes. Overall, these results suggest that deep learning has the potential to provide robust risk stratification that can be used to guide subsequent therapy and surveillance.

SUMMARY

As pathology laboratories continue to embrace digital pathology, powerful AI tools could, be deployed to supplement current reporting of CRC. However, significant barriers to implementation currently exist. In particular, digitization and computing costs as well as AI being perceived as a "black box" make routine implementation difficult in most centers. While some algorithms could be deployed locally, it may be that AI tools are centralized to a few centers with the necessary expertise. A centralized/reference laboratory model could solve some of these issues until it becomes cost-effective to deploy in all centers. In summary, powerful AI tools have been developed that could have tremendous clinical utility in CRC. The number of AI tools is only going to increase as technology improves and the digital pathology revolution accelerates.

CLINICS CARE POINTS

- AI can be used to augment pathologic reporting of colorectal cancer by providing valuable information that can guide clincal decision making.

- Implementation of AI models will remain a challenge in the near future due to cost and lack of expertise.

DISCLOSURE

R.K. Pai reports consulting income from Alimentiv Inc., Eli Lilly, AbbVie, and Allergan outside of the submitted work. K. McHugh reports no financial relationships.

FUNDING SUPPORT

R.K. Pai is funded in part by the National Cancer Institute (NCI) and National Institutes of Health (NIH) (award U01 CA167551).

REFERENCES

1. Siegel RL, Miller KD, Jemal A. Cancer statistics. CA Cancer J Clin 2020;70:7–30.
2. Böckelman C, Engelmann BE, Kaprio T, et al. Risk of recurrence in patients with colon cancer stage II and III: a systematic review and meta-analysis of recent literature. Acta Oncol 2015;54:5–16.
3. Ueno H, Hashiguchi Y, Shimazaki H, et al. Objective criteria for crohn-like lymphoid reaction in colorectal cancer. Am J Clin Pathol 2013;139:434–41.
4. Idos GE, Kwok J, Bonthala N, et al. The Prognostic Implications of Tumor Infiltrating Lymphocytes in Colorectal Cancer: A Systematic Review and Meta-Analysis. Sci Rep 2020;10:3360.
5. Williams DS, Mouradov D, Jorissen RN, et al. Lymphocytic response to tumour and deficient DNA mismatch repair identify subtypes of stage II/III colorectal cancer associated with patient outcomes. Gut 2019;68:465–74.
6. Lee H, Sha D, Foster NR, et al. Analysis of tumor microenvironmental features to refine prognosis by T, N risk group in patients with stage III colon cancer (NCCTG N0147) (Alliance). Ann Oncol 2020;31:487–94.
7. Anon. colon.pdf. Available at: https://www.nccn.org/professionals/physician_gls/pdf/colon.pdf (Accessed July 3, 2020).
8. Shivji S, Conner JR, Barresi V, et al. Poorly differentiated clusters in colorectal cancer: a current review and implications for future practice. Histopathology 2020;77:351–68.
9. Yonemura K, Kajiwara Y, Ao T, et al. Prognostic Value of Poorly Differentiated Clusters in Liver Metastatic Lesions of Colorectal Carcinoma. Am J Surg Pathol 2019;43:1341–8.
10. Lugli A, Kirsch R, Ajioka Y, et al. Recommendations for reporting tumor budding in colorectal cancer based on the International Tumor Budding Consensus Conference (ITBCC) 2016. Mod Pathol 2017;30:1299–311.
11. Trinh A, Lädrach C, Dawson HE, et al. Tumour budding is associated with the mesenchymal colon cancer subtype and RAS/RAF mutations: a study of 1320 colorectal cancers with Consensus Molecular Subgroup (CMS) data. Br J Cancer 2018;119:1244–51.
12. Huijbers A, Tollenaar RaEM, Pelt GW v, et al. The proportion of tumor-stroma as a strong prognosticator for stage II and III colon cancer patients: validation in the VICTOR trial. Ann Oncol 2013;24:179–85.
13. Mesker WE, Junggeburt JMC, Szuhai K, et al. The carcinoma-stromal ratio of colon carcinoma is an independent factor for survival compared to lymph node status and tumor stage. Cell Oncol 2007;29:387–98.
14. Ueno H, Kanemitsu Y, Sekine S, et al. Desmoplastic Pattern at the Tumor Front Defines Poor-prognosis Subtypes of Colorectal Cancer. Am J Surg Pathol 2017;41:1506–12.
15. Ueno H, Kanemitsu Y, Sekine S, et al. A Multicenter Study of the Prognostic Value of Desmoplastic Reaction Categorization in Stage II Colorectal Cancer. Am J Surg Pathol 2019;43:1015–22.
16. Bokhorst JM, Blank A, Lugli A, et al. Assessment of individual tumor buds using keratin immunohistochemistry: moderate interobserver agreement suggests a role for machine learning. Mod Pathol 2020;33:825–33.
17. Harris EI, Lewin DN, Wang HL, et al. Lymphovascular invasion in colorectal cancer: an interobserver variability study. Am J Surg Pathol 2008;32:1816–21.
18. Kirsch R, Messenger DE, Riddell RH, et al. Venous invasion in colorectal cancer: impact of an elastin stain on detection and interobserver agreement among gastrointestinal and nongastrointestinal pathologists. Am J Surg Pathol 2013;37:200–10.
19. Dawson H, Kirsch R, Messenger D, et al. A Review of Current Challenges in Colorectal Cancer Reporting. Arch Pathol Lab Med 2019;143:869–82.
20. Karamchandani DM, Chetty R, King TS, et al. Challenges with colorectal cancer staging: results of an international study. Mod Pathol 2020;33:153–63.
21. Korbar B, Olofson AM, Miraflor AP, et al. Deep Learning for Classification of Colorectal Polyps on Whole-slide Images. J Pathol Inf 2017;8:30.
22. Wei JW, Suriawinata AA, Vaickus LJ, et al. Evaluation of a Deep Neural Network for Automated Classification of Colorectal Polyps on Histopathologic Slides. JAMA Netw Open 2020;3:e203398.
23. Kather JN, Pearson AT, Halama N, et al. Deep learning can predict microsatellite instability directly from histology in gastrointestinal cancer. Nat Med 2019;25:1054–6.
24. Cao R, Yang F, Ma S-C, et al. Development and interpretation of a pathomics-based model for the prediction of microsatellite instability in Colorectal Cancer. Theranostics 2020;10:11080–91.
25. Yamashita R, Long J, Longacre T, et al. Deep learning model for the prediction of microsatellite instability in colorectal cancer: a diagnostic study. Lancet Oncol 2021;22:132–41.
26. Echle A, Grabsch HI, Quirke P, et al. Clinical-Grade Detection of Microsatellite Instability in Colorectal Tumors by Deep Learning. Gastroenterology 2020;159:1406–16.e11.
27. Sirinukunwattana K, Domingo E, Richman SD, et al. Image-based consensus molecular subtype (imCMS)

classification of colorectal cancer using deep learning. Gut 2021;70:544–54.

28. Guinney J, Dienstmann R, Wang X, et al. The consensus molecular subtypes of colorectal cancer. Nat Med 2015;21:1350–6.

29. Bilal M, Raza SEA, Azam A, et al. Development and validation of a weakly supervised deep learning framework to predict the status of molecular pathways and key mutations in colorectal cancer from routine histology images: a retrospective study. Lancet Digit Health 2021;3, e763–e772.

30. Kather JN, Krisam J, Charoentong P, et al. Predicting survival from colorectal cancer histology slides using deep learning: A retrospective multicenter study. PLoS Med 2019;16:e1002730.

31. Wulczyn E, Steiner DF, Moran M, et al. Interpretable survival prediction for colorectal cancer using deep learning. NPJ Digit Med 2021;4:71.

32. Skrede O-J, De Raedt S, Kleppe A, et al. Deep learning for prediction of colorectal cancer outcome: a discovery and validation study. Lancet 2020;395:350–60.

33. Kerr RS, Love S, Segelov E, et al. Adjuvant capecitabine plus bevacizumab versus capecitabine alone in patients with colorectal cancer (QUASAR 2): an open-label, randomised phase 3 trial. Lancet Oncol 2016;17:1543–57.

34. Kleppe A, Skrede O-J, De Raedt S, et al. A clinical decision support system optimising adjuvant chemotherapy for colorectal cancers by integrating deep learning and pathological staging markers: a development and validation study. Lancet Oncol 2022;23:1221–32.

35. Pai RK, Hartman D, Schaeffer DF, et al. Development and initial validation of a deep learning algorithm to quantify histological features in colorectal carcinoma including tumour budding/poorly differentiated clusters. Histopathology 2021;79:391–405.

36. Pai RK, Banerjee I, Shivji S, et al. Quantitative Pathologic Analysis of Digitized Images of Colorectal Carcinoma Improves Prediction of Recurrence-Free Survival. Gastroenterology 2022;163:1531–46.e8.

What Therapeutic Biomarkers in Gastro-Esophageal Junction and Gastric Cancer Should a Pathologist Know About?

Marian Priyanthi Kumarasinghe, MBBS, MD, Dip Cytopath (RCPA), FRCPA[a],*,
Daniel Houghton, FRCPA, BMBS, PhD[b], Benjamin Michael Allanson, MBBS, FRCPA[b],
Timothy J. Price, MBBS, FRACP, DHlthSc (Med)[c,1]

KEYWORDS

• Biomarkers • HER2 • Gastric/GEJ • PD L1 • MMRP

Key points

- Malignancies of upper gastrointestinal tract are aggressive, and most locally advanced unresectable and metastatic cancers are managed by a combination of surgery and neoadjuvant/adjuvant chemotherapy and radiotherapy. Only early tumors with favorable pathological features are managed by endoscopic modalities.

- Current therapeutic recommendations include targeted therapies based on biomarker expression of an individual tumor.

ABSTRACT

Malignancies of upper gastrointestinal tract are aggressive, and most locally advanced unresectable and metastatic cancers are managed by a combination of surgery and neoadjuvant/adjuvant chemotherapy and radiotherapy. Current therapeutic recommendations include targeted therapies based on biomarker expression of an individual tumor. All G/gastro-esophageal junction (GEJ) cancers should be tested for HER2 status as a reflex test at the time of diagnosis. Currently, testing for PDL 1 and mismatch repair protein status is optional. HER2 testing is restricted to adenocarcinomas only and endoscopic biopsies, resections, or cellblocks. Facilities should be available for performing validated immunohistochemical stains and in-situ hybridization techniques, and importantly, pathologists should be experienced with preanalytical and analytical issues and scoring criteria. Genomic profiling via next-generation sequencing (NGS) is another strategy that assess numerous mutations and other molecular events simultaneously, including HER2 amplification, MSS status, tumor mutation burden, and neurotrophic tropomyosin-receptor kinases gene fusions.

---

[a] Anatomical Pathology, PathWest, QEII Medical Centre, School of Pathology and Laboratory Medicine, UWA and Curtin Medical School, J Block, Hospital Avenue, Nedlands, Western Australia 6009, Australia; [b] Department of Anatomical Pathology, PathWest, QEII Medical Centre, J Block, Hospital Avenue, Nedlands, Western Australia 6009, Australia; [c] Department Medical Oncology, The Queen Elizabeth Hospital and University of Adelaide, Adelaide, South Australia, Australia
[1]Present address: 28 Woodville Road, Woodville, South Australia 5022, Australia.
* Corresponding author: Anatomical Pathology, PathWest, QEII Medical Centre, J Block, Hospital Avenue, Nedlands WA 6009, Australia
E-mail address: priyanthi.kumarasinghe@health.wa.gov.au

Surgical Pathology 16 (2023) 659–672
https://doi.org/10.1016/j.path.2023.05.004

- All G/GEJ cancers should be tested for HER2 status as a reflex test at the time of diagnosis. Currently, testing for PD L1 and mismatch repair protein status is optional.
- HER2 testing is restricted to adenocarcinomas only, and endoscopic biopsies, resections, or cellblocks are suitable for testing by immunohistochemical stains (IHC) and in-situ hybridization (ISH).
- Genomic profiling via next-generation sequencing (NGS) is another strategy that assesses numerous mutations and other molecular events.

OVERVIEW

Since the 1930s, incidence of distal GCs has declined, but adenocarcinomas of the gastroesophageal junction (GEJ) and proximal stomach have increased.[1] Since the 1970s, squamous cell carcinomas (SCCs) have decreased while the incidence of adenocarcinoma has increased especially in Caucasian males. SCC and adenocarcinoma account for 93% of all esophageal carcinomas.[2] More than 90% of gastric cancers (GCs) are adenocarcinomas. SCCs now represent a minority of carcinomas even in Asian countries.[3] With these epidemiological changes, gastric, esophageal, and GEJ cancers were considered together for therapy-based research and clinical trials. However, molecular characterization of G/GEJ adenocarcinoma has made remarkable progress with identification of characteristic genetic signatures. There are distinct genomic changes in SCC as opposed to adenocarcinomas and authentic esophageal adenocarcinomas and GC.[4,5] Therefore, since the introduction of targeted therapy and immunotherapy, the therapeutic approach for SCC and adenocarcinoma is distinct. Treatment regimens targeting human epidermal growth factor 2 (trastuzumab) and vascular endothelial growth factor (eg, ramucirumab) are applicable only to adenocarcinoma, whereas immunotherapy appears to be effective for adenocarcinomas and SCCs.

Therapy recommendations are guided by staging and morphological features with early tumors with favorable pathological features managed by endoscopic modalities and more advanced tumors or those with unfavorable features treated with a combination of surgery and neoadjuvant/adjuvant chemotherapy and radiotherapy.[6,7] Targeted therapies currently approved by the Food and Drug Administration (FDA) for use in G/GEJ cancer include HER2 inhibitors (eg, trastuzumab), program cell death 1 (PD-1) checkpoint inhibitors (eg, pembrolizumab, nivolumab, and dostarlimab) and neurotrophic tropomyosin-receptor kinases (NTRK) inhibitors (entrectinib/larotrectinib).

According to their biomarker expression, adenocarcinomas considered for biomarker therapy are placed in 3 categories.

1. HER-2 overexpressed

HER2 overexpressed adenocarcinomas may be treated with additional trastuzumab therapy to other platinum-based cytotoxic chemotherapy.

2. Mismatch repair protein deficient (dMMR)

Immunotherapy-based treatment with nivolumab and pembrolizumab with cytotoxic chemotherapy is considered for those cancers that are MMRP deficient, most of which also show PD L1 overexpression.

3. HER-2 negative, PD-L1 positive, and MMR proficient (pMMR)

Tumors that show PD L1 over expression are considered suitable for immunotherapy with other combination chemotherapy.

Accordingly, a rational approach of biomarker testing to select appropriate therapy for a specific malignancy is needed. All patients who have documented evidence of advanced G/GEJ adenocarcinomas should have the tumor tissue tested for HER2 status as a reflex test at the time of diagnosis. Currently, PD L1 and miss match repair protein (MMRP) testing is often done at clinical request in many centers in the world. Alternatively, testing of all upper-GI cancers for above 3 biomarkers may be done in an algorithmic approach (**Fig. 1**) depending on clinical demands, local logistics, individual health care settings, and professional recommendations.[8] Pathologist is central in decision-making for selection of eligible patients for appropriate therapy.

HER2 STATUS AND TESTING

HER2 overexpression is not demonstrated in SCC; therefore, testing is restricted to adenocarcinomas only. HER2 overexpression is reported in approximately 7% to 42% of G/GEJ adenocarcinomas.[9,10] The reasons for the wide range of positivity are multifactorial including methods and criteria for testing, ethnicity and geography, and the prevalence G/GEJ adenocarcinomas included in individual reports.[11–13] The therapeutic relevance was demonstrated by the 2010 landmark trastuzumab for GC study.[12] Overexpression and/or amplification of HER-2 is also considered as a poor

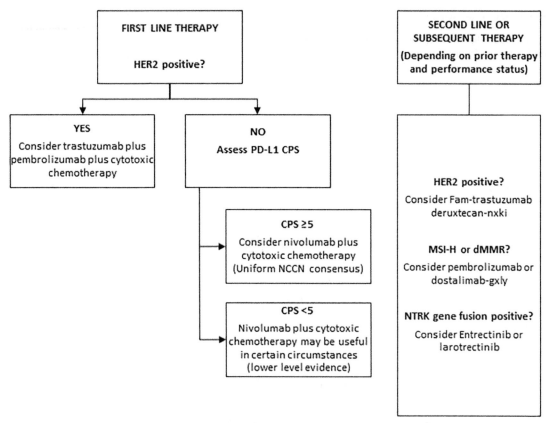

Fig. 1. Biomarker guidance in systemic treatment of advanced/GEJ adenocarcinoma (based on NCCN guidelines).

prognostic marker in several malignancies.[14] Although prognostic significance in the setting of G/GEJ adenocarcinomas is controversial, some studies have documented gene amplification and overexpression of HER2 to be associated with a more aggressive disease and a poor outcome.[15]

Facilities should be available for performing validated immunohistochemical stains (IHC) and in-situ hybridization (ISH) techniques, and importantly, pathologists performing testing should be experienced with preanalytical and analytical issues and scoring criteria. Alternatively, material can be sent for central pathology testing to a laboratory with appropriate facilities and experience. Central testing has shown to reduce interobserver variability.[16,17]

TYPES OF SPECIMENS

Endoscopic biopsies, resection specimens, biopsies of metastatic sites, and cytology samples with cell block preparations can be tested.[18] Testing can be done on archived paraffin-embedded tissue. Dedicated specimens are not required, provided the samples meet adequacy criteria. It is important to avoid preinvasive/dysplastic areas. A minority of tumors may show discordance between the invasive and preinvasive components.[13] Testing of primary

and metastases is equally valid with a high concordance rate of 95% reported in our experience.[19] However, in cases where the primary tumor is HER-2 negative, testing can be repeated on the metastatic site due to the small number of cases that show discordance. If material is to be sent to central laboratory testing, tissue blocks and freshly cut charged slides are suitable. It is advisable that both IHC and ISH be performed in the same laboratory for quality-control and quality-assurance purposes and troubleshooting.

TISSUE FIXATION

Tissue fixation in 10% neutral-buffered formalin as required for routine histopathology analysis is adequate and satisfactory for HER2 testing by IHC and ISH. Prolonged and short duration of fixation has been shown to affect protein expression by immunohistochemistry in general. Some dedicated studies have shown similar experiences in the setting of HER2 testing.[20] Currently, the approach is to follow general principles of tissue fixation as for routine histopathological analysis and special techniques. The time to fixation (cold ischemic time) should be less than 1 hour.

ADEQUACY OF MATERIAL

In an Australia-wide testing program, we found that 5 tumor fragments are optimum for accurate results when endoscopic biopsies are tested.[21] This is due to an increase in the incidence of heterogeneity in G/GEJ adenocarcinomas compared with breast carcinoma.[22] More than one tissue block may be selected if different morphologic patterns are present. Repeat HER2 testing in the primary, metastatic, and recurrent sites has shown to be useful in patients whose primary tumor was initially negative. These patients have had similar treatment benefits compared to cohorts that have shown initial HER-2 positivity.[23]

TESTING METHODS AND SCORING CRITERIA

Testing methods include IHC and ISH. In general, IHC is regarded as a semiquantitative test that is subject to preanalytical and analytical variabilities. ISH techniques are considered superior.

An IHC score of 3+ is strongly predictive of HER2 amplification.[16] Therefore, IHC should be performed first. The approach by American Society of Clinical Oncology (ASCO) and other centers is to consider a tumor with IHC score of 3+ as evidence of amplification.[12,24] However, in addition to amplifications, HER2 mutations have been reported as distinct molecular targets.[25] Interestingly, a recent study has raised the possible therapeutic relevance of a novel HER2 targeted antibody-drug conjugate in HER2-low (as defined by IHC 1 and 2+ without amplification) GCs.[26] Potential false-positive IHC results have been reported in signet-ring cell carcinomas.[27] These factors highlight the importance of further investigation into the mechanisms of protein overexpression, amplification, mutation, and possible other pathways to drive the influence of human epidermal growth factor in carcinogenesis. Hence, in Australia, double testing with ISH is recommended for all cases that are IHC 2 or 3+. This is a requirement for the patients to be eligible for subsidized access to trastuzumab-based therapy via the Pharmaceutical Benefit Scheme in Australia.[21,28] This approach is beneficial to recognize any case with protein overexpression by mechanisms other than amplification while avoiding false-positive results by immunohistochemistry. An IHC score of 0 or 1 is considered as a negative result, and further testing with ISH is not required. This approach appears to be universally practiced.

Fig. 2 shows an inclusive HER2 testing algorithm with immunohistochemistry and ISH. The testing algorithm may be customized to suit individual health-care settings and cost considerations.

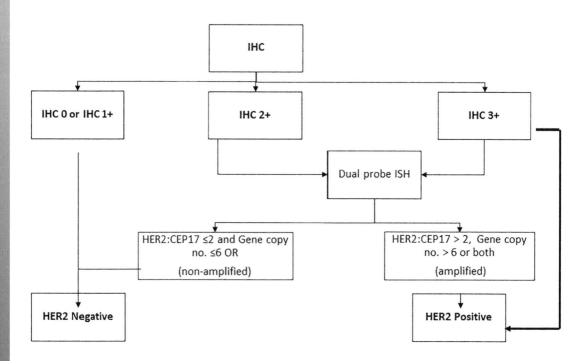

Note IHC3+ may be regarded as confirmative of Amplification without ISH

Fig. 2. A HER2 testing algorithm.

HER2 PROTEIN EXPRESSION BY IMMUNOHISTOCHEMISTRY

TECHNIQUES

Currently available commercial antibodies are the HercepTest and A0485 (Dako, Glostrup, Denmark), SP3 (Labvision; Thermo Fisher Scientific, Fremont, CA), 4B5 (Ventana Medical Systems, Tucson, AZ), and CB11 (Novocastra, Newcastle upon Tyne, England). Although discordant results using different antibodies have been reported, there is general agreement that 4B5 and SP3 have shown comparable results with high accuracy compared to the HercepTest that was used in the trastuzumab for gastric cancer (ToGA) study.[12,22,29,30]

SCORING

The recently validated modified HER2 scoring system for G/GEJ cancers as was used in the TOGA study is shown in Table 1 (Figs. 3–5). Assessment and scoring are based on the intensity of membrane staining. Diffuse cytoplasmic and nuclear staining should not be interpreted as protein expression and should not be scored. Similarly, normal gastric foveolar epithelium may show spurious staining (see Fig. 5). In biopsies, a minimum of 5 positive cells are considered adequate, while in resections, 10% of cells should show positivity. The cell block material is best treated as a small biopsy sample applying similar criteria.

HER2 AMPLIFICATION BY IN- SITU HYBRIDISATION

TECHNIQUES

Amplification can be determined by using chromogenic, silver, or fluorescence techniques (FISH). The former two methods are bright-field (BF) techniques, and slides can be visualized in the conventional microscope while FISH is a dark-field technique that requires a fluorescence microscope. BF examination allows parallel viewing of tumor cells using the light microscope without having to use oil and dark room. The signals in the material can be stored with good preservation in archival material. We routinely use BF techniques considering our experience and established limitations of the FISH technique compared to advantages of BF techniques.[16,21] A further development is using a Dual-probe silver ISH technique with two colors to enumerate both HER2 and CEP17 signals on a single slide (DDISH). We recommend the use of dual probe rather than single probe BF-ISH.

SCORING

At least 20 tumor cells should be examined for counting of HER2 and CEP17 signals (see Figs. 3 and 4). Nontumor cells should not be counted. The average of HER2 signals and CEP17 signals per carcinoma cell should be recorded as mean copy number (CN), and the ratio of HER2 to CEP 17 CN should be calculated. When amplified targets are multiple and clustered, a small cluster is counted as 6 and a larger cluster as 12 signals.[31] If adequate number of cells cannot be enumerated the difficulty should be expressed in the report. Criteria for an amplified or a nonamplified result are given in Fig. 2.

Even with adequate guidelines, discrepancies of HER2 assessment have been reported, and central testing has shown to be associated with significant longer survival rates than local testing and recommended in Australia.[16,17] A recently conducted Varianz study has recommended alternative and more stringent criteria for selection of patients for HER2-directed treatment.[17] Similarly, in Australia, HER2 positivity is defined by an IHC score of 2 or 3+ and HER2 CN > 6 with a ratio greater than 2.[21] Our experience has shown that the HER2 CN differentiated the IHC score better than the ratio alone. This was especially relevant when cases with a score of IHC 1+ and 0 appeared to be amplified by a low ratio and hence deemed HER-2 positive.[32] Coinciding with our experience, it should be noted a subgroup analysis in the ToGA study showed that there was no survival benefit for those cases deemed HER2 amplified but IHC negative.[12] Most recent guidelines recommend consideration of both CN and the ratio without relying on the ratio only.

Artificial intelligence testing algorithms have been tested for breast HER2 interpretation with encouraging results.[33,34] Similar attempts may simplify, supplement, or refine the process of scoring and interpretation in the setting of G/GEJ cancers in the future.

TURNAROUND TIMES

Turnaround times need to be efficient as the objective of treatment is prolongation of survival in an otherwise aggressive malignancy. We recommend a 5-day turnaround time for a result.

Mismatch Repair Protein/Microsatellite Instability Testing

Microsatellite instability (MSI) has been reported in up to 6.6% of invasive adenocarcinomas arising on the background of Barrett's disease and in about 6% to 9% of GC and associated with a better prognosis.[35] The therapeutic

Table 1
Approach to interpretation, scoring, and results of protein overexpression (IHC)

Reactivity Pattern		Score	Result	Next Action
Nuclear staining		Not scored	Spurious/ Negative	No further testing
Staining of foveolar epithelium		Not scored	Spurious/ Negative	No further testing
No reactivity or membranous reactivity		0	Negative	No further testing
Faint/barely perceptible membranous reactivity/ cells are reactive only in part of their membrane		1+	Negative	No further testing
Weak to moderate complete or basolateral membranous reactivity		2+	Equivocal	In situ hybridization for amplification
Moderate to strong complete or basolateral membranous reactivity		3+	Positive	In situ hybridization for amplification or No further testing

Endoscopic in biopsies (and cell blocks), a minimum of 5 positive cells. Resection blocks 10% cells.

relevance has been shown in ongoing studies in relation to the efficacy of immune checkpoint inhibitors (ICIs) in MMR-deficient or MSI-high G/GEJ carcinoma.[36–39]

TESTING AND INTERPRETATION

Testing for MMRP deficiency is performed by immunohistochemistry and MSI by PCR or

Fig. 3. HER2-positive result. (*A*) GEJ adenocarcinoma (hematoxylin and eosin). (*B*) Strong complete or basolateral membranous reactivity: IHC 3+. (*C*) Large clots indicating 6 or more Her 2 signals (inset): Amplification (by SISH).

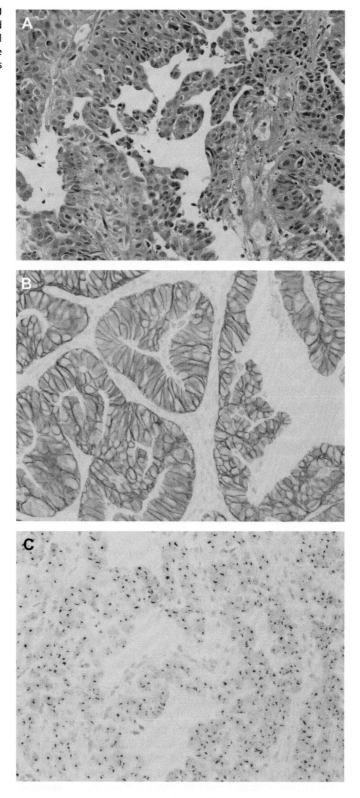

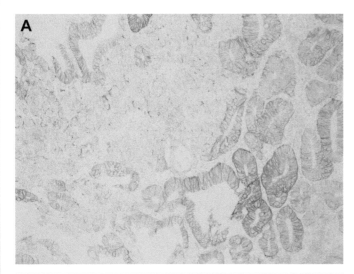

Fig. 4. Heterogeneity. (*A*) Range of protein expression (IHC1-3). (*B*) Similar/concordant amplification by SISH (area marked).

next-generation sequencing (NGS). Testing and interpretation are similar to what is routinely used for colorectal carcinoma.[36] Although not universally practiced, it is recommended that mismatch repair protein (MMRP) immunohistochemistry should be routinely performed.[40]

Programmed Death-Ligand 1 Status and Testing

Programmed death-ligand 1 (PD L1) interacts with the programmed death-1 (PD-1) receptor, that is usually expressed by cytotoxic T cells and other immune cells. Normal tissue uses the PD L1/PD-1 interaction to inhibit, avoid, and protect against immune recognition. The innate and adaptive immune system utilizes T cells to attack pathogens and tumor cells, so the PD L1/PD-1 interaction is a vital checkpoint so that normal tissues are not damaged by the immune response.[41] SCC and

G/GEJ adenocarcinomas can increase expression of PD L1 in tumor cells and in the adjacent peritumoral inflammatory cells to downregulate the action of T cells.[42]

IMMUNOMODULATORY AGENTS

The development of anti-PD-1 immunotherapeutic agents has evolved rapidly with a range of immune checkpoint inhibitors currently used to treat esophageal, GOJ, and GCs including pembrolizumab (Keytruda), nivolumab (Opdivo), and ipilimumab (Yervoy) a CTLA-4 inhibitor. Several KEYNOTE and CheckMate phase III studies have demonstrated pembrolizumab and nivolumab administration to patients with esophageal carcinoma to be associated with prolonged overall survival (OS)[43] and significantly increased disease free survival (DFS) with co-administration of neoadjuvant chemotherapy.[12,43–45]

Fig. 5. Some pitfalls. (*A*) Spurious cytoplasmic and nuclear positivity. (*B*) Spurious positivity in normal gastric foveolar epithelium (4B5 clone).

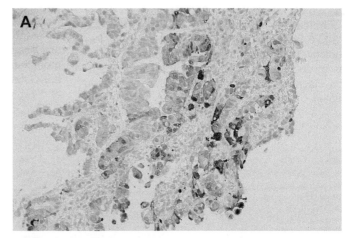

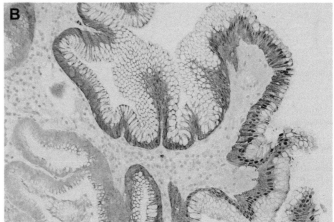

The latest NCCN (National Comprehensive Cancer Network, 5.2022) guidelines for G/GEJ cancers suggest that a PD L1 Combined Positive Score (CPS) may be obtained utilizing an FDA approved test but is not mandatory for access to immunomodulatory agents. The CPS provides information regarding likelihood to respond to immunotherapy to a variety of agents in combination with conventional chemotherapy. Based upon lower-level evidence, there is uniform NCCN consensus that the intervention is appropriate.[7] In Australia, there is currently no requirement for a PD L1 CPS to access a range of immunomodulatory agents.

The landscape of immunotherapy is ever evolving with new data emerging annually without universal agreement or evidence to definitively guide treatment. Different regulatory bodies in different regions adopt different positions and recommendations, such that pathologists should be aware of which local guidelines to follow. Currently PD L1 testing by immunohistochemistry is considered optional.

The following is important to the pathologist who is tasked with providing a PD L1 score in the esophagus, GEJ, or stomach carcinoma.

PROGRAMMED DEATH-LIGAND 1 TESTING

Testing is routinely done by immunohistochemistry. Most of the phase III trials with pembrolizumab were designed utilizing the Dako 22C3 platform, which led the FDA approval of the Dako 22C3 assay as a companion diagnostic test for access to pembrolizumab. Recent harmonization studies in GC show that the analytical performance of 22C3 and SP263 clones on the Ventana platform was close to that of the reference Dako 22C3 assay.[46] Currently there are various standardized PD L1 antibody assays, including Dako 22C3, Dako 28 to 8, Ventana SP263, and Ventana SP142, approved as companion diagnostic devices in a range of tumors for access to various immune checkpoint inhibitors.[47] However, there are different regulatory approvals in different parts of the world, with the Dako 22C3 assay universally accepted and some regions allowing the Dako 28 to 8 assay for esophageal, GEJ, and GC. Pathology laboratories aiming to establish a PD L1 assay should determine the appropriate companion diagnostic assay relevant to the tumor type tested.

PROGRAMMED DEATH-LIGAND 1 SCORING

Different PD L1 scoring systems have been assessed with CPS of GC demonstrated to be a more sensitive biomarker than the Tumor Proportion Score or PD L1% (**Fig. 6**).[48] Accurate, reliable, and reproducible PD L1 scoring in esophageal SCC, GEJ, and GC requires completion of a

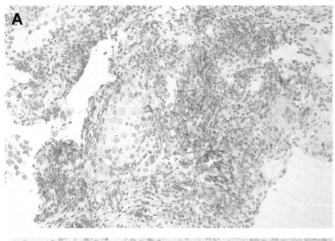

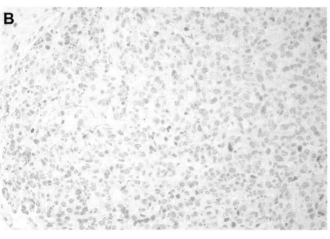

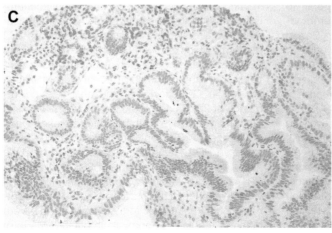

Fig. 6. PD L1 expression (*A*). High PD L1 CPS score of 24.3. (*B*) Positive low-scoring PD L1 of 2. (*C*) PD L1 CPS score of less than 1.

training module.[49] More recently, online training modules by Agilent-Dako and Roche are available. For GEJ and gastric adenocarcinoma, PD L1 scoring requires creating a CPS, which is created by determining the number of PD L1-positive cells (tumor cells, lymphocytes, macrophages) divided by the total number of tumors cells, multiplied by 100.

$$CPS = \frac{\text{\# of PD} - \text{L1 staining cells (tumour cells, lymphocytes, macrophages)}}{\text{Total \# of viable tumour cells}} \times 100$$

Included in the numerator are

- tumor cells showing convincing partial or complete membrane staining (of ANY intensity) that is perceived distinct from cytoplasmic staining and
- Lymphocytes and macrophages (mononuclear inflammatory cells/MIC) *within the tumor nests and/or adjacent supporting stroma* showing convincing membrane and/or cytoplasmic staining (of ANY intensity). The inflammatory cells must be directly associated with the response against the tumor and included within a 20X field of the tumors being assessed.
- All viable invasive tumors cells irrespective of PD L1 staining.

Excluded from the numerator are

- Nonstaining tumor cells, tumors cells with only cytoplasmic staining, carcinoma in situ, and all types inflammatory cells *not within the tumor nests and/or adjacent supporting stroma*

TYPES OF SPECIMENS AND ADEQUACY

Currently, only histology specimens (biopsy and resection) are considered suitable. A minimum of 100 viable tumors cells are required to be present on the PD L1-stained slide for the specimen to be considered adequate. All tissue on the PD L1 stained slide containing tumor needs to be assessed to generate a single CPS. On biopsy, specimens with multiple portions of tumors that present only one CPS are reported.

Other Potential and Emerging Biomarkers

Neurotrophic tropomyosin-receptor kinases overexpression/gene fusion

Oncogenic fusions involving neurotrophic tropomyosin-receptor kinases (NTRK) appear to indicate activity of targeted therapy (inhibition of NTRK signaling), independent of the histological tumor type.[50] Clinical trial data show entrectinib and larotrectinib are feasible and effective treatments for NTRK fusion-positive solid tumors.[51–53] NTRK rearrangements exist at low frequency in G/GOJ adenocarcinoma, and screening for NTRK gene rearrangements may be appropriate when other forms of treatments have failed.[54–57]

Immunohistochemical antibody to screen for alterations in NTRK is commercially available although there is no universally accepted interpretation system. Positive staining may be cytoplasmic, nuclear, or mixed. Some NTRK3 fusion-positive cases show weak and focal staining only, and therefore, any positive staining in at least 1% of cells has been used for the purposes of screening with a sensitivity of 96.9% for NTRK1 and NTRK2 fusions and 79.4% for NTRK3 fusions. Nuclear staining is the most specific (most often associated with NTRK3 fusion, not observed in false-positive cases).[58]

Although published experience is limited, FISH is likely of limited utility as a confirmatory test due to the variety of rearrangements already described, including intrachromosomal rearrangement that would be difficult to detect by FISH. ATP1B1-NTRK1 is an example of intrachromosomal rearrangement that has been detected in GC.[56]

CLAUDIN 18.2 EXPRESSION

Claudin 18.2 (CLDN18.2) is a component of normal gastric epithelial tight junctions, with CLDN18.2 epitopes detectable in G/GEJ carcinoma.[59] In advanced G/GEJ adenocarcinoma, Kubota and colleagues found 24% positive for CLDN18.2 by commercially available immunohistochemistry antibody, defined as moderate to strong membranous staining in equal to or greater than 75% of tumor cells.[60] CLDN18-ARHGAP gene fusion is known to occur in GC, enriched in genomically stable molecular subtype and diffuse carcinomas.[61] CLDN18.2 expression has been reported in most CLDN18-ARHGAP fusion-positive GCs; however, the relationship between the fusion gene and the expression of CLDN18.2 detected on immunohistochemistry requires further investigation.[61]

Primary results from SPOTLIGHT, a global phase 3 trial, demonstrate the addition of zolbetuximab (a monoclonal antibody against CLDN18.2) to chemotherapy statistically significantly prolongs progression free survival and overall survival in patients with previously untreated CLDN18.2-positive/HER2-negative locally advanced unresectable or metastatic G/GEJ.[62]

NEXT-GENERATION SEQUENCING

Genomic profiling via NGS is another strategy that assess numerous mutations and other molecular events simultaneously, including HER2 amplification, MSS status, tumor mutation burden (TMB) and NTRK gene fusions. There may be advantages to this approach if there is limited diagnostic tissue available.[24] High status identifies a subgroup of patients with previously treated recurrent or metastatic solid tumors (including gastric adenocarcinoma) who could have robust tumor responses to pembrolizumab monotherapy.[63]

DISCLOSURE

The authors have nothing to disclose.

REFERENCES

1. Salvon-Harman JC, Cady B, Nikulasson S, et al. Shifting proportions of gastric adenocarcinomas. Arch Surg 1994;129(4):381–8, discussion 8-9.
2. SEER Cancer Stat Facts: Esophageal Cancer Bethesda, MD: National Cancer Institute; Available from: https://seer.cancer.gov/statfacts/html/esoph.html.
3. Xie SH, Lagergren J. Time trends in the incidence of oesophageal cancer in Asia: Variations across populations and histological types. Cancer Epidemiol 2016;44:71–6.
4. Cancer Genome Atlas Research N. Comprehensive molecular characterization of gastric adenocarcinoma. Nature 2014;513(7517):202–9.
5. Cancer Genome Atlas Research, Analysis Working Group, Asan University, et al. Integrated genomic characterization of oesophageal carcinoma. Nature 2017;541(7636):169–75.
6. Japanese Gastric Cancer A. Japanese gastric cancer treatment guidelines 2018 (5th edition). Gastric Cancer 2021;24(1):1–21.
7. Network NCC. Available from: https://www.nccn.org/guidelines/category_1.
8. Tumours of the oesophagus and oesophagogastric junction. 2nd Edition. Royal College of Pathologists of Australasia; 2022. Available from: https://www.rcpa.edu.au/Library/Practising-Pathology/Structured-Pathology-Reporting-of-Cancer/Cancer-Protocols/Gastrointestinal/Protocol-Oesophagus.aspx.
9. Jorgensen JT. Targeted HER2 treatment in advanced gastric cancer. Oncology 2010;78(1):26–33.
10. Gravalos C, Jimeno A. HER2 in gastric cancer: a new prognostic factor and a novel therapeutic target. Ann Oncol 2008;19(9):1523–9.
11. Shan L, Ying J, Lu N. HER2 expression and relevant clinicopathological features in gastric and gastroesophageal junction adenocarcinoma in a Chinese population. Diagn Pathol 2013;8:76.
12. Bang YJ, Van Cutsem E, Feyereislova A, et al. Trastuzumab in combination with chemotherapy versus chemotherapy alone for treatment of HER2-positive advanced gastric or gastro-oesophageal junction cancer (ToGA): a phase 3, open-label, randomised controlled trial. Lancet 2010;376(9742):687–97.
13. Lee S, de Boer WB, Fermoyle S, et al. Human epidermal growth factor receptor 2 testing in gastric carcinoma: issues related to heterogeneity in biopsies and resections. Histopathology 2011;59(5):832–40.
14. Yan M, Schwaederle M, Arguello D, et al. HER2 expression status in diverse cancers: review of results from 37,992 patients. Cancer Metastasis Rev 2015;34(1):157–64.
15. Barros-Silva JD, Leitao D, Afonso L, et al. Association of ERBB2 gene status with histopathological parameters and disease-specific survival in gastric carcinoma patients. Br J Cancer 2009;100(3):487–93.
16. Fox SB, Kumarasinghe MP, Armes JE, et al. Gastric HER2 Testing Study (GaTHER): an evaluation of gastric/gastroesophageal junction cancer testing accuracy in Australia. Am J Surg Pathol 2012;36(4):577–82.
17. Haffner I, Schierle K, Raimundez E, et al. HER2 Expression, Test Deviations, and Their Impact on Survival in Metastatic Gastric Cancer: Results From the Prospective Multicenter VARIANZ Study. J Clin Oncol 2021;39(13):1468–78.
18. Wong DD, de Boer WB, Platten MA, et al. HER2 testing in malignant effusions of metastatic gastric carcinoma: is it feasible? Diagn Cytopathol 2015;43(1):80–5.
19. Wong DD, Kumarasinghe MP, Platten MA, et al. Concordance of HER2 expression in paired primary and metastatic sites of gastric and gastrooesophageal junction cancers. Pathology 2015;47(7):641–6.
20. Yamashita-Kashima Y, Shu S, Yorozu K, et al. Importance of formalin fixing conditions for HER2 testing in gastric cancer: immunohistochemical staining and fluorescence in situ hybridization. Gastric Cancer 2014;17(4):638–47.

21. Kumarasinghe MP, Morey A, Bilous M, et al. HER2 testing in advanced gastric and gastro-oesophageal cancer: analysis of an Australia-wide testing program. Pathology 2017;49(6):575–81.

22. Boers JE, Meeuwissen H, Methorst N. HER2 status in gastro-oesophageal adenocarcinomas assessed by two rabbit monoclonal antibodies (SP3 and 4B5) and two in situ hybridization methods (FISH and SISH). Histopathology 2011;58(3):383–94.

23. Park SR, Park YS, Ryu MH, et al. Extra-gain of HER2-positive cases through HER2 reassessment in primary and metastatic sites in advanced gastric cancer with initially HER2-negative primary tumours: Results of GAStric cancer HER2 reassessment study 1 (GASTHER1). Eur J Cancer 2016;53:42–50.

24. Bartley AN, Washington MK, Colasacco C, et al. HER2 Testing and Clinical Decision Making in Gastroesophageal Adenocarcinoma: Guideline From the College of American Pathologists, American Society for Clinical Pathology, and the American Society of Clinical Oncology. J Clin Oncol 2017;35(4):446–64.

25. Li BT, Ross DS, Aisner DL, et al. HER2 Amplification and HER2 Mutation Are Distinct Molecular Targets in Lung Cancers. J Thorac Oncol 2016;11(3):414–9.

26. Shitara K, Bang YJ, Iwasa S, et al. Trastuzumab Deruxtecan in Previously Treated HER2-Positive Gastric Cancer. N Engl J Med 2020;382(25):2419–30.

27. Woo CG, Ho WJ, Park YS, et al. A potential pitfall in evaluating HER2 immunohistochemistry for gastric signet ring cell carcinomas. Pathology 2017;49(1):38–43.

28. The Pharmaceutical Benefits Scheme: Australian Government; Department of Health and Ageing; 08/01/2023. Available from: https://www.pbs.gov.au/industry/listing/elements/pbac-meetings/psd/2012-07/trastuzumab.pdf.

29. Cho EY, Srivastava A, Park K, et al. Comparison of four immunohistochemical tests and FISH for measuring HER2 expression in gastric carcinomas. Pathology 2012;44(3):216–20.

30. Abrahao-Machado LF, Jacome AA, Wohnrath DR, et al. HER2 in gastric cancer: comparative analysis of three different antibodies using whole-tissue sections and tissue microarrays. World J Gastroenterol 2013;19(38):6438–46.

31. Subasinghe D, Acott N, Kumarasinghe MP. A survival guide to HER2 testing in gastric/gastro-esophageal junction carcinoma. Gastrointest Endosc 2019;90(1):44–54.

32. Kumarasinghe MP, de Boer WB, Khor TS, et al. HER2 status in gastric/gastro-oesophageal junctional cancers: should determination of gene amplification by SISH use HER2 copy number or HER2: CEP17 ratio? Pathology 2014;46(3):184–7.

33. Yue M, Zhang J, Wang X, et al. Can AI-assisted microscope facilitate breast HER2 interpretation? A multi-institutional ring study. Virchows Arch 2021;479(3):443–9.

34. Vandenberghe ME, Scott ML, Scorer PW, et al. Relevance of deep learning to facilitate the diagnosis of HER2 status in breast cancer. Sci Rep 2017;7:45938.

35. Farris AB 3rd, Demicco EG, Le LP, et al. Clinicopathologic and molecular profiles of microsatellite unstable Barrett Esophagus-associated adenocarcinoma. Am J Surg Pathol 2011;35(5):647–55.

36. Dhakras P, Uboha N, Horner V, et al. Gastrointestinal cancers: current biomarkers in esophageal and gastric adenocarcinoma. Transl Gastroenterol Hepatol 2020;5:55.

37. Le DT, Durham JN, Smith KN, et al. Mismatch repair deficiency predicts response of solid tumors to PD-1 blockade. Science 2017;357(6349):409–13.

38. Marabelle A, Le DT, Ascierto PA, et al. Efficacy of Pembrolizumab in Patients With Noncolorectal High Microsatellite Instability/Mismatch Repair-Deficient Cancer: Results From the Phase II KEYNOTE-158 Study. J Clin Oncol 2020;38(1):1–10.

39. Le DT, Uram JN, Wang H, et al. PD-1 Blockade in Tumors with Mismatch-Repair Deficiency. N Engl J Med 2015;372(26):2509–20.

40. Gastric cancer structured reporting protocol. 2nd Edition. Royal College of Pathologists of Australasia; 2020. Available from: https://www.rcpa.edu.au/Library/Practising-Pathology/Structured-Pathology-Reporting-of-Cancer/Cancer-Protocols/Gastrointestinal/Protocol-gastric-cancer.aspx.

41. Keir ME, Butte MJ, Freeman GJ, et al. PD-1 and its ligands in tolerance and immunity. Annu Rev Immunol 2008;26:677–704.

42. Guo W, Wang P, Li N, et al. Prognostic value of PD-L1 in esophageal squamous cell carcinoma: a meta-analysis. Oncotarget 2018;9(17):13920–33.

43. Kojima T, Shah MA, Muro K, et al. Randomized Phase III KEYNOTE-181 Study of Pembrolizumab Versus Chemotherapy in Advanced Esophageal Cancer. J Clin Oncol 2020;38(35):4138–48.

44. Kelly RJ, Ajani JA, Kuzdzal J, et al. Adjuvant Nivolumab in Resected Esophageal or Gastroesophageal Junction Cancer. N Engl J Med 2021;384(13):1191–203.

45. Fuchs CS, Ozguroglu M, Bang YJ, et al. Pembrolizumab versus paclitaxel for previously treated PD-L1-positive advanced gastric or gastroesophageal junction cancer: 2-year update of the randomized phase 3 KEYNOTE-061 trial. Gastric Cancer 2022;25(1):197–206.

46. Dabbagh TZ, Sughayer MA. PD-L1 Expression Harmonization in Gastric Cancer Using 22C3 PharmDx and SP263 Assays. Appl Immunohistochem Mol Morphol 2021;29(6):462–6.

47. (FDA) USFaDA. List of Cleared or Approved Companion Diagnostic Devices (In Vitro and Imaging Tools) Available from: https://www.fda.gov/medical-devices/in-vitro-diagnostics/list-cleared-or-approved-companion-diagnostic-devices-in-vitro-and-imaging-tools.

48. Yamashita K, Iwatsuki M, Harada K, et al. Prognostic impacts of the combined positive score and the tumor proportion score for programmed death ligand-1 expression by double immunohistochemical staining in patients with advanced gastric cancer. Gastric Cancer 2020;23(1):95–104.

49. AgilentDako. The Dako PD-L1 IHC 22C3 pharmDx Interpretation Training Program Available from: https://pdl122c3-learning.dako.com/.

50. Cocco E, Scaltriti M, Drilon A. NTRK fusion-positive cancers and TRK inhibitor therapy. Nat Rev Clin Oncol 2018;15(12):731–47.

51. Doebele RC, Drilon A, Paz-Ares L, et al. Entrectinib in patients with advanced or metastatic NTRK fusion-positive solid tumours: integrated analysis of three phase 1–2 trials. Lancet Oncol 2020;21(2):271–82.

52. Drilon A, Laetsch TW, Kummar S, et al. Efficacy of Larotrectinib in TRK Fusion-Positive Cancers in Adults and Children. N Engl J Med 2018;378(8):731–9.

53. Hong DS, DuBois SG, Kummar S, et al. Larotrectinib in patients with TRK fusion-positive solid tumours: a pooled analysis of three phase 1/2 clinical trials. Lancet Oncol 2020;21(4):531–40.

54. Shi E, Chmielecki J, Tang CM, et al. FGFR1 and NTRK3 actionable alterations in "Wild-Type" gastrointestinal stromal tumors. J Transl Med 2016;14(1):339.

55. Chen Y, Chi P. Basket trial of TRK inhibitors demonstrates efficacy in TRK fusion-positive cancers. J Hematol Oncol 2018;11(1):78.

56. Shinozaki-Ushiku A, Ishikawa S, Komura D, et al. The first case of gastric carcinoma with NTRK rearrangement: identification of a novel ATP1B-NTRK1 fusion. Gastric Cancer 2020;23(5):944–7.

57. Arnold A, Daum S, von Winterfeld M, et al. Analysis of NTRK expression in gastric and esophageal adenocarcinoma (AGE) with pan-TRK immunohistochemistry. Pathol Res Pract 2019;215(11):152662.

58. Solomon JP, Linkov I, Rosado A, et al. NTRK fusion detection across multiple assays and 33,997 cases: diagnostic implications and pitfalls. Mod Pathol 2020;33(1):38–46.

59. Athauda A, Chau I. Claudin 18.2-a FAST-moving target in gastric cancer? Ann Oncol 2021;32(5):584–6.

60. Kubota Y, Kawazoe A, Mishima S, et al. Comprehensive clinical and molecular characterization of claudin 18.2 expression in advanced gastric or gastroesophageal junction cancer. ESMO Open 2023;8(1):100762.

61. Pellino A, Brignola S, Riello E, et al. Association of CLDN18 Protein Expression with Clinicopathological Features and Prognosis in Advanced Gastric and Gastroesophageal Junction Adenocarcinomas. J Pers Med 2021;11(11):1095.

62. Shitara K, Lordick F, Bang YJ, et al. Zolbetuximab + mFOLFOX6 as first-line (1L) treatment for patients (pts) with claudin-18.2+ (CLDN18.2+)/HER2− locally advanced (LA) unresectable or metastatic gastric or gastroesophageal junction (mG/GEJ) adenocarcinoma: Primary results from phase 3 SPOTLIGHT study. J Clin Oncol 2023;41.

63. Marabelle A, Fakih M, Lopez J, et al. Association of tumour mutational burden with outcomes in patients with advanced solid tumours treated with pembrolizumab: prospective biomarker analysis of the multicohort, open-label, phase 2 KEYNOTE-158 study. Lancet Oncol 2020;21(10):1353–65.

Artificial Intelligence-Enabled Gastric Cancer Interpretations: Are We There yet?

Mustafa Yousif, MD[a],*, Liron Pantanowitz, MD, MHA, PhD[b]

KEYWORDS

- Artificial intelligence • Computational pathology • Digital pathology • Whole slide imaging
- Gastric cancer • Machine learning • Deep learning • Cancer diagnosis

---

Key points

- Artificial intelligence (AI) coupled with digital pathology (DP) is driving the use of machine learning in gastric biopsies and has the potential for the evaluation of gastric cancer (GC).
- AI's ability to recognize patterns beyond human perception is valuable for prognostic and predictive purposes in GC.
- AI-based tools have been developed to diagnose gastric carcinoma, detect metastases, automate Ki-67 scoring, quantify tumor-infiltrating lymphocytes, and provide prognostic information.
- The use of AI in DP has the potential to improve workflow, enhance diagnostic accuracy, and lead to novel discoveries in pathology.
- Challenges such as data variability, cost, and limited deployment in clinical practice, highlighting the need for more research and development.

ABSTRACT

The integration of digital pathology and artificial intelligence (AI) is revolutionizing pathology by providing pathologists with new tools to improve workflow, enhance diagnostic accuracy, and undertake novel discovery. The capability of AI to recognize patterns and features in digital images beyond human perception is particularly valuable, thereby providing additional information for prognostic and predictive purposes. AI-based tools diagnose gastric carcinoma in digital images, detect gastric carcinoma metastases in lymph nodes, automate Ki-67 scoring in gastric neuroendocrine tumors, and quantify tumor-infiltrating lymphocytes. This article provides an overview of all of these applications of AI pertaining to gastric cancer.

INTRODUCTION

The examination of tissue samples under a microscope for interpreting histopathology is the gold standard for identifying cancer and is crucial for determining prognostic factors. There are several factors contributing to the increasing need for histopathological diagnoses in addition to the current shortage of pathologists, including an increase in morbidity among an aging population, an increase in the incidence of malignancies among young adults, and an increase in cancer screening programs, which has led to an increase in the number of annual laboratory cases to examine.[1] However, the complexity of working up cases in today's era of personalized medicine places strain on histopathologists and may result in lengthy turnaround times for diagnostic reports in pathology laboratories.[2] An accurate and timely diagnosis is

---

[a] Department of Pathology, University of Michigan, NCRC Building 35, 2800 Plymouth Road, Ann Arbor, MI 48109, USA; [b] Department of Pathology, UPMC Shadyside Hospital, 5150 Centre Avenue Cancer Pavilion, POB2, Suite 3B, Room 347, Pittsburgh, PA 15232, USA
* Corresponding author.
E-mail address: mustafay@med.umich.edu

Surgical Pathology 16 (2023) 673–686
https://doi.org/10.1016/j.path.2023.05.005

especially important for the correct treatment of gastric cancer (GC), the fourth most common tumor in the world that exhibits a high-mortality rate.[3] To address the overwhelming workload and pathologist shortage, advanced technology such as digital pathology (DP) and artificial intelligence (AI) is being leveraged in pathology laboratories.[4] This article aims to provide an overview of the application of AI in the early detection and diagnosis of GC.

DIGITAL IMAGING AND ARTIFICIAL INTELLIGENCE IN PATHOLOGY

Scanning technology in pathology enables the digitization of entire glass slides to generate digital image files called whole-slide images (WSIs). Each digital slide, scanned at approximately 0.25 μm per pixel resolution, contains vast amounts of pixelated data. The large size of WSI files usually requires preprocessing steps such as tessellation, whereby the large image is broken into smaller image patches or "tiles." Smaller image tiles, typically a few hundred pixels, are more amenable to computational analysis.[5] The combination of machine learning (ML), WSI technology, and powerful computing is propelling the use of AI in pathology. The development of newer deep learning (DL) algorithms such as convolutional neural networks (CNNs) have been effectively applied to WSI.[6] DP coupled with AI has been successfully applied to gastric biopsies for the diagnosis of *Helicobacter pylori* and gastritis.[7–9] Despite the application of DP focused on gastric biopsies including GC, there are still few comprehensive reviews that delve into this area.[10–14] This review evaluates the latest research regarding the use of AI in the pathological evaluation of GC and highlights challenges that must be addressed for its successful implementation in gastrointestinal pathology practice (Table 1). Additionally, the review outlines potential future directions to advance the use of AI in this field.

ARTIFICIAL INTELLIGENCE-BASED GASTRIC CARCINOMA DETECTION

The diagnosis of GC, specifically gastric carcinoma, has traditionally involved identifying the morphological characteristics of malignancy by means of histopathological examination using traditional light microscopy. However, this manual method is time consuming, labor intensive, and prone to human error. Although the majority of gastric carcinomas are adenocarcinomas (ADCs), there is heterogeneity with respect to phenotype and genotype. As a result, there has been a push for the use of automatic image analysis to assist in the diagnosis of GC (Figs. 1 and 2), as well as precursor lesions (Fig. 3). Li and colleagues introduced GastricNet, a novel DL-based model for detecting gastric tumors.[15] When analyzing pathology WSIs, the GastricNet model had a classification accuracy of 100%, which was significantly greater than other existing networks, such as DenseNet[16] and ResNet.[17] This method, however, can only perform patch-based as opposed to WSI classification. To detect whether a slide contains GC, a slide-based classification method is suggested. To this end, Sharma and colleagues described a DL approach for computer-aided classification on a limited dataset of 11 hematoxylin and eosin (H&E)-stained histological WSIs of GC.[18] They proposed a CNN architecture for 2 applications: cancer classification based on immunohistochemistry (IHC) staining and necrosis detection based on the presence of tumor necrosis. Their CNN architecture could efficiently evaluate pathological images with a cancer classification accuracy of 0.6990 and a necrosis detection accuracy of 0.8144. Because ground truth data was time-consuming, it was extremely limited in this study. However, this drawback was solved by utilizing data augmentation methodologies. Yoshida and colleagues developed e-Pathologist image analysis software, which can classify digital histological images of gastric biopsy specimens into carcinoma or suspicious for carcinoma (positive), adenoma or suspicion of a neoplastic lesion (caution), or no malignancy (negative), and they compared their results with human pathologists.[19] Although the overall concordance rate for their 3-tier classification was as low as 55.6%, the e-Pathologist AI-based tool correctly identified 90.6% of negative specimens.

Automated image analysis to detect GC in routine practice is feasible, given that the reported diagnostic disagreement rate in gastrointestinal pathology ranges from 1.2% to 3.1%, suggesting that a false-negative rate of 5% could be an appropriate interim target for primary screening.[20–22] Leon and colleagues proposed a computational tool for characterizing gastric histopathological samples using a deep CNN application in the automatic detection of GC pathological images.[23] Two deep CNN-based approaches were presented: one was used to analyze morphological features from entire images, whereas the other independently investigated local characteristic properties. The results of these experiments demonstrated the exquisite performance of the studied model in the detection of GC, with an average accuracy of up to 89.72%. Iizuka and colleagues developed DL models for classifying stomach epithelial

Table 1
Summary of publications regarding artificial intelligence-based applications in gastric cancer pathology

Study (Date)	Task	Computational Approach	Dataset	Results
Li et al,[15] 2018	Classification	GastricNet (DL-based model)	560 slices of GC and 140 slices of normal tissue	100% classification accuracy, patch-based classification
Sharma et al,[18] 2017	Classification	CNN for cancer classification based on IHC response and necrosis detection	11 H&E-stained histological WSIs of GC	Cancer classification accuracy: 0.6990, Necrosis detection accuracy: 0.8144
Yoshida et al,[19] 2018	Classification	e-Pathologist image analysis software	WSIs of 3062 gastric biopsy specimens	Overall concordance rate: 55.6%, Correctly identified 90.6% of negative specimens
Leon et al,[23] 2019	Classification	Deep CNN application for automatic GC detection	40 Gastric histopathological samples	Average accuracy: 89.72%
Iizuka et al,[24] 2020	Classification	DL models for classifying stomach epithelial tumors	4128 WSIs of gastric tumor	AUC for gastric ADC and adenoma: 0.97 and 0.99, respectively
Liang et al,[26] (2019)	Classification	Image segmentation strategy for weakly labeled gastric tumors	100 WSIs of gastric tumor	IoU: 88.3%, Accuracy: 91.1%
Sun et al,[27] 2019	Classification	DL method with deformable and Atrous convolutions	500 WSIs of gastric tumor	Pixel-level accuracy: 91.60%, Mean IoU: 82.65%
Kanavati et al,[28] 2021	Classification	DL models to detect diffuse-type ADC in endoscopic biopsy specimen WSIs	4036 WSIs biopsy cases of human gastric epithelial lesions	ROC AUC in the range of 0.95–0.99
Park et al,[29] 2021	Classification	high-performance DL algorithm	2434 WSIs of gastric tumor	Algorithm-assisted diagnosis reduced review time by 47% and microscopy by 58%. ROC AUC was 0.97–0.99

(continued on next page)

Table 1
(continued)

Study (Date)	Task	Computational Approach	Dataset	Results
Govind et al,[32] 2020	Classification and tumor microenvironment analysis	Automated computational pipelines	50 gastrointestinal neuroendocrine tumors (GI-NETs)	SKIE grading accuracy: 90%. Linear weighted Cohen's kappa 0.62. Deep SKIE (DS) WSI accuracy: 98.4% (training), 90.9% (validation), 91.0% (testing) compared with SS WSI
Hensler et al,[35] 2005	Metastasis predictions	ANNs with QUEEN method	4302 patients, 8 preoperative variables	ANNs had 74.71% sensitivity and 71.65% specificity vs 64.96% sensitivity and 53.73% specificity for established system in predicting lymph node metastasis
Huang et al,[37] 2022	Metastasis predictions	Deep Neural Network (ESCNN)	LNs from gastric carcinoma of 422 studies, consisting of 2422 H&E slides, 125 IHC slides, and 20,000 LN images	Sensitivity of 0.8915, Specificity of 0.9861, Matthew's correlation coefficient of 0.8986 on the main test set; Slide-level ROC AUC of 0.9936
Matsushima et al,[38] 2022	Metastasis predictions	CNN (ResNet-152)	51 metastasis-positive nodes, and 776 metastasis-negative nodes	AUC of 0.9994 and a sensitivity of 0.844 and 0.914, with 1 and 2 false positives per node, respectively
Jagric et al,[39] 2010	Metastasis predictions	Learning Vector Quantization Neural Network	213 patients with liver metastases after GC surgery	Model had a sensitivity of 71% and a specificity of 96.1% in the development group, and a sensitivity of 66.7% and a specificity of 97.1% in the validation group

Kangi et al,[40] 2018	Prognosis predictions	ANN, Bayesian neural network	339 patients with GC	Bayesian NN achieved high accuracy (0.935) and ROC AUC (0.961)
Jiang et al,[41] 2018	Prognosis predictions	GC-SVM classifier	Three separate groups of 251 patients with GC	GC-SVM classifier had better accuracy than TNM stage with AUC of 0.834 and 0.828 for 5-y survival and disease-free survival
Lu et al,[42] 2017	Prognosis predictions	Multi-modal hypergraph approach	WSIs of 939 patients with GC after total gastrectomy	Model outperformed baseline models with an average improvement of 3% in classification accuracy
Liu et al,[44] 2018	Prognosis predictions	SVM classifier on PPI network	432 GC tissue samples	SVM classifier had 92.31% accuracy, identifying 146 nonrecurrence and 94 recurrence samples
Kim et al,[46] 2021	Prognosis predictions	Microarray analysis and ML algorithm	16 IMCs with lymph node metastasis, 12 without metastasis, 7 normal gastric tissue	21 miRNAs linked to metastasis; prediction model built with AUC 0.85. MiRNAs may serve as biomarkers for predicting IMCs metastasis risk
Kather et al,[49] 2019	Prediction of MSI	DL to predict response to immunotherapy based on MSI status	315 patients with TCGA-gastric ADC, 185 patients with GC from Yokohama, Japan	Patient-level AUCs of 0.81 (95% CI, 0.69–0.90) on TCGA dataset, AUC of 0.69 (95% CI, 0.52–0.82) on Japanese cohort
Su et al,[52] 2022	Prediction of MSI	DL system to recognize differentiation grade and MSI status of GC	WSIs from 467 patients	F1 values of 0.8615 and 0.8977 for poorly and well-diff. ADC. Patient-level accuracy of 86.36% for MSI status recognition

(continued on next page)

Table 1
(continued)

Study (Date)	Task	Computational Approach	Dataset	Results
Wang et al,[53] 2022	Prediction of MSI	DL ensemble method to classify 4 subtypes of gastric ADC	WSIs of H&E-stained tissue sections from 332 images from TCGA database	Tile-level AUC: 0.785, 0.668, 0.762, and 0.811 for 4 subtypes. Patient-level AUC: 0.897, 0.764, 0.890, and 0.898 for 4 subtypes
Garcia et al,[55] 2017	Tumor infiltrating lymphocytes	Automated detection and counting of TILs in GC IHC images using deep CNNs	10 GC tissue samples	96.88% accuracy, comparable to human pathologists (11 or less count diff. in 29/35 images)
Challoner et al,[56] 2020	Tumor infiltrating lymphocytes	Study of T-cell subtypes as prognostic markers in GC and GEJ cancers	474 Western GC patients (multicolor immunofluorescence staining)	CD45RO and FOXP3 T cells effectively predict cancer-specific survival. Stomach Cancer Immune Score significantly impacts survival (P < .001)
Li et al,[57] 2023	Tumor infiltrating lymphocytes	Interpretable ML model for detection, enumeration, and classification of TILs in WSIs	1660 WSIs from 1592 TCGA patients and 332 WSIs of independent institution	High accuracy in detecting/classifying TILs (75.6% detection rate in GC, >95% accuracy for 3 TIL maturation states)

Abbreviations: ADC, adenocarcinoma; ANN, artificial neural network; AUC, area under the ROC curve; CNN, convolutional neural network; DL, deep learning; DS, dual stain; ESCNN, enhanced streaming CNN; GC, gastric cancer; GEJ, esophagogastric junction; IHC, immunohistochemistry; IMCs, intramucosal carcinomas; IoU, intersection over union coefficient; ML, machine learning; MSI, microsatellite instability; SVM, support vector machine; TCGA, The Cancer Genome Atlas; TILS, Tumor-infiltrating lymphocytes; TMA, tissue micro array; WSI, whole slide image.

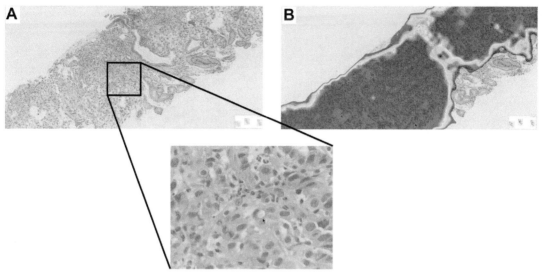

Fig. 1. Gastric biopsy (H&E stained) is shown with a poorly cohesive signet ring cell carcinoma (*A*) that was correctly detected by AI demonstrated as red heatmap that is representative of adenocarcinoma (*B*).

tumors (ADC and adenoma) to aid surgical pathologists in routine histological diagnostics.[24] A total of 4128 WSIs were collected for their study. They used millions of image tiles extracted from these WSIs to train a CNN based on the inception-v3 architecture to classify a tile into one of 3 labels: ADC, adenoma, and nonneoplastic.[25] The predictions from all the tiles in a specific WSI were then pooled to get a final classification using 2 strategies: a simple max-pooling strategy and a recurrent neural network. The area under the curve (AUC) yielded for this algorithm for gastric ADC and adenoma was 0.97 and 0.99, respectively.

DL applications typically require large-scale datasets containing thousands of images for reliable training. If all of these images have to annotated by human experts, then it compounds the complexity of developing a supervised training algorithm. To address this problem, Liang and colleagues proposed an image segmentation strategy for images of weakly labeled gastric tumors.[26] Their proposed reiterative learning framework allows the network to be trained on weakly labeled datasets and achieve excellent results without the need for additional manual annotation. They presented an overlapped region forecast, a new neural network architecture, and an algorithm for detecting GC. Their model met the supervised learning standard with an intersection over union coefficient (IoU) of 88.3% and 91.1% accuracy. Their method could significantly reduce labeling costs and shorten the length of time it takes to develop such an AI-based tool. Newer advances will continue to emerge that can be leveraged to further improve algorithms. For example, Sun and colleagues presented a different DL method that replaces the primary form of convolution in specific layers with deformable and Atrous convolutions,[27] which are better for dealing with geometric variations. Their model achieved pixel-level accuracy of 91.60% and a mean IoU of 82.65%.

Diffuse-type gastric ADC is more challenging to diagnose than other GCs, such as the intestinal

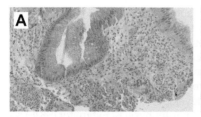
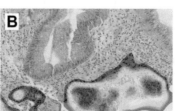
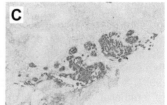

Fig. 2. The application of AI to WSI for detecting gastric NETs. The gastric biopsy (H&E stained) shows a well-differentiated NET (*A*). The heatmap in (*B*) generated by AI is overlaid on the NET of the original image. The NET is confirmed by chromogranin A staining (*C*).

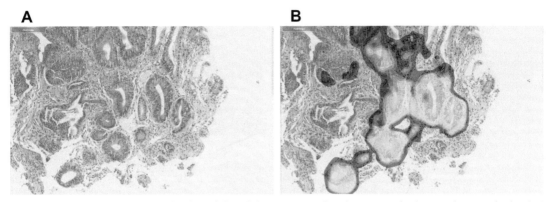

A

B

Fig. 3. Visualization of low-grade dysplasia (*A*) and the corresponding heatmap of adenoma/low-grade dysplasia generated by AI (*B*).

type. Therefore, computer-aided diagnosis to detect this variant of ADC would be a welcome tool for pathologists. Indeed, Kanavati and colleagues trained DL models to detect diffuse-type ADC in WSIs of endoscopic biopsy specimens.[28] A total of 4036 biopsy cases of human gastric epithelial lesions in this study were collected from 5 hospitals. The investigators used partial transfer learning to train their AI-based models and reported an area under the receiver operating characteristic curve (ROC-AUC) in the range of 0.95 to 0.99 for independent test sets. Their best-performing model was the one-stage model at 20× magnification and 512 × 512 pixel tile size. Training at 20× magnification improved performance, where the average ROC-AUC increased from 0.87 to 0.97 for their test sets. Their trained model detected both poorly differentiated type ADC and signet ring cell carcinoma. Most false positives occurred in gastritis cases due to the similarity between diffuse-type ADC and inflammatory cells, especially plasma cells.

Creating an automated screening method that leverages AI tools for the detection of GC can help reduce diagnostic workloads. In this regard, Park and colleagues used a large dataset of 2434 WSIs to develop and test a high-performance DL algorithm for the automated histologic classification of gastric epithelial tumors from biopsy specimens.[29] When compared with a digital image using a viewer alone, the algorithm-assisted diagnosis reduced review time by 47% and microscopy by 58%. The ROC-AUC in this study was used to calculate the algorithm's diagnostic accuracy, which was 0.97–0.99. This particular algorithm was trained to identify epithelial tumors solely; hence, stomach mesenchymal tumors and mucosa-associated lymphoid tissue lymphoma cases for this specific study were labeled as negative for dysplasia.

COMPUTER-ASSISTED KI-67 SCORING FOR GASTRIC NEUROENDOCRINE TUMORS

Gastrointestinal and pancreatic neuroendocrine tumors (NETs) are uncommon neoplasms that may be found incidentally during medical examination. The frequency of their diagnosis is accordingly on the increase.[30] These NETs develop from neural crest cells and can occur in several parts of the digestive system. Gastric NETs, in particular, may have unusual symptoms unrelated to hormone secretion. There are 4 types of gastric NETs, with type 1 being the most common (70%–80%) and related to atrophic gastritis, type 2 (30%) related to Zollinger-Ellison Syndrome and multiple endocrine neoplasia type 1, type 3 (sporadic and aggressive) that is likely to metastasize, and type 4 (poorly differentiated), which is difficult to treat surgically. Ki-67 is a well-known biomarker used in NET diagnosis and has prognostic significance as well as plays a part in the World Health Organization (WHO) grading of these neoplasms. The traditional method for determining the Ki-67 index involves manually counting the proportion of Ki-67 positive cells in a selected region of the tumor tissue. However, this approach has limitations, including the subjective selection of hot spots to count, intraobserver variability, and difficulty in accurately distinguishing between tumor and nontumor (eg, inflammatory) cells, which can result in unreliable Ki-67 indices and thus incorrect tumor grades.[31]

To address the aforementioned drawbacks, image analysis using ML algorithms has been applied to help automate the quantification of Ki-67 immunoreactivity in these NETs. Govind and colleagues developed 2 automated computational pipelines, a Synaptophysin KI Estimator (SKIE) and another deep-SKIE, to accurately assess the Ki-67 index in 50 gastrointestinal NETs.[32] Their pipelines used a double-immunostain (DS) technique utilizing both synaptophysin and Ki-67 antibodies, and performed automated hot spot selection and Ki-67 index quantification. Their first tool, SKIE, is a pipeline that automates the process of Ki-67 index quantitation through WSI analysis. The second tool, deep SKIE, uses a DL approach to generate a Ki-67 index heatmap across the entire tumor. In this study, Ki-67 indices of 50 GI-NETs were quantitated using SKIE and compared with the assessments of 3 pathologists using a microscope and a fourth pathologist using manual counting, which was considered the gold standard. Their results showed that SKIE had a grading accuracy of 90% and yielded substantial agreement (linear weighted Cohen's kappa 0.62). Deep SKIE using DS and WSIs showed significantly higher accuracy levels with training, validation, and resulted in testing accuracies of 98.4%, 90.9%, and 91.0%, respectively, compared with a standard single-immunostain (SS) technique and WSIs. The pipeline these researchers developed relies on an adjacent H&E section to estimate the total number of tumor nuclei, which may cause slight differences in scores. Nevertheless, it is well known that segmentation performance of an algorithm for nuclei counting may vary with image and tissue preparation variables and may accordingly not be robust in all cases, especially when nuclei are clumped together.

ARTIFICIAL INTELLIGENCE-BASED GASTRIC CANCER METASTASIS DETECTION

The detection of lymph node metastases is crucial for the treatment and prognosis of cancer, particularly gastric carcinoma, which has high mortality rates.[33] Sentinel lymph node navigation, a technique originally developed for melanoma and breast cancer, has been proposed for use in GC surgeries to identify metastases.[34] The use of ML algorithms, including DL, applied to digital data has demonstrated potential in detecting metastases in lymph nodes and improving the accuracy and efficiency of DP workflows. Hensler and colleagues developed the QUEEN (QUality-assured Efficient Engineering of Feedforward Neural Networks with Supervised Learning) method for optimizing artificial neural networks (ANNs) and applied this method in the context of improving the preoperative diagnosis of lymph node metastasis in patients with GC.[35] They used a database of 4302 patients and 8 variables known preoperatively using ANNs. Their resulting networks were evaluated on data from patients who had undergone surgery, and the ANNs demonstrated an average sensitivity of 74.71% and an average

specificity of 71.65% in predicting lymph node metastasis.[36] The study by Huang and colleagues found that using a deep neural network trained on high-resolution images, called enhanced streaming CNN (ESCNN), improved the sensitivity of detecting lymph node metastasis in a clinical setting.[37] This specific network was trained using a ResNet50 architecture and achieved a high level of accuracy, with a sensitivity of 0.8915, a specificity of 0.9861, and a Matthew's correlation coefficient of 0.8986 on the main test set. The ESCNN was able to detect tumor cells in GC with a slide-level ROC-AUC of 0.9936. These researchers also found that their ESCNN performed better when applied to down-sampled WSIs at lower magnifications ($5\times$ and $10\times$) but became saturated after application to micrometastasis subset images magnified at $10\times$. However, they noted that the benefits of using $20\times$ magnification required further verification using more isolated tumor cell samples.

Matsushima and colleagues conducted a similar study using an ML algorithm, specifically a CNN (ResNet-152 pretrained on ImageNet), to detect GC metastases in regional lymph nodes with high accuracy.[38] The algorithm had an AUC of 0.9994 and a sensitivity of 0.844 and 0.914, with 1 and 2 false positives per node, respectively. When allowing for approximately 3 false positives per node, the algorithm was able to detect all positive nodes. However, this study did have limitations, including the fact that these authors only focused on one histological subtype of gastric (tubular) ADC and they found a significant number of false positives. Jagric and colleagues conducted a study to determine whether a learning vector quantization neural network could be used to predict liver metastases after GC surgery.[39] They included 213 patients in their study and divided them into a development and validation group. Using an auxiliary regression network, they selected 7 clinicopathological variables to predict liver metastases. Their model was found to have a sensitivity of 71% and a specificity of 96.1% in the development group, and a sensitivity of 66.7% and a specificity of 97.1% in the validation group. This study concluded that the model had a high-negative predictive value and a reasonably high sensitivity for predicting liver metastases but that more patients and possibly biological markers may be necessary to improve sensitivity.

COMPUTATIONAL GASTRIC CANCER PROGNOSTICATION

Although the majority of AI-based studies on GC to date have focused on diagnosis, some studies have shown that AI models can also be useful in evaluating other histopathological parameters such as differentiation and lymphovascular involvement, which are essential in determining survival time,[40–42] recurrence risk,[43,44] predicting metastasis,[35,39,45] and consequently help in the treatment of GC. Indeed, the survival of patients with GC was previously predicted using neural networks. Kangi and colleagues used a 3-layer perceptron neural network and a Bayesian neural network to predict the probability of mortality in 339 patients with GC.[40] The Bayesian neural network achieved high prediction accuracy and ROC-AUC values of 0.935 and 0.961, respectively. The most important predictors of survival for GC were tumor grade, morphology, gender, smoking history, opium consumption, chemotherapy, and radiotherapy. Jiang and colleagues created a classifier called the GC support vector machine (GC-SVM) to improve the ability to predict survival and treatment response in patients with GC.[41] The GC-SVM classifier uses clinicopathologic features (such as age, tumor size, and tumor location) and immunohistochemical features (such as the presence and density of immune cells in the tumor) to make predictions. The GC-SVM classifier was tested on 3 separate groups of patients with GC and was found to have higher predictive accuracy for overall survival and disease-free survival compared with the current standard method of prediction, viz. the TNM stage. In an external validation cohort, the GC-SVM classifier had AUC values of 0.834 and 0.828 for 5-year overall survival and disease-free survival, respectively.

Lu and colleagues developed an ML model using a multimodal hypergraph approach to predict overall survival after total gastrectomy for patients with GC.[42] This model was tested using Random Forest and SVM algorithms and was found to outperform baseline models with an average improvement of 3% in classification accuracy. Liu and colleagues used gene expression data from 432 samples of GC tissue to identify genes associated with the survival time and status of patients with GC.[44] These genes were used to construct a protein–protein interaction (PPI) network, and the top 100 genes with the highest centrality betweenness value were chosen for further analysis. An SVM classifier was then used to classify the tissue samples based on the expression of these GC-related genes. The SVM classifier identified 146 "nonrecurrence" samples and 94 "recurrence" samples with an accuracy of 92.31%. Kim and colleagues conducted a study to identify microRNAs (miRNAs) that could predict the risk of metastasis in intramucosal gastric cancer (IMC).[46] They performed a microarray analysis

on 16 IMCs that resulted in lymph node metastasis, 12 IMCs that did not result in metastasis, and included 7 samples of normal gastric tissue. They identified 21 differentially expressed miRNAs in IMCs with metastasis and used these miRNAs to build a prediction model using an ML algorithm. They found that their model had good performance in classifying these samples, with an AUC of 0.85. Further, they found that the miRNAs identified were associated with pathways related to cancer and metastasis. These results suggest that the miRNAs identified in this study could potentially be used as biomarkers to predict the risk of metastasis in IMC.

COMPUTATIONAL GASTRIC CANCER MOLECULAR SUBTYPING

The WHO currently recognizes 4 types of GC: papillary, tubular, mucinous (colloid), and poorly cohesive carcinomas.[47] However, the Cancer Genome Atlas (TCGA) initiative has identified 4 main subtypes of GC based on molecular characteristics: Epstein-Barr virus (EBV)-infected, those with microsatellite instability (MSI), genomically stable (GS), and chromosomally instable tumors (CIN).[48] These subtypes provide a foundation for patient stratification and targeted therapy trials. However, the process of molecular classification is costly, resource intensive, and requires significant technical and analytical expertise. As an alternative option to address this challenge, Kather and colleagues used DL to predict whether patients with gastrointestinal cancer would respond well to immunotherapy based on MSI status.[49] They retrieved histology images of 315 patients with TCGA-gastric ADC and used these images to train a DL model to detect MSI. When tested on this cohort, the model achieved patient-level AUCs of 0.81 (95% confidence interval, 0.69–0.90). However, when they validated the MSI detector on a separate cohort of 185 patients with GC from Yokohama, Japan,[50] the classifier achieved a lower AUC of 0.69 (95% CI, 0.52–0.82). The lower performance of the classifier on the Japanese cohort may be due to the fact that GC in Asian individuals tends to have different histological and clinical characteristics compared with GC in non-Asian individuals.[51] Of note, the classifier was trained on a dataset primarily composed of non-Asian patients, which may have contributed to its lower performance (generalizability) when tested on an Asian cohort.

Su and colleagues designed a DL system that accurately recognizes differentiation grade and MSI status of GC based on WSIs.[52] The system was trained and tested on WSIs from 467 patients and achieved high performance in both differentiation grade recognition and MSI status recognition. In the test cohort, the system had F1 values of 0.8615 and 0.8977 for poorly and well-differentiated ADC, respectively. This model also had a patient-level accuracy of 86.36% for MSI status recognition. This research team did not have tile-level ground truth for their MSI diagnosis task and had to thus assume that all image tiles from a single patient had the same MSI status. However, tumor tissue can be heterogeneous, and even patients with MSI can have microsatellite-stable tumor tiles.

A study by Wang and colleagues describes a DL ensemble method called DEMoS, which was able to classify the 4 subtypes of gastric ADC (EBV, MSI, GS, and CIN) using WSIs of H&E-stained tissue sections.[53] The model was trained on 332 images from the TCGA database and tested using a 10-fold cross-validation. This model achieved good performance in classifying the 4 tumor subtypes, with tile-level AUC values of 0.785, 0.668, 0.762, and 0.811, respectively, and patient-level AUC values of 0.897, 0.764, 0.890, and 0.898, respectively. The limitations of this model include it not being tested with other architectures, lack of external datasets for generalization evaluation, and needing to consider domain-specific features. Selecting tiles closely associated with molecular subtypes may help improve performance.

TUMOR-INFILTRATING LYMPHOCYTE QUANTIFICATION IN GASTRIC CANCER

Immunotherapy intervenes with tumor immune response instead of directly targeting tumor cells, making it important to understand tumor immunity and identify relevant predictive markers. The advent of anti-PD-1/PD-L1 therapy agents has increased the importance of immunotherapy in GC. These particular biomarkers may enhance patient selection and treatment response, expanding the potential impact of immunotherapy.[54] Garcia and colleagues developed an approach for automatically detecting and counting tumor-infiltrating lymphocytes (TILs) in GC IHC images using deep CNNs.[55] A deep CNN was trained with GC tissue samples and achieved 96.88% accuracy. This model was compared with human pathologists and produced acceptable results, with a count difference of 11 or less in 29 out of 35 images; however, one potential drawback of this study is the limited size of the dataset used for testing, which could impact generalizability of the results.

Challoner and colleagues studied the role of T-cell subtypes as prognostic markers in gastric and gastro-esophageal junction cancers.[56] They used multicolor immunofluorescence staining (antibodies used were cluster of differentiation (CD)8, CD4, CD45RO, forkhead box P3 (FOXP3), and pancytokeratin) to analyze T-cell subtypes in patients with GC and computational image analysis on 474 Western patients with GC, independent of stage, mismatch repair and EBV status, and other pathological features. The study revealed that the concentration of CD45RO and FOXP3 T-cells could effectively predict cancer-specific survival. Combining these 2 markers, known as the Stomach Cancer Immune Score, displayed a notably significant impact on cancer-specific survival ($P < .001$); however, the absence of samples from tumor margins in their tissue microarray prevented the investigation of differences in immune cell populations between the tumor margins and centers. Additionally, the authors emphasized the need for independent validation of their findings in GC cohorts from additional centers.

Li and colleagues proposed an interpretable ML model for the automated detection, enumeration, and classification of TILs in WSIs.[57] Their model incorporated a CNN with deep residual learning (ResNet18) for segmenting tumor versus normal tissue in WSIs and a mask region-based CNN for segmenting and classifying individual nuclei into 3 cell types: lymphocytes, tumor cells, and other nonmalignant cells. The model was trained and evaluated on a dataset of 1660 WSIs from 1592 TCGA patients and 332 images from patients with GC from Nanfang Hospital in Guangzhou, China. The model achieved high accuracy in detecting and classifying TILs, with a detection rate of 75.6% in GC cases and greater than 95% accuracy in identifying the 3 maturation states of TILs in H&E-stained images. The study also found that a quantitative TIL score generated by this model was an independent prognostic factor associated with patient survival in gastrointestinal tumors.

SUMMARY

AI-based tools, often in conjunction with DP, have the potential to transform pathology, which includes improved diagnosis and prognostication for GC. AI-based tools applied to GC also offer novel methods to improve biomarker discovery. In recent years, the development of several AI-based tools has shown promising results. In the United States, the Food and Drug Administration has proposed a regulatory framework for AI/ML-based medical devices that emphasizes safety, quality, efficiency, and continuous improvement. However, challenges such as data variability, cost, limited deployed solution in clinical practice, lack of published evidence showing positive outcomes, and the negative mindset of many pathologists regarding this emerging technology still exist. The success of AI applied to GC requires more research and development. Moreover, as these AI tools advance, they are likely to be more palatable to pathologists if they are designed to augment and not replace pathologists.

CLINICS CARE POINTS

- AI and DP: AI-based tools and DP have the potential to revolutionize pathology. These tools can lead to more accurate diagnoses and prognostication for GC, thus clinicians should stay informed about the latest advancements in AI-based diagnostic technologies.

- Biomarker Discovery: AI has the potential to significantly improve biomarker discovery for GC. In conjunction with other medical developments, these could greatly assist in early detection and targeted therapy.

- Regulatory Framework: The FDA has proposed a regulatory framework for AI/ML-based medical devices, with a focus on safety, quality, and efficiency. Clinicians need to be aware of the regulatory landscape as they consider integrating AI-based tools into their practice.

- Barriers to AI Adoption: Despite the potential benefits, there are challenges to AI adoption in pathology, such as data variability, cost, and limited deployed solutions in clinical practice. Clinicians should be prepared for these potential barriers when considering AI-based tools.

- Evidence and Perception: There is a lack of published evidence showing positive outcomes from AI-based tools and a negative mindset among many pathologists regarding this emerging technology. Encouraging robust studies and open dialogue can help address these issues.

- Augmentation Not Replacement: As AI tools continue to advance, it is crucial to communicate that these are meant to augment, not replace, the skills of pathologists. Ensuring pathologists feel comfortable and supported with these tools will be critical to their successful adoption.

DISCLOSURES

L. Pantanowitz is on the scientific advisory board for Ibex and NTP and serves as a consultant for AIxMed and Hamamatsu.

ACKNOWLEDGMENTS

The authors thank Ibex Medical Analytics and Maccabi Healthcare Services in Israel for providing the images.

REFERENCES

1. Kamel HM. Trends and Challenges in Pathology Practice: Choices and necessities. Sultan Qaboos Univ Med J 2011;11(1):38–44.
2. Ribé A, Ribalta T, Lledó R, et al. Evaluation of turn-around times as a component of quality assurance in surgical pathology. Int J Qual Health Care J Int Soc Qual Health Care 1998;10(3):241–5.
3. Van Cutsem E, Sagaert X, Topal B, et al. Gastric cancer. Lancet Lond Engl 2016;388(10060):2654–64.
4. Bui MM, Asa SL, Pantanowitz L, et al. Digital and Computational Pathology: Bring the Future into Focus. J Pathol Inform 2019;10:10.
5. Pantanowitz L, Sharma A, Carter AB, et al. Twenty Years of Digital Pathology: An Overview of the Road Travelled, What is on the Horizon, and the Emergence of Vendor-Neutral Archives. J Pathol Inform 2018;9. https://doi.org/10.4103/jpi.jpi_69_18.
6. Tomaszewski JE. Chapter 11 - Overview of the role of artificial intelligence in pathology: the computer as a pathology digital assistant. In: Cohen S, editor. Artificial intelligence and deep learning in pathology. Elsevier; 2021. p. 237–62. https://doi.org/10.1016/B978-0-323-67538-3.00011-7.
7. Liscia DS, D'Andrea M, Biletta E, et al. Use of digital pathology and artificial intelligence for the diagnosis of Helicobacter pylori in gastric biopsies. Pathologica 2022;114(4):295–303.
8. Steinbuss G, Kriegsmann K, Kriegsmann M. Identification of Gastritis Subtypes by Convolutional Neuronal Networks on Histological Images of Antrum and Corpus Biopsies. Int J Mol Sci 2020; 21(18):6652.
9. Franklin MM, Schultz FA, Tafoya MA, et al. A Deep Learning Convolutional Neural Network Can Differentiate Between Helicobacter Pylori Gastritis and Autoimmune Gastritis With Results Comparable to Gastrointestinal Pathologists. Arch Pathol Lab Med 2022;146(1):117–22.
10. Deng Y, Qin HY, Zhou YY, et al. Artificial intelligence applications in pathological diagnosis of gastric cancer. Heliyon 2022;8(12). https://doi.org/10.1016/j.heliyon.2022.e12431.
11. Barmpoutis P, Waddingham W, Yuan J, et al. A digital pathology workflow for the segmentation and classification of gastric glands: Study of gastric atrophy and intestinal metaplasia cases. PLoS One 2022;17(12):e0275232.
12. Ko YS, Choi YM, Kim M, et al. Improving quality control in the routine practice for histopathological

interpretation of gastrointestinal endoscopic biopsies using artificial intelligence. PLoS One 2022; 17(12):e0278542.

13. Jeong Y, Cho CE, Kim JE, et al. Deep learning model to predict Epstein–Barr virus associated gastric cancer in histology. Sci Rep 2022;12(1):18466.

14. Lee SH, Lee Y, Jang HJ. Deep learning captures selective features for discrimination of microsatellite instability from pathologic tissue slides of gastric cancer. Int J Cancer 2023;152(2):298–307.

15. Li Y, Li X, Xie X, et al. Deep learning based gastric cancer identification. In: 2018 IEEE 15th International Symposium on Biomedical imaging (ISBI 2018). 2018:182–5. doi:10.1109/ISBI.2018.8363550.

16. Huang G, Liu Z, Van Der Maaten L, et al. Densely Connected Convolutional Networks. In: 2017 IEEE Conference on computer vision and pattern recognition (CVPR). 2017:2261–69. doi:10.1109/CVPR.2017.243.

17. He K, Zhang X, Ren S, et al. Deep Residual Learning for Image Recognition. In: 2016 IEEE Conference on computer vision and pattern recognition (CVPR). 2016:770–8. doi:10.1109/CVPR.2016.90.

18. Sharma H, Zerbe N, Klempert I, et al. Deep convolutional neural networks for automatic classification of gastric carcinoma using whole slide images in digital histopathology. Comput Med Imaging Graph 2017;61:2–13.

19. Yoshida H, Shimazu T, Kiyuna T, et al. Automated histological classification of whole-slide images of gastric biopsy specimens. Gastric Cancer 2018; 21(2):249–57.

20. Renshaw AA, Gould EW. Measuring errors in surgical pathology in real-life practice: defining what does and does not matter. Am J Clin Pathol 2007; 127(1):144–52.

21. Renshaw AA, Gould EW. Comparison of disagreement and amendment rates by tissue type and diagnosis: identifying cases for directed blinded review. Am J Clin Pathol 2006;126(5):736–9.

22. Kronz JD, Westra WH, Epstein JI. Mandatory second opinion surgical pathology at a large referral hospital. Cancer 1999;86(11):2426–35.

23. Leon F, Gelvez M, Jaimes Z, et al. Supervised Classification of Histopathological Images Using Convolutional Neuronal Networks for Gastric Cancer Detection. In: 2019 XXII Symposium on image, signal processing and artificial vision (STSIVA). 2019:1–5. doi:10.1109/STSIVA.2019.8730284.

24. Iizuka O, Kanavati F, Kato K, et al. Deep Learning Models for Histopathological Classification of Gastric and Colonic Epithelial Tumours. Sci Rep 2020;10(1):1504.

25. Szegedy C, Vanhoucke V, Ioffe S, et al. Rethinking the Inception Architecture for Computer Vision. In: 2016 IEEE Conference on computer vision and pattern recognition (CVPR). 2016:2818–26. doi:10.1109/CVPR.2016.308.

26. Liang Q, Nan Y, Coppola G, et al. Weakly Supervised Biomedical Image Segmentation by Reiterative Learning. IEEE J Biomed Health Inform 2019; 23(3):1205–14.

27. Sun M, Zhang G, Dang H, et al. Accurate Gastric Cancer Segmentation in Digital Pathology Images Using Deformable Convolution and Multi-Scale Embedding Networks. IEEE Access 2019;7: 75530–41.

28. Kanavati F, Tsuneki M. A deep learning model for gastric diffuse-type adenocarcinoma classification in whole slide images. Sci Rep 2021;11(1):20486.

29. Park J, Jang BG, Kim YW, et al. A Prospective Validation and Observer Performance Study of a Deep Learning Algorithm for Pathologic Diagnosis of Gastric Tumors in Endoscopic Biopsies. Clin Cancer Res 2021;27(3):719–28.

30. Bonds M, Rocha FG. Neuroendocrine Tumors of the Pancreatobiliary and Gastrointestinal Tracts. Surg Clin North Am 2020;100(3):635–48.

31. Canakis A, Lee LS. Current updates and future directions in diagnosis and management of gastroenteropancreatic neuroendocrine neoplasms. World J Gastrointest Endosc 2022;14(5):267–90.

32. Govind D, Jen KY, Matsukuma K, et al. Improving the accuracy of gastrointestinal neuroendocrine tumor grading with deep learning. Sci Rep 2020; 10(1):11064.

33. Japanese Gastric Cancer Association. Japanese gastric cancer treatment guidelines 2014 (ver. 4). Gastric Cancer 2017;20(1):1–19.

34. Hayashi H, Ochiai T, Mori M, et al. Sentinel lymph node mapping for gastric cancer using a dual procedure with dye- and gamma probe-guided techniques. J Am Coll Surg 2003;196(1):68–74.

35. Hensler K, Waschulzik T, Mönig SP, et al. Quality-assured Efficient Engineering of Feedforward Neural Networks (QUEEN): Pretherapeutic Estimation of Lymph Node Status in Patients with Gastric Carcinoma. Methods Inf Med 2005;44(05):647–54.

36. Kampschöer GH, Maruyama K, van de Velde CJ, et al. Computer analysis in making preoperative decisions: a rational approach to lymph node dissection in gastric cancer patients. Br J Surg 1989; 76(9):905–8.

37. Huang SC, Chen CC, Lan J, et al. Deep neural network trained on gigapixel images improves lymph node metastasis detection in clinical settings. Nat Commun 2022;13(1):3347.

38. Matsushima J, Sato T, Ohnishi T, et al. The Use of Deep Learning-Based Computer Diagnostic Algorithm for Detection of Lymph Node Metastases of Gastric Adenocarcinoma. Int J Surg Pathol 2022; 27. https://doi.org/10.1177/10668969221113475, 106689692211134.

39. Jagric T, Potrc S, Jagric T. Prediction of Liver Metastases After Gastric Cancer Resection with the Use of

Learning Vector Quantization Neural Networks. Dig Dis Sci 2010;55(11):3252–61.

40. Korhani Kangi A, Bahrampour A. Predicting the Survival of Gastric Cancer Patients Using Artificial and Bayesian Neural Networks. Asian Pac J Cancer Prev 2018;19(2):487–90.

41. Jiang Y, Xie J, Han Z, et al. Immunomarker Support Vector Machine Classifier for Prediction of Gastric Cancer Survival and Adjuvant Chemotherapeutic Benefit. Clin Cancer Res 2018;24(22):5574–84.

42. Lu F, Chen Z, Yuan X, et al. MMHG: Multi-modal Hypergraph Learning for Overall Survival After D2 Gastrectomy for Gastric Cancer. In: 2017 IEEE 15th Intl Conf on Dependable, Autonomic and Secure Computing, 15th Intl Conf on Pervasive Intelligence and Computing, 3rd Intl Conf on Big Data Intelligence and Computing and Cyber Science and Technology Congress(DASC/PiCom/DataCom/CyberSciTech). 2017:164-169. doi:10.1109/DASC-PICom-DataCom-CyberSciTec.2017.40.

43. Zhang W, Fang M, Dong D, et al. Development and validation of a CT-based radiomic nomogram for preoperative prediction of early recurrence in advanced gastric cancer. Radiother Oncol 2020;145:13–20.

44. Liu B, Tan J, Wang X, et al. Identification of recurrent risk-related genes and establishment of support vector machine prediction model for gastric cancer. Neoplasma 2018;65(03):360–6.

45. Bollschweiler EH, Mönig SP, Hensler K, et al. Artificial Neural Network for Prediction of Lymph Node Metastases in Gastric Cancer: A Phase II Diagnostic Study. Ann Surg Oncol 2004;11(5):506–11.

46. Kim S, Bae WJ, Ahn JM, et al. MicroRNA signatures associated with lymph node metastasis in intramucosal gastric cancer. Mod Pathol 2021;34(3):672–83.

47. FT B, F C, RH H, ND T. WHO Classification of Tumours of the Digestive System. https://publications.iarc.fr/Book-And-Report-Series/Who-Classification-Of-Tumours/WHO-Classification-Of-Tumours-Of-The-Digestive-System-2010. Accessed January 8, 2023.

48. Cancer Genome Atlas Research Network. Comprehensive molecular characterization of gastric adenocarcinoma. Nature 2014;513(7517):202–9.

49. Kather JN, Pearson AT, Halama N, et al. Deep learning can predict microsatellite instability directly from histology in gastrointestinal cancer. Nat Med 2019;25(7):1054–6.

50. Aoyama T, Hutchins G, Arai T, et al. Identification of a high-risk subtype of intestinal-type Japanese gastric cancer by quantitative measurement of the luminal tumor proportion. Cancer Med 2018;7(10):4914–23.

51. Rahman R, Asombang AW, Ibdah JA. Characteristics of gastric cancer in Asia. World J Gastroenterol 2014;20(16):4483–90.

52. Su F, Li J, Zhao X, et al. Interpretable tumor differentiation grade and microsatellite instability recognition in gastric cancer using deep learning. Lab Invest 2022;102(6):641–9.

53. Wang Y, Hu C, Kwok T, et al. DEMoS: a deep learning-based ensemble approach for predicting the molecular subtypes of gastric adenocarcinomas from histopathological images. Bioinformatics 2022;38(17):4206–13.

54. Kwak Y, Seo AN, Lee HE, et al. Tumor immune response and immunotherapy in gastric cancer. J Pathol Transl Med 2019;54(1):20–33.

55. Garcia E, Hermoza R, Castanon CB, et al. Automatic Lymphocyte Detection on Gastric Cancer IHC Images Using Deep Learning. In: 2017 IEEE 30th International Symposium on computer-based medical systems (CBMS). 2017:200–204.

56. Challoner BR, von Loga K, Woolston A, et al. Computational Image Analysis of T-Cell Infiltrates in Resectable Gastric Cancer: Association with Survival and Molecular Subtypes. JNCI J Natl Cancer Inst 2020;113(1):88–98.

57. Li Z, Jiang Y, Li B, et al. Development and Validation of a Machine Learning Model for Detection and Classification of Tertiary Lymphoid Structures in Gastrointestinal Cancers. JAMA Netw Open 2023;6(1):e2252553.

Characteristics, Reporting, and Potential Clinical Significance of Nonconventional Dysplasia in Inflammatory Bowel Disease

Won-Tak Choi, MD, PhD

KEYWORDS

- Colorectal cancer • Dysplasia • Inflammatory bowel disease • Nonconventional
- Primary sclerosing cholangitis

Key points

- Nonconventional dysplasia in inflammatory bowel disease has distinct morphologic, clinicopathologic, molecular, and risk profiles compared with conventional dysplasia.

- There are seven nonconventional dysplastic subtypes, including (1) hypermucinous dysplasia; (2) crypt cell dysplasia; (3) dysplasia with increased Paneth cell differentiation; (4) goblet cell-deficient dysplasia; (5) sessile serrated lesion-like dysplasia; (6) traditional serrated adenoma-like dysplasia; and (7) serrated dysplasia, not otherwise specified.

- Growing evidence supports that hypermucinous, crypt cell, and goblet cell-deficient dysplasias represent high-risk subtypes for advanced neoplasia, as they often present as invisible/flat dysplasia, show molecular alterations characteristic of advanced neoplasia (eg, aneuploidy and *KRAS* mutations), and more frequently develop advanced neoplasia than conventional dysplasia on follow-up.

- The high-risk subtypes are frequently associated with primary sclerosing cholangitis and account for greater than half of all dysplastic lesions found in this high-risk patient group.

- The risk of nonconventional dysplasia, in particular the high-risk subtypes, is positively correlated with increased histologic inflammation in the colon.

ABSTRACT

The term nonconventional dysplasia has been coined to describe several underrecognized morphologic patterns of epithelial dysplasia in inflammatory bowel disease (IBD), but to date, the full recognition of these newly characterized lesions by pathologists is uneven. The identification of nonconventional dysplastic subtypes is becoming increasingly important, as they often present as invisible/flat dysplasia and are more frequently associated with advanced neoplasia than conventional dysplasia on follow-up. This review describes the morphologic, clinicopathologic, and molecular characteristics of seven nonconventional subtypes known to date, as well as their potential significance in the clinical management of IBD patients.

OVERVIEW

Although pathologists are familiar with the morphologic criteria of conventional (intestinal type) dysplasia,[1] the most common form of dysplasia,

Conflicts of Interest and Source of Funding: None Declared.
Department of Pathology, University of California at San Francisco, 505 Parnassus Avenue, M552, Box 0102, San Francisco, CA 94143, USA
E-mail address: Won-Tak.Choi@ucsf.edu

Surgical Pathology 16 (2023) 687–702
https://doi.org/10.1016/j.path.2023.05.006
1875-9181/23/© 2023 Elsevier Inc. All rights reserved.

surgpath.theclinics.com

several underrecognized morphologic patterns of epithelial dysplasia (collectively known as nonconventional dysplasia) have been recently described in inflammatory bowel disease (IBD).[2–13] The recognition of these nonconventional subtypes is becoming increasingly important, as they are often endoscopically invisible or flat and have a higher risk of developing advanced neoplasia (high-grade dysplasia [HGD] or colorectal cancer [CRC]) than conventional dysplasia on follow-up.[3–5,8,9] Also despite the lack of high-grade morphologic features, they frequently demonstrate molecular alterations characteristic of advanced neoplasia (eg, aneuploidy and KRAS mutations).[3,4,6,7] As such, it is crucial for pathologists to have a good grasp of the morphologic criteria of different nonconventional subtypes as well as recent advances in our understanding of their clinicopathologic and molecular features that can assist in the diagnosis, risk stratification, and clinical management. This review summarizes their distinct morphologic, clinicopathologic, and molecular features compared with conventional dysplasia as well as their potential significance in the clinical management of IBD patients. The review is divided into three major sections.

1. Diagnosis, characteristics, and management of invisible/flat dysplasia
2. Diagnosis, characteristics, and reporting of nonconventional dysplastic subtypes
   a. Hypermucinous dysplasia
   b. Crypt cell dysplasia
   c. Dysplasia with increased Paneth cell differentiation
   d. Goblet cell-deficient dysplasia
   e. Serrated dysplasia, including sessile serrated lesion (SSL)-like dysplasia, traditional serrated adenoma (TSA)-like dysplasia, and serrated dysplasia, not otherwise specified (NOS)
3. Potential clinical significance of nonconventional dysplasia

DIAGNOSIS, CHARACTERISTICS, AND MANAGEMENT OF INVISIBLE/FLAT DYSPLASIA

Patients with long-standing IBD, including ulcerative colitis (UC) and Crohn's disease, are at a higher risk of developing dysplasia and/or CRC compared with the general population.[14–18] Established risk factors for colorectal neoplasia in IBD include male gender, younger age, longer disease duration, increased colonic inflammation, and primary sclerosing cholangitis (PSC).[8,10,17,19–25] Surveillance

colonoscopy typically begins at 8 years after IBD diagnosis,[25] but IBD patients with concomitant PSC (termed PSC-IBD) undergo an annual colonoscopy from the time of PSC diagnosis, regardless of IBD duration.[26–28] Indeed, compared with those with IBD alone, PSC-IBD patients have a two to fivefold higher risk of developing colorectal neoplasia,[8,20,29–33] more commonly in the right/proximal colon,[8,31,33,34] and they often develop CRC at a much younger age compared with IBD controls (median: 39 vs 59 years, respectively).[35]

Traditionally, the detection of IBD-associated dysplasia has relied on extensive random biopsies throughout the colon (ie, four-quadrant biopsies every 10 cm) to identify invisible dysplasia as well as targeted biopsies of endoscopically visible lesions.[36,37] However, thanks to advances in both endoscopic visualization (ie, high-definition endoscopy and chromoendoscopy) and resection techniques, the vast majority of IBD-associated dysplastic lesions are now endoscopically visible[38,39] and can be safely removed with endoscopic resection, obviating the need for colectomy.[40–43] Distinguishing IBD-associated visible/polypoid dysplasia from sporadic adenomas is no longer necessary from a therapeutic standpoint, as complete endoscopic resection followed by continued surveillance is sufficient either way. In fact, the annual incidence of CRC was reported to be only 0.5% in IBD patients with endoscopically resectable visible/polypoid dysplasia.[40] Also, a randomized controlled trial in UC patients demonstrated similar rates of dysplasia detected by targeted (11.4%) versus random (9.3%) biopsies,[44] leading to some experts advocating that targeted biopsies alone may be sufficient for dysplasia surveillance.[25,45,46]

In light of these findings, the Surveillance for Colorectal Endoscopic Neoplasia Detection and Management in Inflammatory Bowel Disease Patients: International Consensus Recommendations guidelines currently recommend that visible/polypoid dysplasia be managed with complete endoscopic resection followed by continued surveillance every 1 to 2 years, regardless of the histologic grade of dysplasia.[25] Colectomy should be reserved for invisible/flat dysplasia, especially HGD[25] due to its frequent association with synchronous CRC (50–67%) following a diagnosis of invisible/flat HGD (Fig. 1A).[47–50] Although the management of invisible/flat low-grade dysplasia (LGD) remains controversial due to its highly variable progression rates to advanced neoplasia ranging from 0% to greater than 50%,[48,51–62] colectomy is often recommended to manage multifocal invisible/flat LGD (Fig. 1A).[25] It is worth noting that these recommendations are based on

Fig. 1. Conventional dysplasia. (*A*) Guidelines for the management of invisible/flat dysplasia in IBD patients undergoing surveillance colonoscopy. (*B*) Low-grade conventional dysplasia shows crowded, penicillate, hyperchromatic nuclei limited to the basal half of the cytoplasm, involving both crypts and surface epithelial cells. Goblet cells are reduced but easily identified. (*C*) High-grade conventional dysplasia demonstrates more severe cytologic and architectural atypia.

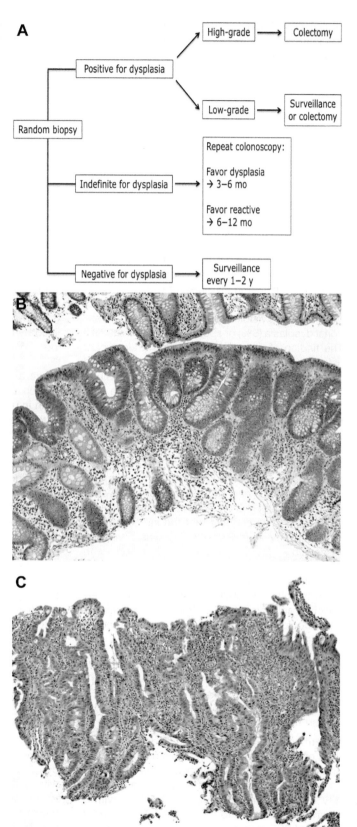

finding conventional dysplasia, which is categorized into either LGD or HGD based on cytologic and/or architectural atypia. As defined by the Riddell grading system,[1] LGD is characterized by crowded, elongated, hyperchromatic nuclei that are confined to the basal half of the cytoplasm, involving both crypts and surface epithelial cells (Fig. 1B), whereas HGD demonstrates more severe cytologic (ie, pleomorphic, enlarged, rounder nuclei, and loss of nuclear polarity) and/or architectural atypia (such as cribriform formation) (Fig. 1C).

Interestingly, recent molecular data on invisible/flat dysplasia in IBD seem to support the current aggressive surgical approach for patients with invisible/flat dysplasia. For instance, based on the analysis of cellular DNA content by flow cytometry, the rate of aneuploidy was reported to be significantly higher in invisible/flat dysplasia (41% for invisible/flat LGD and 93% for invisible/flat HGD)[62] than in visible/polypoid low-grade conventional dysplasia (8%) or sporadic adenomas (9%).[4] The finding of aneuploidy was also a significant risk factor for subsequent detection of advanced neoplasia in IBD patients with baseline invisible/flat LGD, with the univariate and multivariate hazard ratios of 5.3 ($P = 0.006$) and 4.5 ($P = 0.040$), respectively.[62] Similarly, using next-generation sequencing, Wanders and colleagues[63] recently reported that IBD-associated dysplastic lesions that are often invisible or flat have more DNA copy number alterations (average number of gains and losses of 4.3 and 3.2, respectively) than sporadic adenomas (1.5 and 0.5, respectively). Overall, these results suggest that the increased rate of aneuploidy in invisible/flat dysplasia may be responsible for its higher association with advanced neoplasia compared with visible/polypoid dysplasia, supporting the viewpoint that patients with invisible/flat dysplasia would likely benefit from colectomy and/or more aggressive endoscopic surveillance with increased random biopsies.

DIAGNOSIS, CHARACTERISTICS, AND REPORTING OF NONCONVENTIONAL DYSPLASTIC SUBTYPES

Hypermucinous Dysplasia

Hypermucinous dysplasia is an underrecognized form of nonconventional dysplasia accounting for approximately 2% of all dysplastic lesions in IBD patients (Table 1).[4] Most patients have a long history of IBD, more commonly UC (57%), with a mean duration of 21 to 23 years.[4,5] A concurrent history of PSC is found in up to 29% of patients,[4,5] with hypermucinous dysplasia being the second most common nonconventional subtype (25%) detected in this patient group.[8] Hypermucinous dysplasia most often presents as a large polypoid lesion (58%) with a mean size of 2.1 to 2.5 cm, but up to 42% of cases are endoscopically invisible or flat.[4,5] Indeed, in a recent retrospective analysis of 207 consecutive IBD patients who underwent a total colectomy or proctocolectomy and had at least one high-definition colonoscopy before colectomy, 15 (31%) of 49 previously undetected dysplastic lesions found only at colectomy showed features of hypermucinous dysplasia.[9] Although not uncommonly associated with conventional dysplasia, often in the same colonic segment (23%), hypermucinous dysplasia may be the only dysplastic subtype found in up to 57% of patients.[5] It shows a predilection for the left colon (57–64%).[4,5]

Morphologically, hypermucinous dysplasia most often demonstrates a tubulovillous/villous growth (76% vs 24% for a tubular architecture) lined by tall, prominent mucinous cells representing greater than 50% of the lesion (Fig. 2).[2,4,5,8–13] Cytologic atypia is usually low grade and typically more prominent in the lower portion of crypts (Fig. 2A, B), but HGD can be seen in up to 29% of cases.[4] Owing to prominent mucinous differentiation, especially in the surface epithelium, the degree of nuclear atypia tends to decrease toward the surface of the lesion (Fig. 2A) and may be focal or minimal in the surface epithelium (Fig. 2C). So, one must be careful not to miss hypermucinous dysplasia, if an initial biopsy is superficial and demonstrates fragments of hypermucinous epithelium but without significant cytologic or architectural atypia (Fig. 2D). Conversely, hypermucinous features may be associated with ulceration or pseudopolyps; however, cytologic and architectural anomalies are typically absent in these settings. In challenging situations, a descriptive diagnosis (eg, "hypermucinous features" or "hypermucinous epithelium") is recommended, with a follow-up colonoscopy within 3 to 6 months (similar to the management of indefinite for dysplasia [IND]; Fig. 1A), especially if a biopsy is from a clinically and/or endoscopically suspicious area of the colon. Approximately 33% to 50% of cases may demonstrate aberrant p53 expression (null or overexpression),[5,7] which can be useful in supporting a diagnosis of hypermucinous dysplasia. Of note, hypermucinous dysplasia frequently presents as a "mixed type" with either conventional or another nonconventional subtype (67% vs 33% for "pure type"), but to be categorized as the mixed type, the hypermucinous component should account for greater than 50% of the lesion.[2]

Table 1
Morphologic, clinicopathologic, and molecular features of nonconventional dysplastic subtypes

Characteristics	Hypermucinous Dysplasia	Crypt Cell Dysplasia	Dysplasia with Increased Paneth Cell Differentiation	Goblet Cell-Deficient Dysplasia	Sessile Serrated Lesion-Like Dysplasia	Traditional Serrated Adenoma-Like Dysplasia	Serrated Dysplasia, Not Otherwise Specified
Morphologic features	Tall, prominent mucinous cells with typically mild cytologic atypia predominantly involving the lower portion of crypts	Crowded, mildly enlarged, round-to-oval (or slightly elongated), non-stratified nuclei limited to the crypt base without surface involvement	Increased Paneth cell differentiation (either diffuse or patchy) involving at least two contiguous dysplastic crypts in two different foci	Complete or near-complete absence of goblet cells, often resulting in intensely eosinophilic cytoplasm	Dilatation and/or lateral spread of the crypt base (ie, dilated L- or inverted T-shaped crypts)	Ectopic crypts and columnar cells with elongated nuclei and eosinophilic cytoplasm	Complex serrated profile without features of sessile serrated lesion-like dysplasia or traditional serrated adenoma-like dysplasia
Most common histologic architecture (%)	Tubulovillous/villous (76%)	Flat (100%)	Tubular (>50%)	Tubular (92%)	Tubular (>50%)	Tubulovillous/villous (>50%)	Unknown
Incidence (% of all dysplastic lesions)	Rare (2%)	Rare (4%)	Relatively common (13%)	Rare (3%)	Rare (1%)	Rare (1%)	Rare (<1%)
Most common IBD subtype (%)	UC (57%)	UC (89–100%)	UC (71%)	UC (71–74%)	UC (75%)	UC (67–72%)	Likely UC
Association with PSC (%)	Common (29%)	Common (43%)	Infrequent (9%)	Not uncommon (14%)	Rare (0–1%)	Rare (0–6%)	Rare (1%)
Most common location (%)	Left colon (57–64%)	Left colon (79%), but more common in the right colon in PSC-IBD patients	Right colon (45%)	Equally common in both right and left colon (40–50% each)	Right colon (>50%)	Left colon (>50%)	Unknown

(continued on next page)

Table 1
(continued)

Characteristics	Hypermucinous Dysplasia	Crypt Cell Dysplasia	Dysplasia with Increased Paneth Cell Differentiation	Goblet Cell-Deficient Dysplasia	Sessile Serrated Lesion-Like Dysplasia	Traditional Serrated Adenoma-Like Dysplasia	Serrated Dysplasia, Not Otherwise Specified
Invisible/flat endoscopic appearance (%)	Common (42%)	Common (96–100%)	Not uncommon (30%)	Common (65%)	Rare (<25%)	Rare (<25%)	Unknown
Mean size (cm) of visible/polypoid dysplasia	2.1–2.5	Not applicable	1.0	1.7–1.9	1.2	1.2	Unknown
Rate of advanced neoplasia compared with conventional dysplasia (%)	Higher (49–57%)	Higher (72–86%)	Similar (15%)	Higher (59%)	At least comparable (≥17%)	At least comparable (≥17%)	Likely at least comparable (≥17%)
Reported molecular alterations	Aneuploidy, *KRAS, TP53*	Aneuploidy, *TP53, KRAS*	Aneuploidy	Aneuploidy, *PIK3CA, TP53, KRAS*	*BRAF, TP53*	*KRAS, BRAF, TP53*, aneuploidy	Unknown

Abbreviations: IBD, inflammatory bowel disease; PSC, primary sclerosing cholangitis; UC, ulcerative colitis.

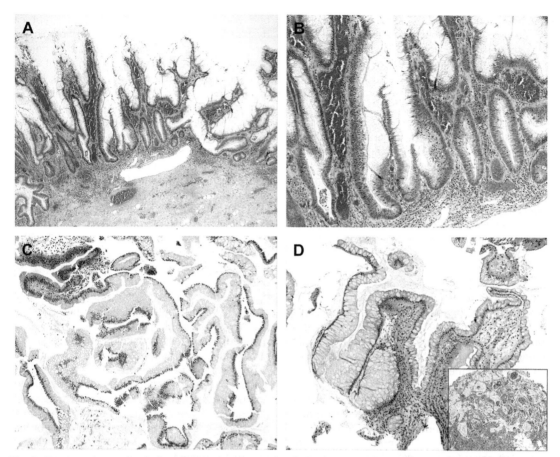

Fig. 2. Hypermucinous dysplasia. (*A*) Hypermucinous dysplasia shows a tubulovillous architecture lined by tall, prominent mucinous cells. (*B*) At high-power, low-grade nuclear atypia predominantly involves the lower portion of crypts. (*C*) Superficial fragments of hypermucinous dysplasia demonstrate prominent mucinous cells with focal low-grade dysplasia (top left corner). (*D*) Another superficial biopsy of hypermucinous dysplasia shows no nuclear atypia; however, a follow-up biopsy demonstrates mucinous adenocarcinoma (*inset*).

There is increasing evidence to support that hypermucinous dysplasia is a high-risk marker for advanced neoplasia (Table 1). First, Andersen and colleagues[6] demonstrated a higher frequency of *KRAS* mutations (61%) in hypermucinous dysplasia, even for hypermucinous epithelium without cytologic atypia, than in conventional LGD (4%; $P < 0.001$) or HGD (29%; $P > 0.05$). This is consistent with the previous report that *KRAS* mutations in sporadic adenomas are significantly associated with larger adenomas ≥ 2.0 cm (odd ratio [OR] 3.3), tubulovillous/villous histology (OR 3.2), and HGD (OR 3.0).[64] Similarly, it was reported that the rate of aneuploidy in low-grade hypermucinous dysplasia (80%) is similar to that of invisible/flat HGD (93%) but is significantly higher than that of visible/polypoid low-grade conventional dysplasia (8%) or sporadic adenomas (9%) ($P < 0.001$).[4,62] These results indicate that akin to conventional dysplasia, hypermucinous

dysplasia most likely develops via the chromosomal instability pathway involving multiple genetic (eg, *KRAS* and *TP53*) and large-scale chromosomal alterations.[4,6,7,65–67] Second, in line with these high-risk molecular features, a significant proportion (49–57%) of hypermucinous dysplastic lesions are correlated with subsequent detection of advanced neoplasia on follow-up.[4,5,8] In support of this, in a multi-institutional analysis, 19 (49%) of 39 low-grade hypermucinous dysplastic lesions were correlated with subsequent detection of HGD ($n = 9$; 23%) or CRC ($n = 10$; 26%) at the site of previous biopsy or in the same colonic segment within a mean follow-up time of 11 months.[5] In another study, 57% of hypermucinous dysplastic lesions developed advanced neoplasia on follow-up, whereas only 19% of conventional LGD did ($P < 0.001$).[4] Last, hypermucinous dysplasia was the most common nonconventional subtype (42%) found in a cohort of 58 IBD patients with CRC, further underscoring its high malignant potential.[2] Overall, these findings suggest that despite having low-grade morphology, hypermucinous dysplasia may represent at least a high-risk low-grade lesion, if not already HGD. Therefore, it is recommended that hypermucinous dysplasia be reported as "(polypoid) low- (or high)-grade dysplasia, hypermucinous variant," with a comment stating that it is frequently associated with advanced neoplasia on follow-up (Fig. 2D, inset) and thus complete excision and/or careful follow-up is recommended. Of note, the histologic grading of hypermucinous dysplasia and other dysplastic subtypes should be based on cytologic and/or architectural atypia, as defined by the Riddell grading system.[1]

Crypt Cell Dysplasia

Crypt cell dysplasia is another underrecognized variant of nonconventional dysplasia and accounts for approximately 4% of all dysplastic lesions in IBD patients (Table 1).[4] It is frequently associated with PSC (up to 43% of patients)[3] and represents the most common nonconventional subtype found in PSC-IBD patients (49%).[8] The vast majority of these lesions are found in UC patients (89–100%) with a long history of disease (mean duration: 14–15 years).[3–5] Crypt cell dysplasia usually shows a propensity for the left colon (up to 79%),[3–5] but in PSC-IBD patients, it is predominantly found in the right/proximal colon.[8] It almost exclusively presents as invisible/flat dysplasia (96–100%).[3–5] In a multi-institutional analysis, 43 (96%) of 45 crypt cell dysplastic lesions were endoscopically normal (n = 40; 89%) or showed subtle flat mucosal abnormalities such as "erythema," "edema," "pale," or "mild inflammation" (n = 3; 7%).[5] Although crypt cell dysplasia may be associated with conventional dysplasia, greater than half of these lesions (52%) may occur as isolated dysplastic lesions in IBD patients,[5] underscoring the importance of recognizing this challenging lesion by pathologists.

Unlike conventional and other nonconventional subtypes that show surface involvement by dysplastic changes, crypt cell dysplasia is defined by the presence of mild enlargement and hyperchromasia of mostly round-to-oval (or slightly elongated), non-stratified nuclei limited to the crypt base without surface involvement or significant architectural atypia (Fig. 3A).[3–5,8–13] Increased mitoses are common at the base of crypts. To avoid confusion with reactive changes, significant neutrophilic inflammation involving multiple crypts and/or ulceration should be absent, if one wishes to make a diagnosis of crypt cell dysplasia purely based on its morphologic features. Although a few scattered cells may demonstrate more than mild nuclear enlargement and/or focal loss of nuclear polarity (Fig. 3B, C), the degree of atypia does not represent unequivocal evidence of HGD. In practice, it may be difficult to diagnose crypt cell dysplasia in a consistent manner on histologic grounds alone.[3] Therefore, p53 staining is strongly recommended to assist in the diagnosis of crypt cell dysplasia, as strong and diffuse p53 nuclear staining can be present in up to 63% of cases (Fig. 3B, inset).[3] If p53 staining is strong and diffuse, it is recommended that crypt cell dysplasia be reported as "(at least) low-grade dysplasia, crypt cell variant," with a comment stating that it is frequently associated with advanced neoplasia on follow-up (Fig. 3D) and thus complete excision and/or careful follow-up is recommended. If p53 staining is weak or patchy (wild-type pattern), a descriptive diagnosis (eg, "crypt cell atypia") or IND diagnosis is recommended, with a follow-up colonoscopy within 3 to 6 months.

Similar to hypermucinous dysplasia, growing evidence indicates that crypt cell dysplasia is another high-risk marker for advanced neoplasia (Table 1). In favor of this, in spite of having at most low-grade morphology, all 14 crypt cell dysplastic lesions from 7 IBD patients were reported to present as invisible/flat dysplasia and demonstrated aneuploidy,[3] suggesting that crypt cell dysplasia represents at least a high-risk low-grade lesion, if not already HGD. Of note, six (86%) of the seven patients developed HGD (n = 4; 67%) or CRC (n = 2; 33%) in the same colonic segment within a mean follow-up time of 27 months.[3,4] This is consistent with the previous results that IBD-associated invisible/flat dysplasia frequently demonstrates aneuploidy (41% for invisible/flat LGD and 93% for invisible/flat HGD), and that the presence of aneuploidy in the setting of invisible/flat LGD is significantly correlated with subsequent detection of advanced neoplasia on follow-up.[62] Other investigators also demonstrated that crypt cell dysplasia often contains TP53 (43%) and KRAS (14%) mutations, further confirming its dysplastic nature.[7] In line with these earlier findings, in a larger cohort study, 26 (72%) of 36 crypt cell dysplastic lesions were associated with subsequent detection of HGD (n = 21; 58%) or CRC (n = 5; 14%) at the site of previous biopsy or in the same colonic segment within a mean follow-up time of 16 months.[5] Furthermore, it was recently demonstrated that crypt cell dysplasia is the most common nonconventional subtype found in PSC-IBD patients (49% vs 16%

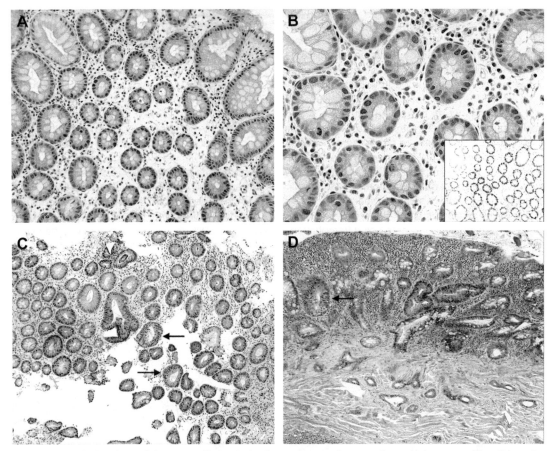

Fig. 3. Crypt cell dysplasia. (*A*) Crypt cell dysplasia demonstrates clusters of atypical crypts with mild nuclear enlargement, crowding, and hyperchromasia limited to the crypt base without surface involvement. Increased mitoses are present, but there is no significant active inflammation. (*B*) At high-power, nuclei are mostly round-to-oval and mildly enlarged, but no significant loss of nuclear polarity or architectural atypia is identified. The dysplastic crypts show strong and diffuse p53 positivity (*inset*). (*C*) A follow-up biopsy shows more elongated, crowded nuclei with areas of nuclear stratification (*arrows*). (*D*) A subsequent colectomy specimen demonstrates a very well-differentiated adenocarcinoma infiltrating the submucosa, consistent with low-grade tubuloglandular adenocarcinoma. A similar dysplastic crypt (*arrow*) identified in the prior biopsy (*C, arrows*) is still present in the overlying mucosa.

for non-PSC IBD patients; $P < 0.001$), likely contributing to a nearly twofold increase in the rate of advanced neoplasia in the PSC-IBD group (37%) compared with the non-PSC IBD group (22%) ($P = 0.035$).[8]

Dysplasia with Increased Paneth Cell Differentiation

Dysplasia with increased Paneth cell differentiation is a relatively common nonconventional subtype accounting for approximately 13% of all dysplastic lesions in IBD patients (**Table 1**).[4] Most patients have a long history of IBD (mean duration: 17 years), more commonly UC (71%), and present with a small polypoid lesion (mean size: 1 cm).[4] However, up to 30% of cases are

endoscopically invisible or flat.[4] Compared with hypermucinous and crypt cell dysplasias, dysplasia with increased Paneth cell differentiation is more common in the right colon (45%), shows male predominance (82%), and is infrequently associated with PSC (9%).[4] Indeed, in a recent retrospective analysis of dysplastic lesions in PSC-IBD patients, dysplasia with increased Paneth differentiation accounted for only 8% of nonconventional dysplastic lesions (vs 49% for crypt cell dysplasia and 25% for hypermucinous dysplasia).[8]

Dysplasia with increased Paneth cell differentiation is morphologically similar to conventional dysplasia or sporadic adenomas, but its defining feature is increased Paneth cell differentiation (either diffuse or patchy) involving at least two contiguous dysplastic crypts in two different foci (**Fig.** 4A, B).[2,4,8–13] It most often shows a tubular architecture (>50%) lined by crowded, elongated, hyperchromatic nuclei involving both crypts and surface epithelial cells. Although goblet cells may be reduced, they are not completely absent in most cases. It is worth noting that although scattered or rare Paneth cells may be present in other dysplastic subtypes, they are not present in multiple crypts and in multiple foci as in dysplasia with increased Paneth cell differentiation, and the same degree of Paneth cell differentiation is always present in adjacent, non-dysplastic mucosa.

Unlike hypermucinous and crypt cell dysplasias, dysplasia with increased Paneth cell differentiation may be a low-risk marker for advanced neoplasia (**Table** 1). In support of this, dysplasia with

increased Paneth cell differentiation was reported to have a low rate of aneuploidy (12%) similar to that of visible/polypoid low-grade conventional dysplasia (8%; $P = 0.715$) or sporadic adenomas (9%; $P = 0.823$).[4] Its risk of harboring advanced neoplasia (15%) was also comparable to that of low-grade conventional dysplasia (19%) ($P = 0.523$).[4] Furthermore, dysplasia with increased Paneth cell differentiation was a relatively rare nonconventional subtype found in IBD patients with CRC (11%)[2] or PSC-IBD patients (8%),[8] further supporting its apparent low malignant potential.

Interestingly, a similar entity (so called "Paneth cell-rich" adenomas) has been described in the sporadic setting with the reported frequency of 0.2% to 39%.[68–71] Although varying definitions were used to characterize these lesions, with some defining the presence of even one Paneth

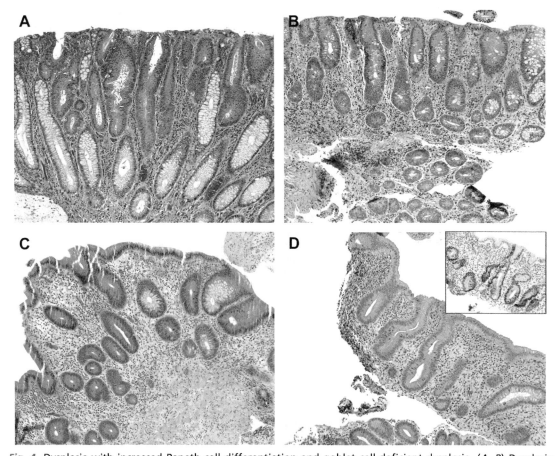

Fig. 4. Dysplasia with increased Paneth cell differentiation and goblet cell-deficient dysplasia. (*A, B*) Dysplasia with increased Paneth cell differentiation is characterized by increased Paneth cell differentiation involving multiple dysplastic crypts. The distribution of Paneth cells in the dysplastic crypts can be either diffuse (*A*) or patchy (*B*). Low-grade dysplasia (LGD) involves both crypts and surface epithelial cells. (*C*) Low-grade goblet cell-deficient dysplasia shows a complete or near-complete absence of goblet cells, leading to intensely bright eosinophilic cytoplasm. Mild nuclear atypia meeting the criteria of LGD involves both crypts and surface epithelial cells. (*D*) Another example of low-grade goblet cell-deficient dysplasia demonstrates multiple mitotic figures at the base of crypts as well as strong and diffuse p53 positivity (*inset*).

cell as histologic evidence of increased Paneth cell differentiation, Paneth cell-rich adenomas demonstrated similar clinicopathologic features to their IBD-associated counterpart. For instance, Paneth cell-rich adenomas showed a predilection for the right colon (85% vs 56% for non-Paneth cell-containing adenomas; $P = 0.006$) and male predominance (89% vs 56% for non-Paneth cell-containing adenomas; $P = 0.002$).[71] Also, regardless of their location, Paneth cell-rich adenomas were not significantly associated with subsequent development of CRC compared with sporadic adenomas devoid of Paneth cells.[69] As such, it is recommended that dysplasia with increased Paneth cell differentiation be reported as "(polypoid) low-(or high)-grade dysplasia" without specifying its subtype, as dysplasia with increased Paneth cell differentiation seems to share similar clinical and molecular features with its sporadic counterpart. Nonetheless, the recognition of this particular nonconventional subtype can be potentially helpful in identifying a subtle focus of dysplasia characterized by increased Paneth cell differentiation, which could be misinterpreted as benign metaplastic changes by pathologists.

Goblet Cell-Deficient Dysplasia

Goblet cell-deficient dysplasia accounts for approximately 3% of all dysplastic lesions in IBD patients, but it is likely underdiagnosed (Table 1).[4] Most patients have a long history of IBD with a mean duration of 16 to 17 years, more commonly UC (71–74%), and a concurrent history of PSC is found in up to 14%.[4,5] Goblet cell-deficient dysplasia is detected throughout the colon (40–50% each in the right and left colon) and often presents as invisible/flat dysplasia.[4,5] In a multi-institutional analysis, 17 (65%) of 26 goblet cell-deficient dysplastic lesions were endoscopically normal ($n = 14$; 54%) or showed subtle flat mucosal abnormalities ($n = 3$; 12%).[5] When endoscopically visible, it frequently presents as a large polypoid lesion with a mean size of 1.7 to 1.9 cm.[4,5] Also, goblet cell-deficient dysplasia is more commonly associated with conventional dysplasia (74%; $P = 0.044$), often in the same colonic segment (61%), compared with hypermucinous (43%) and crypt cell (48%) dysplasias.[5]

The defining histologic feature of goblet cell-deficient dysplasia is a complete or near-complete absence of goblet cells, often resulting in intensely eosinophilic cytoplasm (Fig. 4C, D).[2,4,5,8–13] It predominantly demonstrates a tubular architecture (92%) with mild nuclear atypia meeting the criteria of LGD involving both crypts and surface epithelial cells, along with increased mitoses at the base of crypts.[5] However, up to 40% of cases may demonstrate HGD at diagnosis, often with eosinophilic luminal secretion.[4] In challenging cases, p53 stain may assist in the diagnosis of goblet cell-deficient dysplasia, as aberrant p53 expression (null or overexpression) can be seen in 29% to 44% of cases (Fig. 4D, inset).[5,7]

Similar to hypermucinous and crypt cell dysplasias, goblet cell-deficient dysplasia may be a marker of increased risk for advanced neoplasia (Table 1). Indeed, 10 (59%) of 17 low-grade goblet cell-deficient dysplastic lesions were reported to be associated with subsequent detection of HGD ($n = 4$; 24%) or CRC ($n = 6$; 35%) at the site of previous biopsy or in the same colonic segment within a mean follow-up time of 13 months.[5] Also, 61% of patients with goblet cell-deficient dysplasia had a history of conventional dysplasia in the same colonic segment, supporting the potential role of field effect or cancerization in the development of advanced neoplasia in these patients. Furthermore, low-grade goblet cell-deficient dysplasia had a higher rate of aneuploidy (25%) than visible/polypoid low-grade conventional dysplasia (8%) or sporadic adenomas (9%).[4] This is further corroborated by the previous finding that goblet cell-deficient dysplasia has high rates of PIK3CA (56%), TP53 (44%), and KRAS (22%) mutations.[7] Thus, it is recommended that goblet cell-deficient dysplasia be reported as "(polypoid) low- (or high)-grade dysplasia, goblet cell-deficient variant," with a comment stating that it is frequently associated with advanced neoplasia on follow-up and thus complete excision and/or careful follow-up is recommended. In challenging situations, a descriptive diagnosis (eg, "atypia with loss of goblet cells") or IND diagnosis is recommended, with a follow-up colonoscopy within 3 to 6 months. Additional biopsies at the site of previous biopsy or in the same colonic segment may reveal more convincing dysplastic features and/or nearby conventional dysplasia.

Serrated Dysplasia

Serrated dysplasia in IBD includes three distinct subtypes, including SSL-like dysplasia, TSA-like dysplasia, and serrated dysplasia NOS.[2,4,8–13] Even as a group, they seem to be rare and account for only 2% of all dysplastic lesions in IBD patients (Table 1).[4] Most patients have UC (67–75%) with a long history of disease (mean duration: > 10 years), but they seldom have a concurrent history of PSC (~1%).[4,8,72] In a recent analysis of PSC-IBD patients, serrated dysplasia, as a group, accounted for only 5% of nonconventional dysplastic lesions.[8] They most often have a polypoid endoscopic appearance (mean size: 1.2 cm) and less than 25% of cases present as invisible/flat dysplasia.[4,8,9,72] Although the characteristics of serrated dysplasia NOS are yet to be defined, SSL-like and TSA-like dysplasias share similar clinicopathologic and molecular features with their respective sporadic counterparts.[4,72–74] For instance, SSL-like dysplasia shows a propensity for the right colon, whereas TSA-like dysplasia is more common in the left colon.[4,72,73] SSL-like dysplasia also lacks aneuploidy, supporting that a serrated (rather than chromosomal instability) pathway is responsible for its development.[4,74] Furthermore, TSA-like dysplasia frequently demonstrates KRAS mutations (45% vs 18% for BRAF mutations) similar to its sporadic counterpart.[72]

Morphologically, SSL-like and TSA-like dysplasias are essentially identical to their respective sporadic counterparts.[2,4,8–13] SSL-like dysplasia is characterized by dilatation and/or lateral spread of the crypt base (ie, dilated L- or inverted T-shaped crypts) at the interface with muscularis mucosa (Fig. 5A). TSA-like dysplasia often demonstrates a tubulovillous/villous architecture lined by columnar cells with elongated nuclei and eosinophilic cytoplasm, along with ectopic crypts (Fig. 5B). Serrated dysplasia NOS has no definite features of SSL-like or TSA-like dysplasia (Fig. 5C, D,E). By definition, all three serrated subtypes should demonstrate morphologic evidence of dysplasia, in addition to their characteristic serrated profiles representing greater than 50% of the lesion. To avoid confusion, it is recommended that the terms "SSL-like dysplasia," "TSA-like dysplasia," or "serrated dysplasia NOS" be used to describe dysplastic serrated lesions that are endoscopically invisible or flat, because endoscopically visible/polypoid serrated lesions might be sporadic serrated polyps. These terms could also be used to describe dysplastic serrated lesions with ambiguous morphologic features. Although the differential diagnosis of endoscopically invisible/flat serrated lesions in IBD includes "serrated epithelial change (SEC)," this is a distinct entity characterized by hyperplastic polyp-like mucosal change found on random biopsy without morphologic evidence of dysplasia (Fig. 5F).[74–77]

The natural history of IBD-associated serrated dysplasia, in particular invisible/flat serrated dysplasia, is not well-defined. However, Ko and colleagues[72] reported that mostly visible/polypoid low-grade serrated dysplasia (which often resembled sporadic TSA) was associated with higher rates of advanced neoplasia (17% within 10 years; $P = 0.020$) and prevalent conventional neoplasia (76%; $P < 0.001$) than non-dysplastic serrated lesions (0% and 11%, respectively), although its risk of having advanced neoplasia (17%) was similar to that of low-grade conventional dysplasia (23%). However, in another study, serrated dysplasia (42%), as a group, was as common as hypermucinous dysplasia (42%) in a cohort of 58 IBD patients with CRC, with TSA-like dysplasia being the most common serrated subtype (28%) followed serrated dysplasia NOS (11%) and SSL-like dysplasia (3%).[2] Taken together, these findings suggest that low-grade serrated dysplasia has at least a similar risk of developing advanced neoplasia compared with low-grade conventional dysplasia, but a subset of serrated dysplastic lesions (eg, serrated dysplasia NOS and invisible/flat serrated dysplasia) may be associated with an increased risk for advanced neoplasia. Additional studies are necessary to further characterize serrated dysplasia in IBD.

POTENTIAL CLINICAL SIGNIFICANCE OF NONCONVENTIONAL DYSPLASIA

Nonconventional dysplasia has distinct morphologic, clinicopathologic, molecular, and risk profiles compared with conventional dysplasia (Table 1). Growing evidence supports that hypermucinous, crypt cell, and goblet cell-deficient dysplasias represent high-risk subtypes for advanced neoplasia, as they often present as invisible/flat dysplasia (42–100%), and although morphologically low grade, show molecular alterations characteristic of advanced neoplasia (eg, aneuploidy and KRAS mutations), and are more frequently correlated with advanced neoplasia (49–86%) than conventional dysplasia on follow-up.[3–8] Also, these high-risk subtypes are frequently associated with PSC and account for greater than half (53%) of all dysplastic lesions found in PSC-IBD patients,[8] likely contributing to the increased risk of advanced neoplasia in this high-risk patient group. Overall, these findings suggest that in spite of the development of newer endoscopic techniques, performing only targeted biopsies in IBD patients (as advocated by some investigators) may miss some of these high-risk, nonconventional dysplastic lesions, and that IBD patients, particularly those diagnosed with nonconventional dysplasia, would likely benefit from increased random biopsy sampling or even preventive colectomy. This is further corroborated by the recent finding that previously undetected dysplastic lesions found only at colectomy are more likely to have nonconventional dysplastic features (76%) compared with previously detected dysplastic lesions (13%) ($P < 0.05$).[9] This also underscores the importance of recognizing different nonconventional subtypes by pathologists.

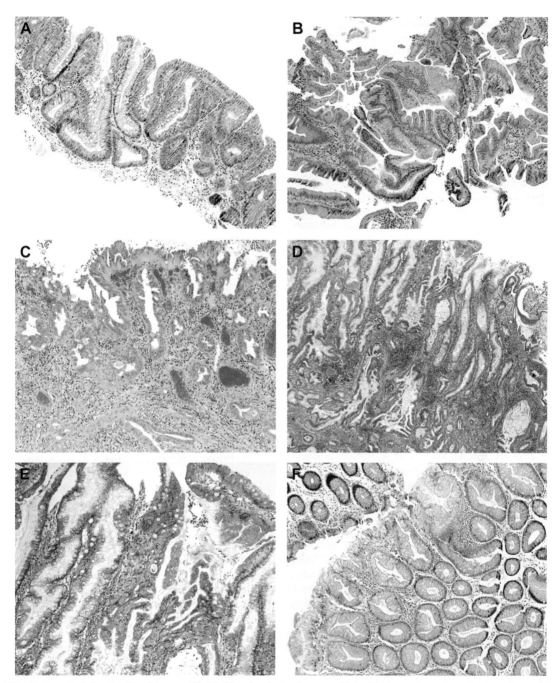

Fig. 5. Serrated dysplastic subtypes. (*A*) SSL-like dysplasia shows a dilated L-shaped crypt at the interface with muscularis mucosa. Low-grade dysplasia involves both crypts and surface epithelial cells. (*B*) TSA-like dysplasia demonstrates a tubulovillous architecture lined by low-grade columnar cells with eosinophilic cytoplasm. Characteristic ectopic crypts are also present. (*C*) Serrated dysplasia NOS lacks features of either SSL-like or TSA-like dysplasia. It shows full-thickness nuclear atypia and cribriform formation and is associated with invasive adenocarcinoma. (*D, E*) Another example of serrated dysplasia NOS shows a complex serrated architecture without features of SSL-like or TSA-like dysplasia. Despite having minimal to mild nuclear atypia (*E*, at high-power), it is architecturally complex and associated with invasive adenocarcinoma. (*F*) Serrated epithelial change demonstrates hyperplastic polyp-like mucosal change, but there is no histologic evidence of dysplasia, distinguishing it from the serrated dysplastic subtypes.

Of note, it is recently demonstrated that the risk of nonconventional dysplasia, in particular the high-risk subtypes, is positively correlated with increased histologic inflammation in the colon.[10] In multivariate analyses, higher mean and maximum scores (calculated from all biopsies taken during each colonoscopy before the initial detection of dysplasia) increased the odds of nonconventional dysplasia by 2.7 and 4.9, respectively, compared with conventional dysplasia ($P < 0.05$). There was a stronger association between these two scores and the high-risk subtypes (ORs 4.0 and 7.5, respectively, $P < 0.05$). From a clinical perspective, these results suggest that increasingly severe histologic inflammation may contribute to higher rates of genomic instability and nonconventional dysplasia, especially the high-risk subtypes, in IBD patients. Therefore, more severely active disease should prompt consideration of intensive surveillance strategies to identify these high-risk lesions earlier as well as more aggressive therapeutic management to control inflammation.

REFERENCES

1. Riddell RH, Goldman H, Ransohoff DF, et al. Dysplasia in inflammatory bowel disease: standardized classification with provisional clinical applications. Hum Pathol 1983;14:931–68.
2. Choi WT, Yozu M, Miller G, et al. Non-conventional dysplasia in patients with inflammatory bowel disease and colorectal carcinoma: a multicenter clinicopathologic study. Mod Path 2020;33:933–43.
3. Wen KW, Umetsu SE, Goldblum JR, et al. DNA flow cytometric and interobserver study of crypt cell atypia in inflammatory bowel disease. Histopathology 2019;75:578–88.
4. Lee H, Rabinovitch PS, Mattis AN, et al. Non-conventional dysplasia in inflammatory bowel disease is more frequently associated with advanced neoplasia and aneuploidy than conventional dysplasia. Histopathology 2021;78:814–30.
5. Choi WT, Salomao M, Zhao L, et al. Hypermucinous, goblet cell deficient, and crypt cell dysplasias in inflammatory bowel disease are often associated with flat/invisible endoscopic appearance and advanced neoplasia on follow-up. J Crohns Colitis 2022;16:98–108.
6. Andersen SN, Lovig T, Clausen OP, et al. Villous, hypermucinous mucosa in long standing ulcerative colitis shows high frequency of K-ras mutations. Gut 1999;45:686–92.
7. Gui X, Köbel M, Ferraz JG, et al. Histological and molecular diversity and heterogeneity of precancerous lesions associated with inflammatory bowel diseases. J Clin Pathol 2020;73:391–402.
8. Zhang R, Lauwers GY, Choi WT. Increased risk of non-conventional and invisible dysplasias in patients with primary sclerosing cholangitis and inflammatory bowel disease. J Crohns Colitis 2022;16:1825–34.
9. Bahceci D, Lauwers GY, Choi WT. Clinicopathologic features of undetected dysplasia found in total colectomy or proctocolectomy specimens of patients with inflammatory bowel disease. Histopathology 2022;81:183–91.
10. Nguyen ED, Wang D, Lauwers GY, et al. Increased histologic inflammation is an independent risk factor for nonconventional dysplasia in ulcerative colitis. Histopathology 2022;81:644–52.
11. Choi WT. Non-conventional dysplastic subtypes in inflammatory bowel disease: a review of their diagnostic characteristics and potential clinical implications. J Pathol Transl Med 2021;55:83–93.
12. Choi WT, Kővári BP, Lauwers GY. The significance of flat/invisible dysplasia and nonconventional dysplastic subtypes in inflammatory bowel disease: a review of their morphologic, clinicopathologic, and molecular characteristics. Adv Anat Pathol 2022;29:15–24.
13. Pereira D, Kővári B, Brown I, et al. Non-conventional dysplasias of the tubular gut: a review and illustration of their histomorphological spectrum. Histopathology 2021;78:658–75.
14. Ekbom A, Helmick C, Zack M, et al. Ulcerative colitis and colorectal cancer. A population-based study. N Engl J Med 1990;323:1228–33.
15. Söderlund S, Brandt L, Lapidus A, et al. Decreasing time-trends of colorectal cancer in a large cohort of patients with inflammatory bowel disease. Gastroenterology 2009;136:1561–7.
16. Bernstein CN, Blanchard JF, Kliewer E, et al. Cancer risk in patients with inflammatory bowel disease: a population-based study. Cancer 2001;91:854–62.
17. Jess T, Rungoe C, Peyrin-Biroulet L. Risk of colorectal cancer in patients with ulcerative colitis: a meta-analysis of population-based cohort studies. Clin Gastroenterol Hepatol 2012;10:639–45.
18. Ekbom A, Helmick C, Zack M, et al. Increased risk of large-bowel cancer in Crohn's disease with colonic involvement. Lancet 1990;336:357–9.
19. Eaden JA, Abrams KR, Mayberry JF. The risk of colorectal cancer in ulcerative colitis: a meta-analysis. Gut 2001;48:526–35.
20. Soetikno RM, Lin OS, Heidenreich PA, et al. Increased risk of colorectal neoplasia in patients with primary sclerosing cholangitis and ulcerative colitis: a meta-analysis. Gastrointest Endosc 2002;56:48–54.
21. Beaugerie L, Svrcek M, Seksik P, et al. Risk of colorectal high-grade dysplasia and cancer in a prospective observational cohort of patients with inflammatory bowel disease. Gastroenterology 2013;145:166–75.

22. Rutter M, Saunders B, Wilkinson K, et al. Severity of inflammation is a risk factor for colorectal neoplasia in ulcerative colitis. Gastroenterology 2004;126:451–9.

23. Gupta RB, Harpaz N, Itzkowitz S, et al. Histologic inflammation is a risk factor for progression to colorectal neoplasia in ulcerative colitis: a cohort study. Gastroenterology 2007;133:1099–105.

24. Choi CR, Al Bakir I, Ding NJ, et al. Cumulative burden of inflammation predicts colorectal neoplasia risk in ulcerative colitis: a large single-centre study. Gut 2019;68:414–22.

25. Laine L, Kaltenbach T, Barkun A, et al. SCENIC international consensus statement on surveillance and management of dysplasia in inflammatory bowel disease. Gastrointest Endosc 2015;81:489–501.

26. Rubin DT, Ananthakrishnan AN, Siegel CA, et al. ACG clinical guideline: ulcerative colitis in adults. Am J Gastroenterol 2019;114:384–413.

27. Farraye FA, Odze RD, Eaden J, et al. AGA technical review on the diagnosis and management of colorectal neoplasia in inflammatory bowel disease. Gastroenterology 2010;138:746–74.

28. American Society for Gastrointestinal Endoscopy Standards of Practice Committee, Shergill AK, Lightdale JR, et al. The role of endoscopy in inflammatory bowel disease. Gastrointest Endosc 2015;81:1101–21.e1-e13.

29. Torres J, Pineton de Chambrun G, Itzkowitz S, et al. Review article: colorectal neoplasia in patients with primary sclerosing cholangitis and inflammatory bowel disease. Aliment Pharmacol Ther 2011;34:497–508.

30. Zheng HH, Jiang XL. Increased risk of colorectal neoplasia in patients with primary sclerosing cholangitis and inflammatory bowel disease: a meta-analysis of 16 observational studies. Eur J Gastroenterol Hepatol 2016;28:383–90.

31. Cordes F, Laumeyer T, Gerß J, et al. Distinct disease phenotype of ulcerative colitis in patients with coincident primary sclerosing cholangitis: evidence from a large retrospective study with matched cohorts. Dis Colon Rectum 2019;62:1494–504.

32. Brentnall TA, Haggitt RC, Rabinovitch PS, et al. Risk and natural history of colonic neoplasia in patients with primary sclerosing cholangitis and ulcerative colitis. Gastroenterology 1996;110:331–8.

33. Shetty K, Rybicki L, Brzezinski A, et al. The risk for cancer or dysplasia in ulcerative colitis patients with primary sclerosing cholangitis. Am J Gastroenterol 1999;94:1643–9.

34. Claessen MM, Lutgens MW, van Buuren HR, et al. More right-sided IBD-associated colorectal cancer in patients with primary sclerosing cholangitis. Inflamm Bowel Dis 2009;15:1331–6.

35. Boonstra K, Weersma RK, van Erpecum KJ, et al. Population-based epidemiology, malignancy risk, and outcome of primary sclerosing cholangitis. Hepatology 2013;58:2045–55.

36. Farraye FA, Odze RD, Eaden J, et al. AGA medical position statement on the diagnosis and management of colorectal neoplasia in inflammatory bowel disease. Gastroenterology 2010;138:738–45.

37. Leighton JA, Shen B, Baron TH, et al. ASGE guideline: endoscopy in the diagnosis and treatment of inflammatory bowel disease. Gastrointest Endosc 2006;63:558–65.

38. Rutter MD, Saunders BP, Wilkinson KH, et al. Most dysplasia in ulcerative colitis is visible at colonoscopy. Gastrointest Endosc 2004;60:334–9.

39. Rubin DT, Rothe JA, Hetzel JT, et al. Are dysplasia and colorectal cancer endoscopically visible in patients with ulcerative colitis? Gastrointest Endosc 2007;65:998–1004.

40. Wanders LK, Dekker E, Pullens B, et al. Cancer risk after resection of polypoid dysplasia in patients with longstanding ulcerative colitis: a meta-analysis. Clin Gastroenterol Hepatol 2014;12:756–64.

41. Blonski W, Kundu R, Furth EF, et al. High-grade dysplastic adenoma-like mass lesions are not an indication for colectomy in patients with ulcerative colitis. Scand J Gastroenterol 2008;43:817–20.

42. Odze RD, Farraye FA, Hecht JL, et al. Long-term follow-up after polypectomy treatment for adenoma-like dysplastic lesions in ulcerative colitis. Clin Gastroenterol Hepatol 2004;2:534–41.

43. Kisiel JB, Loftus EVJ, Harmsen WS, et al. Outcome of sporadic adenomas and adenoma-like dysplasia in patients with ulcerative colitis undergoing polypectomy. Inflamm Bowel Dis 2012;18:226–35.

44. Watanabe T, Ajioka Y, Mitsuyama K, et al. Comparison of targeted vs random biopsies for surveillance of ulcerative colitis-associated colorectal cancer. Gastroenterology 2016;151:1122–30.

45. Murthy SK, Feuerstein JD, Nguyen GC, et al. AGA clinical practice update on endoscopic surveillance and management of colorectal dysplasia in inflammatory bowel diseases: expert review. Gastroenterology 2021;161:1043–51.e4.

46. Rabinowitz LG, Kumta NA, Marion JF. Beyond the SCENIC route: updates in chromoendoscopy and dysplasia screening in patients with inflammatory bowel disease. Gastrointest Endosc 2022;95:30–7.

47. Choi CH, Rutter MD, Askari A, et al. Forty-year analysis of colonoscopic surveillance program for neoplasia in ulcerative colitis: an updated overview. Am J Gastroenterol 2015;110:1022–34.

48. Connell WR, Lennard-Jones JE, Williams CB, et al. Factors affecting the outcome of endoscopic surveillance for cancer in ulcerative colitis. Gastroenterology 1994;107:934–44.

49. Friedman S, Rubin PH, Bodian C, et al. Screening and surveillance colonoscopy in chronic Crohn's colitis. Gastroenterology 2001;120:820–6.

50. Hata K, Watanabe T, Kazama S, et al. Earlier surveillance colonoscopy programme improves survival in patients with ulcerative colitis associated colorectal cancer: results of a 23-year surveillance programme in the Japanese population. Br J Cancer 2003;89:1232–6.

51. Bernstein CN, Shanahan F, Weinstein WM. Are we telling patients the truth about surveillance colonoscopy in ulcerative colitis? Lancet 1994;343:71–4.

52. Thomas T, Abrams KA, Robinson RJ, et al. Meta-analysis: cancer risk of low-grade dysplasia in chronic ulcerative colitis. Aliment Pharmacol Ther 2007;25:657–68.

53. Jess T, Loftus EVJ, Velayos FS, et al. Incidence and prognosis of colorectal dysplasia in inflammatory bowel disease: a population-based study from Olmsted County, Minnesota. Inflamm Bowel Dis 2006;12:669–76.

54. Ullman T, Croog V, Harpaz N, et al. Progression of flat low-grade dysplasia to advanced neoplasia in patients with ulcerative colitis. Gastroenterology 2003;125:1311–9.

55. Ullman TA, Loftus EVJ, Kakar S, et al. The fate of low grade dysplasia in ulcerative colitis. Am J Gastroenterol 2002;97:922–7.

56. van Schaik FD, ten Kate FJ, Offerhaus GJ, et al. Misclassification of dysplasia in patients with inflammatory bowel disease: consequences for progression rates to advanced neoplasia. Inflamm Bowel Dis 2011;17:1108–16.

57. Befrits R, Ljung T, Jaramillo E, et al. Low-grade dysplasia in extensive, long-standing inflammatory bowel disease: a follow-up study. Dis Colon Rectum 2002;45:615–20.

58. Venkatesh PG, Jegadeesan R, Gutierrez NG, et al. Natural history of low grade dysplasia in patients with primary sclerosing cholangitis and ulcerative colitis. J Crohns Colitis 2013;7:968–73.

59. Pekow JR, Hetzel JT, Rothe JA, et al. Outcome after surveillance of low-grade and indefinite dysplasia in patients with ulcerative colitis. Inflamm Bowel Dis 2010;16:1352–6.

60. Zisman TL, Bronner MP, Rulyak S, et al. Prospective study of the progression of low-grade dysplasia in ulcerative colitis using current cancer surveillance guidelines. Inflamm Bowel Dis 2012;18:2240–6.

61. Navaneethan U, Jegadeesan R, Gutierrez NG, et al. Progression of low-grade dysplasia to advanced neoplasia based on the location and morphology of dysplasia in ulcerative colitis patients with extensive colitis under colonoscopic surveillance. J Crohns Colitis 2013;7:e684–91.

62. Tsai JH, Rabinovitch PS, Huang D, et al. Association of aneuploidy and flat dysplasia with development of high-grade dysplasia or colorectal cancer in patients with inflammatory bowel disease. Gastroenterology 2017;153:1492–5.

63. Wanders LK, Cordes M, Voorham Q, et al. IBD-Associated dysplastic lesions show more chromosomal instability than sporadic adenomas. Inflamm Bowel Dis 2020;26:167–80.

64. Maltzman T, Knoll K, Martinez ME, et al. Ki-ras proto-oncogene mutations in sporadic colorectal adenomas: relationship to histologic and clinical characteristics. Gastroenterology 2001;121:302–9.

65. Vogelstein B, Fearon ER, Hamilton SR, et al. Genetic alterations during colorectal-tumor development. N Engl J Med 1988;319:525–32.

66. Ried T, Knutzen R, Steinbeck R, et al. Comparative genomic hybridization reveals a specific pattern of chromosomal gains and losses during the genesis of colorectal tumors. Genes Chromosomes Cancer 1996;15:234–45.

67. Meijer GA, Hermsen MA, Baak JP, et al. Progression from colorectal adenoma to carcinoma is associated with non-random chromosomal gains as detected by comparative genomic hybridisation. J Clin Pathol 1998;51:901–9.

68. Joo M, Shahsafaei A, Odze RD. Paneth cell differentiation in colonic epithelial neoplasms: evidence for the role of the Apc/beta-catenin/Tcf pathway. Hum Pathol 2009;40:872–80.

69. Mahon M, Xu J, Yi X, et al. Paneth cell in adenomas of the distal colorectum is inversely associated with synchronous advanced adenoma and carcinoma. Sci Rep 2016;6:26129.

70. Bansal M, Fenoglio CM, Robboy SJ, et al. Are metaplasias in colorectal adenomas truly metaplasias? Am J Pathol 1984;115:253–65.

71. Pai RK, Rybicki LA, Goldblum JR, et al. Paneth cells in colonic adenomas: association with male sex and adenoma burden. Am J Surg Pathol 2013;37:98–103.

72. Ko HM, Harpaz N, McBride RB, et al. Serrated colorectal polyps in inflammatory bowel disease. Mod Pathol 2015;28:1584–93.

73. Yang C, Tarabishy Y, Dassopoulos T, et al. Clinical, histologic, and immunophenotypic features of serrated polyps in patients with inflammatory bowel disease. Gastroenterology Res 2018;11:355–60.

74. Choi WT, Wen KW, Rabinovitch PS, et al. DNA content analysis of colorectal serrated lesions detects an aneuploid subset of inflammatory bowel disease-associated serrated epithelial change and traditional serrated adenomas. Histopathology 2018;73:464–72.

75. Kilgore SP, Sigel JE, Goldblum JR. Hyperplastic-like mucosal change in Crohn's disease: an unusual form of dysplasia? Mod Pathol 2000;13:797–801.

76. Parian A, Koh J, Limketkai BN, et al. Association between serrated epithelial changes and colorectal dysplasia in inflammatory bowel disease. Gastrointest Endosc 2016;84:87–95.

77. Parian AM, Limketkai BN, Chowdhury R, et al. Serrated epithelial change is associated with high rates of neoplasia in ulcerative colitis patients: a case-controlled study and systematic review with meta-analysis. Inflamm Bowel Dis 2021;27:1475–81.

Histopathologic Manifestations of Immune Checkpoint Inhibitor Therapy-Associated Gastrointestinal Tract Injury: A Practical Review

James Michael Mitchell, MD,
Dipti M. Karamchandani, MD*

KEYWORDS

- Immune checkpoint inhibitors • Immune-related adverse events • Programmed death (PD)-1
- Programmed death ligand (PD-L1) • Cytotoxic T lymphocyte antigen (CTLA)-4

Key points

- Immune checkpoint inhibitor therapy has the propensity to cause immune-related adverse events (irAEs).
- The irAEs commonly affect the gastrointestinal (GI) tract and can produce a spectra of histologic findings mimicking many well-known inflammatory, infectious, or other drug-related etiologies.
- The colon, a commonly affected site in the GI tract, can show active colitis, chronic active colitis, microscopic colitis, apoptotic colopathy, or a mixed pattern of injury on histologic examination.
- Some cases exclusively involve the upper GI tract and can mimic celiac disease in duodenal biopsies or *Helicobacter pylori* gastritis or Crohn disease in gastric biopsies.
- Accurate diagnosis necessitates awareness of the histopathologic spectra of these drugs and clinico-pathologic correlation.

ABSTRACT

Immune checkpoint inhibitors have revolutionized the management of many advanced cancers by producing robust remissions. They mostly target two immune regulatory pathways: cytotoxic T lymphocyte antigen-4 and programmed death-1 or its ligand. However, a flip side is the immune-related adverse events (irAEs) commonly affecting the gastrointestinal (GI) tract that can cause treatment interruptions or discontinuation. This practical review discusses the clinical and histopathologic findings of irAEs encountered in the luminal GI tract, along with histopathologic differentials that can mimic varied inflammatory, infectious, or other medication-associated etiologies and the importance of clinico-pathologic correlation for an accurate diagnosis.

INTRODUCTION

Immune checkpoint inhibitors (ICIs) are being increasingly incorporated into the armamentarium of treatment options for advanced stage tumors,

Department of Pathology, University of Texas Southwestern Medical Center, 5323 Harry Hines Boulevard, Dallas, TX 75390, USA
* Corresponding author.
E-mail address: dipti.karamchandani@utsouthwestern.edu
Twitter: @GIJamesMD (J.M.M.)

Surgical Pathology 16 (2023) 703–718
https://doi.org/10.1016/j.path.2023.05.007

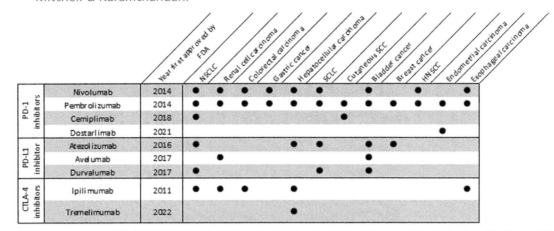

Fig. 1. Food and Drug Administration (FDA)-approved indications for programmed cell death-1 (PD-1), anti-PD ligand 1 (PD-L1), and cytotoxic T-lymphocyte antigen-4 (CTLA-4) inhibitors for selected pertinent tumors. NSCLC, non-small-cell lung cancer; SCC, squamous cell carcinoma; SCLC, small cell lung cancer.

either as monotherapy or as part of a combination therapy. These wonder drugs have been shown to produce robust responses with prolonged survival rates.[1–11] There are an ever-growing number of Food and Drug Administration (FDA)-approved ICIs—the broad categories include monoclonal antibodies that block the programmed cell death-1 (PD-1), antiprogrammed cell death-ligand 1 (PD-L1), and/or cytotoxic T-lymphocyte antigen-4 (CTLA-4) antibodies. The pertinent examples of ICIs under each category, the year of FDA approval, and selected applicable indications are depicted in **Fig. 1.**[1,2,6,10,12,13]

Given the present escalating use of ICIs, pathologists are seeing increasing number of specimens retrieved from these patients. This practical review discusses the mechanism of action of these novel drugs, the clinical, endoscopic, and histopathologic features of the immune-related adverse events (irAEs) that may be seen in the luminal gastrointestinal (GI) tract, the importance of clinicopathologic correlation while making this diagnosis, and awareness about the varied spectra of histopathologic mimics in the differential.

MECHANISM OF ACTION

PD-1, a cell surface coinhibitory receptor, is expressed on the surface of immune cells, including activated T cells, B cells, and monocytes. Its ligands, PD-L1 and PD-L2, are expressed on antigen-presenting cells (APCs) as well as tumor cells. The binding of PD-L1 on the tumor cells to PD-1 on the T-cell surface causes deactivation of T cells, hence allowing the tumor cells to evade the immune surveillance. The PD-1 and PD-L1 inhibitors inhibit this binding, and hence facilitate the cytotoxic T-cell activation against the tumor cells. Tumors that upregulate

PD-L1 can escape the immune surveillance and antitumor T-cell response, and hence, the PD-1/PD-L1 inhibitors act to block the immune system's tolerance to tumor cells.[3,10,14–16]

CTLA-4, an immune regulatory protein on the surface of T cells, results in inhibition of T cells by binding to B7 ligand present on antigen-presenting cells. The tumor cell is able to evade the immune system as the CTLA-4/B7 checkpoint suppresses the cytotoxic T-cell immune response. Some studies suggest that other mechanisms by which CTLA-4 suppresses T-cell activation include the inhibition of T-cell receptor (TCR) signaling, alteration of CD28 localization, and sequestration of B7 ligands from APCs. CTLA-4 inhibitors block T-cell inhibitory signals resulting in T-cell activation and expansion, ultimately augmenting T cells' response to cancer cells.[17–21]

IMMUNE RELATED ADVERSE EVENTS: MECHANISM AND CLINICAL FEATURES

Although these wonder drugs are effective therapeutically by reviving the host antitumor immune response, the flip side is that they have the potential to cause irAEs, presumably by triggering an anti-"self" immune response through the activation of T cells. Emerging data also suggest that gut microbiome features play an important role in the development of GI-irAEs by causing disturbances in microbiota-gut barrier equilibrium due to intraepithelial lymphocyte-mediated apoptosis of the gut epithelial cells.[22] The GI-irAE are one of the most common complications of ICI therapy and a frequent reason for treatment interruption, discontinuation, and associated morbidity.[5,23,24]

Colitis, typically manifesting as diarrhea, is the most common GI-irAE and is reported to affect

Table 1
Histomorphologic patterns and differentials of Immune checkpoint inhibitor (ICI)-associated injury in esophagus

Pattern of Injury	Histologic Features	Differential Diagnoses	Pearls
Acute/ulcerative esophagitis	• Intraepithelial neutrophils • ± Erosions • ± Ulcers	• GERD • Infections, for example, CMV, HSV, fungi • Pill-induced esophagitis • Radiation injury	• Diagnosis of exclusion • Presence of GERD prior to therapy would favor GERD over ICI esophagitis
Lymphocytic-predominant esophagitis/Lichenoid pattern of injury	• Intraepithelial lymphocytosis • Variable apoptotic keratinocytes	• Crohn disease • Infections • GVHD • Autoimmune diseases • Reflux esophagitis • Motility disorders	• Typically lack granulomas • Granulomas support Crohn's disease in patient with known/suspected history)

Abbreviations: CMV, cytomegalovirus; GERD, gastroesophageal reflux disease; GVHD; graft-versus-host disease; HSV; herpes simplex virus.

up to 40% of patients and can occur with or without associated enteritis and upper GI symptoms.[23–25] The median time interval between initiation of therapy and onset of colitis has been reported to be 6 to 8 weeks, with a range of 1 to 32 weeks.[2,10,26–28] These adverse events could appear at any time, including sometimes months to years after treatment cessation, making the diagnosis of these GI-irAEs even more challenging.[22] Hence, a high index of suspicion along with the awareness of delayed onset and prolonged duration of these events is crucial for accurate diagnosis and optimal patient management. Common Terminology Criteria for Adverse Events, Version 5 (CTCAE), a grading system established for oncology clinical trials, grades enterocolitis on a scale from grade 1 (mild) to grade 5 (death), although the clinical value of this grading system has not been well-proven for irAEs. Anti-CTLA-4 therapy is more commonly associated with severe enterocolitis necessitating treatment interruptions, reported in about 10% of patients, while therapies that target only PD-1/PD-L1 have been reported to cause severe disease in about 2%–5% of patients.[5,23,25,29]

Of note, about a quarter of patients with diarrhea have been reported to lack histologic evidence of colitis, and the majority of these have been reported to exhibit histologic evidence of injury in the upper GI tract, underscoring the importance of evaluation of concurrent upper- and lower-GI biopsies when suspecting this diagnosis.[30] Limited data report that about 5% of patients may show mucosal injury limited to the upper-GI tract, and patients usually present with symptoms

such as nausea, vomiting, dyspepsia, dysphagia, and/or low-grade fever starting about 4 months after therapy initiation.[25,31,32] ICI-associated esophagitis is rare and reported in about 3% of patients on therapy, and isolated esophageal involvement is extremely unusual and reported in about 0.5% patients.[32] The majority of patients with esophageal involvement have concurrent involvement of the stomach, duodenum, or both.[32]

IMMUNE RELATED ADVERSE EVENTS: ENDOSCOPIC AND HISTOPATHOLOGIC FEATURES WITH HISTOPATHOLOGIC DIFFERENTIALS

ESOPHAGUS

The endoscopic findings seen in esophagus include erythema, ulceration, edema, and stricture/stenosis. Existing limited data suggest that ICI-associated esophagitis is more commonly associated with anti-PD-1/PD-L1 monotherapy (71%), compared to combination (24%), or anti-CTLA-4 (5%) therapy.[1,32–34]

The main histopathologic patterns of ICI-associated esophageal injury (Table 1) include

1. *Acute/ulcerative esophagitis* characterized by neutrophilic inflammation of the squamous mucosa with variable foci of erosion and ulceration (Fig. 2A).[1,6,10,32,35] These histologic findings are nonspecific, and ICI -associated acute esophagitis is a diagnosis of exclusion. Identical findings can be seen with gastroesophageal reflux disease (GERD) (Fig. 2B). In fact, the presence

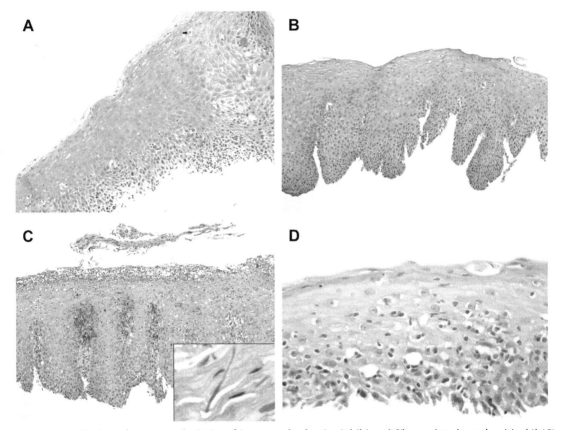

Fig. 2. Histopathologic features and mimics of immune checkpoint inhibitor (ICI)-associated esophagitis. (*A*) ICI esophagitis with neutrophilic inflammation of squamous epithelium (*arrow*) along with increased intraepithelial lymphocytes, these features mimic reflux disease. (*B*) Reflux esophagitis exhibiting basal cell hyperplasia, reactive changes, and scattered inflammatory cells, mimicking ICI esophagitis. (*C*) Candida-associated acute esophagitis with prominent intraepithelial neutrophils and superficial desquamation. Inset shows *Candida* organisms. (*D*) Lymphocytic esophagitis showing increased intraepithelial lymphocytes, superficial apoptotic keratinocytes, and spongiosis. (Hematoxylin & Eosin x200 [*A*], x100 [*B, C*], x400 [*C inset, D*]).

of GERD pretherapy would favor GERD over ICI-associated esophagitis. Infectious esophagitis can present with a similar histologic picture (Fig. 2C), and given that these patients are often immunosuppressed, exclusion of infectious etiologies is essential in this setting. Ancillary immunostains for the detection of cytomegalovirus (CMV) or herpes simplex virus viral inclusions and periodic acid Schiff or Grocott methenamine silver staining for the detection of fungal organisms can be helpful. Pill esophagitis can exhibit similar features; however, it may show polarizable pill fragments.

2. *Lymphocytic predominant esophagitis/lichenoid pattern of injury*, the other main pattern of injury, is characterized by increased intraepithelial lymphocytes (predominantly CD3+ T lymphocytes) with variable apoptotic keratinocytes.[1,6,10,32,34,36] This pattern of ICI-associated injury recapitulates the features of

so-called lymphocytic esophagitis (Fig. 2D) and encompasses a broad differential diagnosis, including dysmotility, GERD, infections, Crohn's disease, immune-mediated diseases, among other causes.[37,38] Finding granulomas in a patient with suspected or known Crohn disease would support a diagnosis of Crohn disease.

The symptoms of ICI-associated esophagitis are usually mild and typically respond well to non-immunosuppressive therapies,[32] with rare reported severe complications.[35]

STOMACH

Variable endoscopic findings can be seen ranging from unremarkable appearance to erythema with or without erosions; ulcers and polyps have also been rarely described.[30] Studies have shown no correlation between the endoscopic findings and

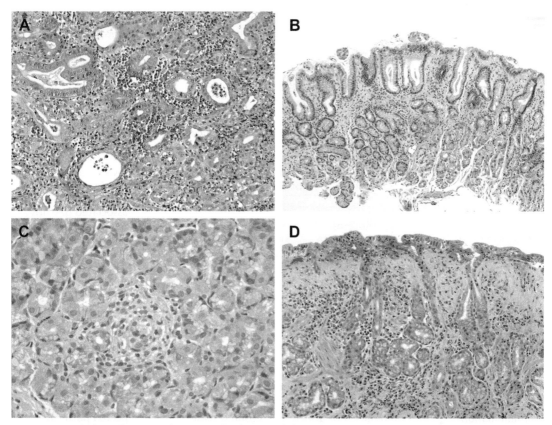

Fig. 3. Histopathologic features of immune checkpoint inhibitor (ICI)-associated gastritis. (*A*) Active gastritis with neutrophil-mediated epithelial injury and neutrophilic abscesses. (*B*) Chronic inactive gastritis with the expansion of lamina propria by lymphoplasmacytic infiltrates. Note that the infiltrates are mild and lack lymphoid aggregates. (*C*) Periglandular inflammation pattern seen as aggregates of lymphocytes, surrounding a gastric gland. (*D*) Microscopic gastritis pattern of injury with increased intraepithelial lymphocytes. This case also showed an increased subepithelial collagen layer with entrapment of capillaries and inflammatory cells, reminiscent of collagenous gastritis pattern of injury (hematoxylin & eosin ×200 [*A, D*], ×100 [*B*], ×400 [*C*]).

therapy-related histologic changes.[30] Patients receiving a combination of anti-PD-1/PD-L1 and anti-CTLA4 drugs are more likely to show gastric injury than PD-1 monotherapy.[30]

The histologic changes seen in ICI-associated gastric injury affects both gastric body/fundic and antral compartments, without any zonal predilection.[30] The common patterns of injury (Fig. 3A–D, Table 2) reported in gastric biopsies include

1. *Chronic gastritis with or without activity*, which is the most common form of ICI-associated gastritis (see Fig. 3A, B) and is characterized by an expansion of the lamina propria by lymphoplasmacytic infiltrates.[1,6,26,30,39] Diffuse mild lymphoplasmacytic infiltrates (see Fig. 3B) have been reported in about 36% of cases, and moderate or severe infiltrates in 13% of cases.[30] Intraepithelial neutrophils are seen in cases with activity,[30,31] and active gastritis with neutrophilic abscesses has been

reported in 13% of cases (see Fig. 3A).[6,30,31] Accompanying intraepithelial lymphocytosis and apoptotic bodies are frequently seen.[26,30,31,39,40] The main histologic differential (Fig. 4A–D) includes infections such as *Helicobacter pylori* (*H. pylori*)-gastritis (see Fig. 4A) or CMV gastritis (see Fig. 4D). Identification of organisms or viral inclusions on H&E stain or with the help of ancillary immunostains can aid in distinction. As compared to *H. pylori*-gastritis, ICI-associated gastritis usually shows a less-dense lymphoplasmacytic infiltrate, fewer lymphoid aggregates and plasma cells, and more prevalent intraepithelial lymphocytosis.[40] However, infectious causes always need to be excluded before making a diagnosis of ICI-gastritis in this histologic setting. It may also be difficult to distinguish these findings from mild chronic nonspecific gastritis commonly seen in adult gastric biopsies.

Table 2
Histomorphologic patterns and differentials of immune checkpoint inhibitor (ICI)-associated injury in stomach

Pattern of Injury	Histologic Features	Differential Diagnoses	Pearls
Chronic gastritis with or without activity	• Lamina propria expanded by lympho-plasmacytic infiltrate • Increased intraepithelial neutrophils and/or glandular abscesses (in cases with activity) • ± Epithelial apoptotic bodies • ± Intraepithelial lymphocytosis • ± Granulomata	• Infections, for example, *H. pylori*, CMV, EBV • Mild chronic nonspecific gastritis	• Most common pattern of ICI -gastric injury • Intraepithelial lymphocytosis and apoptotic bodies with fewer plasma cells and fewer lymphoid aggregates favor ICI-associated gastritis (over *H.pylori* gastritis) • Exclude infectious causes before making this diagnosis
Peri-glandular inflammation	• Lymphocytic infiltrates, generally localized to the pit/isthmus/neck region • ± Intraepithelial lymphocytosis • ± Nonnecrotizing granulomata	• Focally enhanced gastritis, typically seen in Crohn disease	• Compared to Crohn's disease gastritis, periglandular inflammation tends to lack plasma cells and histiocytes
Granulomatous inflammation	• Nonnecrotizing granulomata (not associated with glandular rupture)	• Infections • Crohn disease • Sarcoidosis	• Less common reported patterns • Non-caseating granulomas often seen in conjunction with periglandular inflammation
Lymphocytic gastritis pattern of injury	• Intraepithelial lymphocytosis with surface epithelial injury	• De novo lymphocytic gastritis • Celiac disease	
Reactive gastropathy	• Mucin loss • Foveolar hyperplasia • Fibromuscular and capillary hyperplasia	• Medications, for example, NSAIDS	

Abbreviations: CMV, cytomegalovirus; EBV, Epstein-Barr virus; NSAIDs, nonsteroidal anti-inflammatory drugs.

2. *Periglandular inflammation* described as aggregates of lymphocytes (see **Fig. 3**C) and typically devoid of histiocytes and plasma cells surrounding the gastric pit/isthmus/neck regions have been reported in around 40% cases.[30] A recent study showed that finding greater than 5 foci of periglandular inflammation correlated with a clinical diagnosis of GI-irAE.[30] The main histopathologic mimic includes "focally enhanced gastritis," typically seen in gastric involvement by Crohn disease; however, the latter typically shows a mixed periglandular infiltrate that also includes histiocytes, plasma cells, and occasional neutrophils and eosinophils (see **Fig. 4**B).[30]

3. *Other patterns of injury* seen in gastric biopsies include noncaseating granulomas (unrelated to glandular rupture), often seen in conjunction with periglandular inflammation and reported in about 30% of patients.[30] This pattern of injury is more commonly reported with anti–CTLA-4 or a combination of anti–CTLA-4/anti–PD-1 therapy than with anti-PD-1 monotherapy and requires correlation with clinical history and ancillary staining to exclude entities with granulomas in histologic differential including infections, sarcoidosis, and Crohn disease. Reactive gastropathy (reported in about 13% of cases)[30] and an occasional case of microscopic (lymphocytic) gastritis pattern of injury

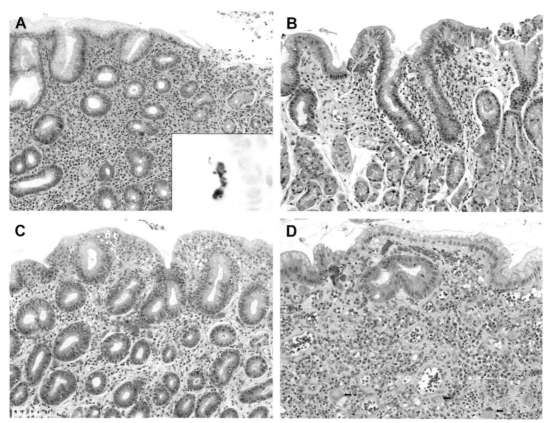

Fig. 4. Histopathologic mimics of immune checkpoint inhibitor-associated gastritis. (*A*) *Helicobacter pylori (H. py-lori)*-associated chronic active gastritis. Inset highlights organisms on immunostain. (*B*) Focally enhanced gastritis in Crohn disease with mixed lymphocytes, plasma cells, and histiocytes (*C*) De novo lymphocytic gastritis characterized by increased intraepithelial lymphocytes with associated epithelial injury, (*D*) Cytomegalovirus (CMV)-associated chronic active gastritis with crypt atrophy, apoptotic bodies, and diagnostic viral inclusions (highlighted by *arrow*). (Hematoxylin & Eosin x200 [*A–D*], H. pylori immunolabeling x400 [*A inset*]).

are other less commonly reported patterns of gastric injury (see **Fig. 3**D).[41] The latter can mimic de novo lymphocytic gastritis and requires correlation with clinical history for accurate diagnosis (see **Fig. 4**C).

DUODENUM/SMALL INTESTINE

The endoscopic findings are variable and range from unremarkable appearance to exhibiting erythema with or without erosions, ulcers, mucosal flattening, white exudate, and benign stricture.[30] Akin to gastric biopsies, patients receiving a combination of anti-PD-1/PD-L1 and anti-CTLA4 drugs are more likely to show duodenal injury than PD-1 monotherapy, as well as no correlation is seen between the endoscopic and histologic findings associated with therapy.[30]

Villous blunting with an associated increased number of lamina propria inflammatory cells and increase in intraepithelial lymphocytes is the most common pattern of injury, reported in about 40%

of cases (**Fig. 5**A, **Table 3**). In the absence of clinical history, this pattern of injury is virtually histologically indistinguishable from celiac disease. However, these cases are typically associated with neutrophilic activity as well as an increase in intraepithelial lymphocytes, which usually shows a patchy distribution and variable apoptosis.[26,30] The duodenal epithelium often shows a loss of brush border and reduced goblet cells. Nonnecrotizing granulomas have been reported in 18% of cases, and these cases have been negative for infections or systemic granulomatous diseases such as sarcoidosis on follow-up.[30] The authors of this article have seen a case of "collagenous sprue" pattern of injury in duodenum biopsy characterized by villous blunting, increased lamina propria infiltrates with increased intraepithelial lymphocytes along with thickened subepithelial collagen table with associated epithelial detachment (**Fig. 5**B).

When compared to celiac disease (**Fig. 5**C), ICI-associated duodenitis usually shows patchy

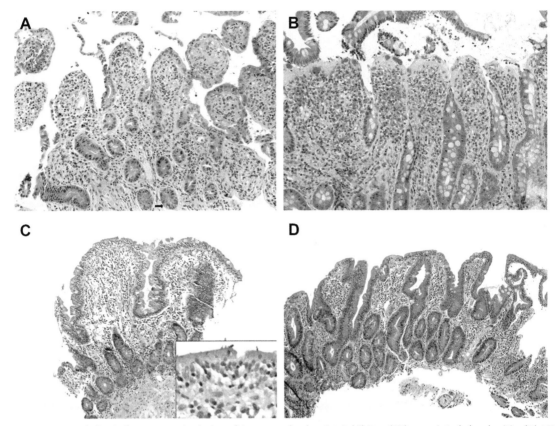

Fig. 5. Histopathologic features and mimics of immune checkpoint inhibitor (ICI)-associated duodenitis. (*A*) ICI duodenitis with patchy villous blunting and increased intraepithelial lymphocytes. Scattered apoptosis (highlighted by *arrow*) and interspersed neutrophilic inflammation is also seen. (*B*) ICI-associated collagenous sprue-like changes, characterized by villus blunting, increased lymphocytes, and thickened subepithelial collagen table with epithelial detachment (*C*) De novo celiac disease and (*D*) Olmesartan-associated duodenal injury, both show villous blunting with increased lymphocytes and increased lamina propria inflammation and can mimic ICI duodenitis. Inset (*C*) highlights increased intraepithelial lymphocytes (hematoxylin & eosin ×200 [*A, B, C inset*], ×100 [*C, D*]).

intraepithelial lymphocytosis, variable apoptosis, as well as associated neutrophilic inflammation and may show granulomas in a small subset of cases. However, these features are subtle and lack specificity and the distinction of ICI-related duodenitis from de novo celiac disease (including cases in which ICI may have unmasked latent celiac disease or induced "real" celiac disease) and necessitates correlation with clinical history and serologic markers for celiac disease, as the latter would respond favorably to a gluten-free diet.[42–44]

Other drugs causing a similar pattern of duodenal injury (ie, angiotensin receptor blockers, **Fig. 5**D) are also in the histologic differential, as is Crohn disease or infections, especially when encountered with granulomas in this setting. Special stains for fungal organisms and acid-fast bacilli would be negative in ICI-associated duodenitis. The absence of clinical history of ICI therapy, along with the absence of goblet cells and paneth cells on histologic sections and serologic testing for auto-antibodies, such as antienterocyte brush border antibodies, and the right clinical context would be helpful to distinguish ICI-associated duodenitis from de novo autoimmune enteropathy.[45]

COLON

Endoscopic findings can be normal in about 30% of patients, and in others, they may mimic other colitides, that is, exhibit erythema, loss of vascular pattern, mucosal friability, erosions, and ulcers and hence the findings are pretty nonspecific. Endoscopic examination with biopsies remains the gold standard for the diagnosis of ICI-

Table 3
Histomorphologic patterns and differentials of Immune checkpoint inhibitor (ICI)-associated injury in duodenum/small bowel

Pattern of Injury	Histologic Features	Differential Diagnoses	Pearls
Duodenitis/enteritis with villous blunting	• Villous blunting • Lamina propria expansion by lymphoplasmacytic infiltrate • Usually increased intraepithelial lymphocytes • ± Increased neutrophils • ± Increased apoptotic bodies • ± Non-necrotizing granulomata	• Celiac disease • Medications, for example, ARBs • Infections • Autoimmune enteropathy • Crohn disease	Features favoring ICI-associated injury (over celiac disease): • Neutrophilic inflammation • Patchy intraepithelial lymphoplasmacytosis(vs diffuse in celiac) • Granulomata
Granulomatous inflammation	• Nonnecrotizing granulomata • ± Villous blunting	• Crohn disease • Sarcoidosis • Infections	

Abbreviation: ARBs, angiotensin receptor blockers.

associated enterocolitis; however, endoscopic findings are not significantly associated with the severity of ICI colitis.[22,23,46] ICI-associated colitis can show a wide range of histomorphologic features (**Fig. 6A–F, Table 4**), including

Active Colitis

Active Colitis, the most common pattern of ICI-associated colonic injury, typically exhibits neutrophil-induced epithelial injury characterized by cryptitis and/or crypt abscesses with associated mixed lamina propria inflammatory cell infiltrates (see **Fig. 6A**).[1–3,6,10,26,30,33,47] Features of chronic mucosal injury are typically lacking in this pattern of injury. Crypt atrophy and dropout may be seen. This pattern of injury is variably associated with increased intraepithelial lymphocytes and increased apoptosis. Crypt rupture granulomas may be present, but well-formed granulomas are typically not seen in colonic biopsies.[22,26] A recent study reported that patients on ipilimumab (about 57%) are more likely to show a diffuse active colitis pattern of injury, in contrast to about 22% patients on pembrolizumab and 5% on nivolumab therapy.[48] The main histologic differential includes acute infections (**Fig. 7A**) and other medication-induced injury, and these can be histologically indistinguishable from ICI-associated active colitis. Correlation with clinical and drug history and ancillary staining for infectious etiologies are necessary. Concurrent assessment of upper-GI biopsies showing a constellation of granulomas or celiac-disease-like appearance in duodenum or periglandular gastric inflammation can be helpful.

Given that these patients are mostly immunosuppressed, ICI-associated active colitis can show coexisting infectious etiology in the same biopsy, and pathologists should have a low threshold for ordering ancillary stains. The absence of chronic injury supports a diagnosis of ICI injury over inflammatory bowel disease (IBD).

Chronic Active Colitis

Chronic active colitis: This pattern of injury (see **Fig. 6B**) is histologically indistinguishable from IBD, that is, exhibits one or more features of chronicity, including basilar lymphoplasmacytosis, crypt architectural distortion, Paneth cell metaplasia, increased lamina propria lymphoplasmacytosis, along with associated activity (cryptitis and crypt abscesses) (**Fig. 7B**).[1,6,10,46,48–50] Some have proposed ICI-associated colitis as a peculiar form of IBD and have shown successful treatment of these cases with IBD therapy.[49,51] Granulomas, however, are very rare in colon and are seen more often in upper-GI-tract biopsies.[30,51] This pattern of injury is more commonly (45%) described in patients on nivolumab therapy, and a recent study showed that these patients received more ICI doses and were on ICI therapy longer than other treatment groups.[48] In contrast, chronic active colitis is seen less commonly in patients with ipilimumab (22%) or pembrolizumab (17%) therapy.[48]

Microscopic Colitis

Microscopic colitis secondary to ICI therapy has been well described, with lymphocytic colitis (see **Fig. 6C**) comprising most cases of this subgroup,

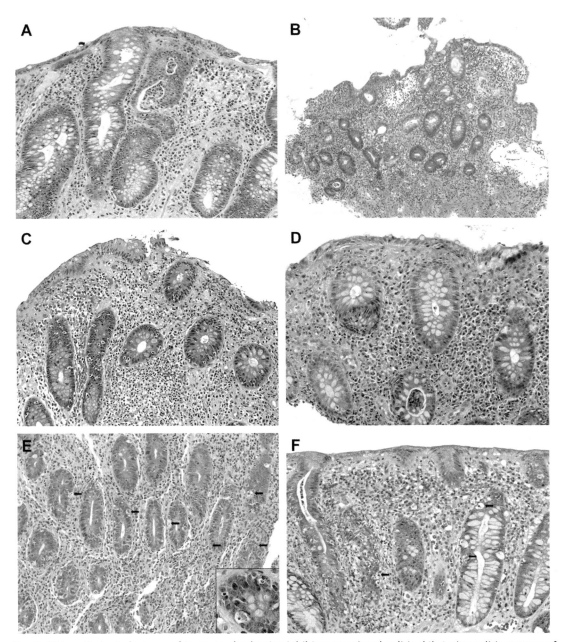

Fig. 6. Histopathologic features of immune checkpoint inhibitor-associated colitis. (*A*) Active colitis pattern of injury with acute cryptitis, and crypt abscess and generally preserved crypt architecture. (*B*) Chronic active colitis pattern of injury with crypt architectural distortion, basilar and lamina propria lymphoplasmacytosis, along with active injury and accompanying crypt destruction. (*C*) Lymphocytic colitis pattern of injury with increased intraepithelial lymphocytes and associated surface epithelial injury. (*D*) Collagenous colitis pattern of injury with thickened subepithelial collagen table with entrapped capillaries and inflammatory cells and epithelial injury. (*E*) Apoptotic colopathy pattern of injury demonstrating lamina propria lymphoplasmacytosis and numerous apoptotic bodies (highlighted by *arrows*).Inset shows apoptotic bodies. (*F*) Active colitis with apoptotic colopathy showing intraepithelial neutrophils, crypt abscesses, and prominent epithelial apoptotic bodies (highlighted by *arrows*). (Hematoxylin & Eosin ×100 (*A*, *B*), ×200 (*C–F*), x400× (*E inset*).

while rare cases showing a collagenous colitis pattern of injury (see **Fig. 6**D).[52] The former manifests as increased intraepithelial lymphocytes with associated epithelial injury and increased lamina propria mononuclear inflammatory infiltrates in a top-heavy distribution.[1,6,10,30,46,47,53] Collagenous colitis shows thickened subepithelial collagen table with entrapped capillaries and

Table 4
Histomorphologic patterns and differentials of immune checkpoint inhibitor (ICI)-associated injury in colon

Pattern of Injury	Histologic Features	Differential Diagnoses	Pearls
Active colitis	• Acute cryptitis and/or crypt abscesses • Lamina propria neutrophilic infiltrate • ± Lamina propria expanded by mixed inflammation • ± Increased crypt apoptotic bodies • ± Crypt atrophy and/or crypt dropout • ± Intraepithelial lymphocytes	• Infections, for example, CMV • Medications	• Most frequently observed pattern of injury • Coexisting prominent crypt apoptotic bodies favor ICI-associated colitis • More commonly seen with ipilimumab therapy
Chronic active colitis	• Chronic mucosal injury (ie, crypt architectural distortion, basal plasmacytosis, Paneth cell metaplasia, increased lamina propria lymphoplasmacytosis) • Active injury (cryptitis and/or crypt abscesses) • ± Increased crypt apoptotic bodies	• IBD • Infections • Medications • Chronic ischemia	• More commonly seen with nivolumab therapy • Granulomata very rare
Lymphocytic colitis	• Intraepithelial lymphocytosis • Epithelial injury • ± Lamina propria expansion by mononuclear inflammation • ± Acute cryptitis and/or crypt abscesses • ± Increased crypt apoptotic bodies	• De novo microscopic colitis • Medications, for example, ARBs, NSAIDs, histamine H_2 receptor blockers, PPI, gold salts • Infections	• Mixed active and lymphocytic colitis patterns of injury with endoscopic mucosal abnormalities favor ICI-associated colitis • More commonly associated with nivolumab and pembrolizumab
Collagenous colitis	• Increased subepithelial collagen layer with		

(continued on next page)

Table 4
(continued)

Pattern of Injury	Histologic Features	Differential Diagnoses	Pearls
	entrapment of capillaries and inflammatory cells • ± Intraepithelial lymphocytosis		
Apoptotic colopathy	• Apoptotic bodies (typically > 5 crypt apoptotic bodies per 10 HPF) • ± Intraepithelial lymphocytosis • Acute cryptitis and/or crypt abscesses	• Acute GVHD • Medications (such as MMF) • Infections (such as CMV)	• Can present as a mixed pattern of injury (apoptotic bodies, with active injury, and lymphocytosis) • Generally lacking granulomata and features of chronicity
Ischemic colitis	• Mucin depletion ("withered" crypts) • Reactive epithelial changes • Lamina propria hyalinization	• Ischemia • Infections • Medications	• Infrequent

Abbreviations: ARBs, angiotensin receptor blockers; CMV, cytomegalovirus; GVHD, graft-versus-host disease; IBD, inflammatory bowel disease; MMF, mycophenolate mofetil; NSAIDs, nonsteroidal anti-inflammatory drugs; PPI; proton pump inhibitors.

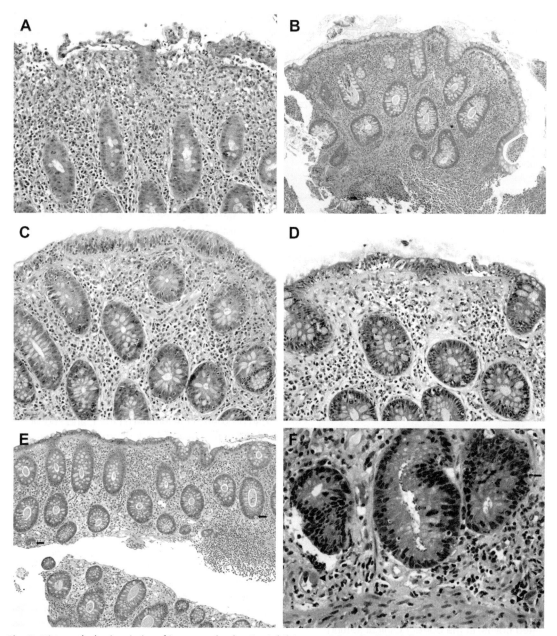

Fig. 7. Histopathologic mimics of immune checkpoint inhibitor-associated colitis. (*A*) Acute infectious colitis characterized by active neutrophil-mediated epithelial injury. (*B*) Inflammatory bowel disease showing chronic active colitis characterized by architectural distortion, basilar lymphoplasmacytosis, and active injury. (*C*) De novo lymphocytic colitis characterized by increased intraepithelial lymphocytes with epithelial injury. (*D*) De novo collagenous colitis with thickened subepithelial collagen table and associated epithelial injury. (*E*) Mycophenolate mofetil-associated colitis showing prominent apoptosis (*arrows*) along with mixed lamina propria infiltrates with eosinophils. (*F*) Infectious colitis with prominent apoptosis (*black arrow*), patchy acute inflammation and with cytomegalovirus viral inclusions (*arrow head*, lower part of figure) and cryptosporidium (*open arrow*, center of figure). (Hematoxylin & Eosin x200 [*A, C, D*], x100 [*B, E*], x400 [*F*]).

inflammatory cells.[30,54,55] Microscopic colitis has been more commonly reported in patients on nivolumab (45%) and pembrolizumab (48%) therapy and less likely (7%) with ipilimumab therapy, than other ICIs.[48] De novo microscopic colitis (Fig. 7C, D) is in the histologic differential; however, ICI associated microscopic colitis usually shows co-existing neutrophilic injury in almost half the patients, which can sometimes be prominent with associated crypt abscesses, and that is unusual for de novo microscopic colitis.[30] A recent study showed that ICI-associated microscopic colitis usually shows mucosal abnormality on endoscopy (vs normal findings in the de novo group), and the former also had a more aggressive disease course necessitating more treatments with immunosuppressive agents and a greater rate of hospitalization.[56] Other medication-induced microscopic colitis are also in the differential, and correlation with clinical setting (most importantly history of malignancy and drug history) is required.

Apoptotic Colopathy or Graft Versus Host Disease (GVHD)-Like Colitis

Isolated crypt epithelial apoptosis (typically >5 apoptosis per 10 high power fields) is another injury pattern seen with ICI-associated colitis. Increased apoptosis can be seen alone in the absence of associated active or chronic injury or can be seen in conjunction with other patterns of injury such as active colitis or microscopic colitis (see **Fig. 6**E, F).[1,3,6,33,57,58] The differential diagnosis for this pattern of injury is broad and includes other drug-related injury, such as idelalisib, or mycophenolate mofetil (**Fig. 7**E), acute GVHD, infections such as CMV or cryptosporidiosis (**Fig. 7**F), autoimmune enterocolitis, among other causes.[45]

Mixed Patterns and Other Less Common Patterns of Injury

Lastly, ICI-associated colitis can present histologically with a mixed pattern of injury, consisting of varying combinations of active colitis and/or increased intraepithelial lymphocytes and/or epithelial cell apoptosis. Hence, ICI colitis should be considered in the differential diagnosis of all the common inflammatory patterns of colitis, or a mixed colitis pattern of injury (see **Fig. 6**F). In fact, co-existence of multiple histologic patterns of injury in colonic biopsies would favor ICI-related colitis, in the correct clinical setting.[1,59]

The other less commonly described patterns of injury include ischemic colitis and nonspecific reactive changes. The former is characterized by variable active inflammation, atrophic crypts, and lamina propria hyalinization, and the latter is characterized by attenuation of epithelium and mucin depletion. Reactive epithelial changes are seen in both.[22,26]

For clinical sign-out purposes, in the presence of a corroborative history of ICI therapy, it may be best to describe the histologic pattern of injury with a comment that this pattern of injury has been well described in association with ICIs, attempt to exclude other etiologies in histologic differential (wherever indicated), such as by performing ancillary stains for excluding infections, and suggest correlation with clinical findings.

CLINICAL MANAGEMENT

Mild diarrhea is common on ICIs and is typically managed with empiric, symptom-directed treatment. Systemic glucocorticoids are the recommended first-line therapy; however, the severity of ICI colitis should be considered before the initiation of high-dose systemic steroids. Infliximab and vedolizumab are therapeutic approaches for the treatment of steroid refractory colitis. Patients who develop ICI colitis may be retreated with immunotherapy under select conditions.[23]

SUMMARY

To conclude, the escalating use of ICIs in clinical practice with associated GI-irAEs accounts for growing number of retrieved specimens from these patients. Even when the clinical history of ICI therapy is not provided by the clinician, a high index of clinical suspicion in a patient with a history of advanced malignancy, a review of medical record to confirm the ICI use, being cognizant of the wide spectra of histopathologic findings that can be seen in the luminal GI tract, and knowledge of the varied histopathologic mimics is crucial for accurate diagnosis and optimal patient management. Clinico-pathologic correlation is the key to exclude diagnostic mimics. Since these patients are immunosuppressed and may be on multiple drugs, excluding dual or multiple etiologies such as co-existing infections and other drug-induced injury is crucial. Lastly, with increasing ICIs being approved for use in clinical practice, we expect that the spectra of reported histopathologic findings encountered with these drugs would expand to possibly embrace "yet unreported" other patterns of injury secondary to these drugs in the future.

CLINICS CARE POINTS

- Immune Checkpoint Inhibitors can cause clinically significant immune related adverse events (irAEs) in the gastrointestinal (GI) tract.

- GI-irAEs can show varied spectra of histopathologic injury patterns in the GI tract.

- Clinico-pathologic correlation is crucial for a definitive diagnosis and optimal patient management.

DISCLOSURE

The authors have nothing to disclose.

REFERENCES

1. Alruwaii ZI, Montgomery EA. Gastrointestinal and Hepatobiliary Immune-related Adverse Events: A Histopathologic Review. Adv Anat Pathol 2022. https://doi.org/10.1097/PAP.0000000000000346.

2. Assarzadegan N, Montgomery E, Anders RA. Immune checkpoint inhibitor colitis: the flip side of the wonder drugs. Virchows Arch 2018;472(1):125–33.

3. Karamchandani DM, Chetty R. Immune checkpoint inhibitor-induced gastrointestinal and hepatic injury: pathologists' perspective. J Clin Pathol 2018;71(8):665–71.

4. Naidoo J, Page DB, Li BT, et al. Toxicities of the anti-PD-1 and anti-PD-L1 immune checkpoint antibodies. Ann Oncol 2015;26(12):2375–91.

5. Wang DY, Salem JE, Cohen JV, et al. Fatal Toxic Effects Associated With Immune Checkpoint Inhibitors: A Systematic Review and Meta-analysis. JAMA Oncol 2018;4(12):1721–8.

6. Zhang ML, Deshpande V. Histopathology of Gastrointestinal Immune-related Adverse Events: A Practical Review for the Practicing Pathologist. Am J Surg Pathol 2022;46(1):e15–26.

7. Hodi FS, O'Day SJ, McDermott DF, et al. Improved survival with ipilimumab in patients with metastatic melanoma. N Engl J Med 2010;363(8):711–23.

8. Topalian SL, Hodi FS, Brahmer JR, et al. Safety, activity, and immune correlates of anti-PD-1 antibody in cancer. N Engl J Med 2012;366(26):2443–54.

9. Brahmer JR, Tykodi SS, Chow LQ, et al. Safety and activity of anti-PD-L1 antibody in patients with advanced cancer. N Engl J Med 2012;366(26):2455–65.

10. Karamchandani DM, Westbrook L, Arnold CA. Drug-induced digestive tract injury: decoding some invisible offenders. Hum Pathol 2022. https://doi.org/10.1016/j.humpath.2022.06.014.

11. Brahmer JR, Drake CG, Wollner I, et al. Phase I study of single-agent anti-programmed death-1 (MDX-1106) in refractory solid tumors: safety, clinical activity, pharmacodynamics, and immunologic correlates. J Clin Oncol 2010;28(19):3167–75.

12. Iranzo P, Callejo A, Assaf JD, et al. Overview of Checkpoint Inhibitors Mechanism of Action: Role of Immune-Related Adverse Events and Their Treatment on Progression of Underlying Cancer. Front Med 2022;9:875974.

13. Lee JB, Kim HR, Ha SJ. Immune Checkpoint Inhibitors in 10 Years: Contribution of Basic Research and Clinical Application in Cancer Immunotherapy. Immune Netw 2022;22(1):e2.

14. Azuma T, Yao S, Zhu G, et al. B7-H1 is a ubiquitous antiapoptotic receptor on cancer cells. Blood 2008;111(7):3635–43.

15. Keir ME, Butte MJ, Freeman GJ, et al. PD-1 and its ligands in tolerance and immunity. Annu Rev Immunol 2008;26:677–704.

16. Pardoll DM. The blockade of immune checkpoints in cancer immunotherapy. Nat Rev Cancer 2012;12(4):252–64.

17. Oyewole-Said D, Konduri V, Vazquez-Perez J, et al. Beyond T-Cells: Functional Characterization of CTLA-4 Expression in Immune and Non-Immune Cell Types. Front Immunol 2020;11:608024.

18. Gaikwad S, Agrawal MY, Kaushik I, et al. Immune checkpoint proteins: Signaling mechanisms and molecular interactions in cancer immunotherapy. Semin Cancer Biol 2022;86(Pt 3):137–50.

19. Korman AJ, Garrett-Thomson SC, Lonberg N. The foundations of immune checkpoint blockade and the ipilimumab approval decennial. Nat Rev Drug Discov 2022;21(7):509–28.

20. Walker LS, Sansom DM. Confusing signals: recent progress in CTLA-4 biology. Trends Immunol 2015;36(2):63–70.

21. Wei SC, Duffy CR, Allison JP. Fundamental Mechanisms of Immune Checkpoint Blockade Therapy. Cancer Discov 2018;8(9):1069–86.

22. Tang L, Wang J, Lin N, et al. Immune Checkpoint Inhibitor-Associated Colitis: From Mechanism to Management. Front Immunol 2021;12:800879.

23. Dougan M, Wang Y, Rubio-Tapia A, et al. AGA Clinical Practice Update on Diagnosis and Management of Immune Checkpoint Inhibitor Colitis and Hepatitis: Expert Review. Gastroenterology 2021;160(4):1384–93.

24. Pauken KE, Dougan M, Rose NR, et al. Adverse Events Following Cancer Immunotherapy: Obstacles and Opportunities. Trends Immunol 2019;40(6):511–23.

25. Beck KE, Blansfield JA, Tran KQ, et al. Enterocolitis in patients with cancer after antibody blockade of cytotoxic T-lymphocyte-associated antigen 4. J Clin Oncol 2006;24(15):2283–9.

26. Gonzalez RS, Salaria SN, Bohannon CD, et al. PD-1 inhibitor gastroenterocolitis: case series and appraisal of 'immunomodulatory gastroenterocolitis. Histopathology 2017;70(4):558–67.

27. Hofmann L, Forschner A, Loquai C, et al. Cutaneous, gastrointestinal, hepatic, endocrine, and renal side-effects of anti-PD-1 therapy. Eur J Cancer 2016;60:190–209.

28. Mooradian MJ, Wang DY, Coromilas A, et al. Mucosal inflammation predicts response to systemic steroids in immune checkpoint inhibitor colitis. J Immunother Cancer 2020;8(1). https://doi.org/10.1136/jitc-2019-000451.

29. Dougan M. Checkpoint Blockade Toxicity and Immune Homeostasis in the Gastrointestinal Tract. Front Immunol 2017;8:1547.

30. Zhang ML, Neyaz A, Patil D, et al. Immune-related adverse events in the gastrointestinal tract: diagnostic

utility of upper gastrointestinal biopsies. Histopathology 2020;76(2):233–43.

31. Johncilla M, Grover S, Zhang X, et al. Morphological spectrum of immune check-point inhibitor therapy-associated gastritis. Histopathology 2020;76(4):531–9.

32. Panneerselvam K, Amin RN, Wei D, et al. Clinicopathologic Features, Treatment Response, and Outcomes of Immune Checkpoint Inhibitor-Related Esophagitis. J Natl Compr Canc Netw 2021;19(8):896–904.

33. Patil PA, Zhang X. Pathologic Manifestations of Gastrointestinal and Hepatobiliary Injury in Immune Checkpoint Inhibitor Therapy. Arch Pathol Lab Med 2021;145(5):571–82.

34. Onuki T, Morita E, Sakamoto N, et al. Severe upper gastrointestinal disorders in pembrolizumab-treated non-small cell lung cancer patient. Respirol Case Rep 2018;6(6):e00334.

35. Acero Brand FZ, Suter N, Adam JP, et al. Severe immune mucositis and esophagitis in metastatic squamous carcinoma of the larynx associated with pembrolizumab. J Immunother Cancer 2018;6(1):22.

36. Horisberger A, La Rosa S, Zurcher JP, et al. A severe case of refractory esophageal stenosis induced by nivolumab and responding to tocilizumab therapy. J Immunother Cancer 2018;6(1):156.

37. Pittman ME, Hissong E, Katz PO, et al. Lymphocyte-predominant Esophagitis: A Distinct and Likely Immune-mediated Disorder Encompassing Lymphocytic and Lichenoid Esophagitis. Am J Surg Pathol 2020;44(2):198–205.

38. Lisovsky M, Westerhoff M, Zhang X. Lymphocytic esophagitis: a histologic pattern with emerging clinical ramifications. Ann N Y Acad Sci 2016;1381(1):133–8.

39. Tang T, Abu-Sbeih H, Luo W, et al. Upper gastrointestinal symptoms and associated endoscopic and histological features in patients receiving immune checkpoint inhibitors. Scand J Gastroenterol 2019;54(5):538–45.

40. Irshaid L, Robert ME, Zhang X. Immune Checkpoint Inhibitor-Induced Upper Gastrointestinal Tract Inflammation Shows Morphologic Similarities to, but Is Immunologically Distinct From, Helicobacter pylori Gastritis and Celiac Disease. Arch Pathol Lab Med 2021;145(2):191–200.

41. Yip RHL, Lee LH, Schaeffer DF, et al. Lymphocytic gastritis induced by pembrolizumab in a patient with metastatic melanoma. Melanoma Res 2018;28(6):645–7.

42. Badran YR, Shih A, Leet D, et al. Immune checkpoint inhibitor-associated celiac disease. J Immunother Cancer 2020;8(1). https://doi.org/10.1136/jitc-2020-000958.

43. Alsaadi D, Shah NJ, Charabaty A, et al. A case of checkpoint inhibitor-induced celiac disease. J Immunother Cancer 2019;7(1):203.

44. Gentile NM, D'Souza A, Fujii LL, et al. Association between ipilimumab and celiac disease. Mayo Clin Proc 2013;88(4):414–7.

45. Masia R, Peyton S, Lauwers GY, et al. Gastrointestinal biopsy findings of autoimmune enteropathy: a review of 25 cases. Am J Surg Pathol 2014;38(10):1319–29.

46. Wang Y, Abu-Sbeih H, Mao E, et al. Endoscopic and Histologic Features of Immune Checkpoint Inhibitor-Related Colitis. Inflamm Bowel Dis 2018;24(8):1695–705.

47. Chen JH, Pezhouh MK, Lauwers GY, et al. Histopathologic Features of Colitis Due to Immunotherapy With Anti-PD-1 Antibodies. Am J Surg Pathol 2017;41(5):643–54.

48. Isidro RA, Ruan AB, Gannarapu S, et al. Medication-specific variations in morphological patterns of injury in immune check-point inhibitor-associated colitis. Histopathology 2021;78(4):532–41.

49. Yamauchi R, Araki T, Mitsuyama K, et al. The characteristics of nivolumab-induced colitis: an evaluation of three cases and a literature review. BMC Gastroenterol 2018;18(1):135.

50. Verschuren EC, van den Eertwegh AJ, Wonders J, et al. Clinical, Endoscopic, and Histologic Characteristics of Ipilimumab-Associated Colitis. Clin Gastroenterol Hepatol 2016;14(6):836–42.

51. Marthey L, Mateus C, Mussini C, et al. Cancer Immunotherapy with Anti-CTLA-4 Monoclonal Antibodies Induces an Inflammatory Bowel Disease. J Crohns Colitis 2016;10(4):395–401.

52. Collins M, Michot JM, Danlos FX, et al. Inflammatory gastrointestinal diseases associated with PD-1 blockade antibodies. Ann Oncol 2017;28(11):2860–5.

53. Khan J, Katona T. Immune Checkpoint Inhibitor-Induced Colitis Presenting As Lymphocytic Colitis. Cureus 2021;13(9):e18085.

54. Baroudjian B, Lourenco N, Pages C, et al. Anti-PD1-induced collagenous colitis in a melanoma patient. Melanoma Res 2016;26(3):308–11.

55. Janela-Lapert R, Bouteiller J, Deschamps-Huvier A, et al. Anti-PD-1 induced collagenous colitis in metastatic melanoma: a rare severe adverse event. Melanoma Res 2020;30(6):603–5.

56. Choi K, Abu-Sbeih H, Samdani R, et al. Can Immune Checkpoint Inhibitors Induce Microscopic Colitis or a Brand New Entity? Inflamm Bowel Dis 2019;25(2):385–93.

57. Randomised trial comparing tacrolimus (FK506) and cyclosporin in prevention of liver allograft rejection. European FK506 Multicentre Liver Study Group. Lancet 1994;344(8920):423–8.

58. Karamchandani DM, Chetty R. Apoptotic colopathy: a pragmatic approach to diagnosis. J Clin Pathol 2018;71(12):1033–40.

59. Adler BL, Pezhouh MK, Kim A, et al. Histopathological and immunophenotypic features of ipilimumab-associated colitis compared to ulcerative colitis. J Intern Med 2018;283(6):568–77.

Lymphomas and Amyloid in the Gastrointestinal Tract

Alisha D. Ware, MD[a], Laura M. Wake, MD[b],
Yuri Fedoriw, MD[c],*

KEYWORDS

- Lymphoma • Gastrointestinal lymphoma • B-cell lymphoma • T-cell lymphoma
- Lymphoproliferative disorder

Key points

- Lymphoproliferative disorders involving the gastrointestinal tract are a heterogeneous group of neoplasms with varying clinical, morphologic, immunophenotypic, and genetic characteristics.
- There can be significant morphologic, immunophenotypic, and genetic overlap between lymphoproliferative disorders involving the gastrointestinal tract.
- Genetic correlation is important for the diagnosis, management, and prognostication of many lymphomas that are identified in the gastrointestinal tract.

ABSTRACT

Lymphoproliferative disorders are a heterogeneous group of neoplasms with varying clinical, morphologic, immunophenotypic, and genetic characteristics. A subset of lymphomas have a proclivity for the gastrointestinal tract, although this region may also be involved by systemic lymphomas. In addition, a number of indolent lymphoproliferative disorders of the gastrointestinal tract have been defined over the past decade, and it is important to accurately differentiate these neoplasms to ensure that patients receive the proper management. Here, the authors review lymphoid neoplasms that show frequent gastrointestinal involvement and provide updates from the recent hematolymphoid neoplasm classification systems.

OVERVIEW

Lymphoproliferative disorders (LPDs) involving the gastrointestinal (GI) tract are a heterogeneous group of neoplasms with varied clinical outcomes and diagnostic features. These tumors are broadly defined as either B-lineage or T-cell/NK-cell neoplasms, and immunophenotypic evaluation remains a key in identifying and accurately classifying these tumors. Recent classification systems have increasingly emphasized the importance of cytogenetic and molecular correlation in diagnosing lymphoid neoplasms, including entities that are defined by cytogenetic/molecular abnormalities.[1–3] Although systemic lymphomas can present as tissue masses in virtually any organ system, the environment or region gives rise to other lymphoproliferations unique to the GI tract. Here, the authors provide an overview of LPDs involving the GI system, focusing on entities defined in the 5th *edition of the WHO Classification of Haematolymphoid Tumours* (WHO-HAEM5).[3] Where appropriate, the authors provide comparison with *The International Consensus Classification* (ICC) *of Mature Lymphoid Neoplasms.*[2]

[a] Department of Pathology & Laboratory Medicine, University of North Carolina School of Medicine, 160 Medical Drive, Brinkhous-Bullitt Building, CB#7525, Chapel Hill, NC 27599, USA; [b] Department of Pathology, Johns Hopkins University School of Medicine, 600 North Wolfe Street, Pathology Building, Room 401, Baltimore, MD 21287, USA; [c] Department of Pathology & Laboratory Medicine, Lineberger Comprehensive Cancer Center, University of North Carolina School of Medicine, 160 Medical Drive, Brinkhous-Bullitt Building, CB#7525, Chapel Hill, NC 27599, USA
* Corresponding author.
E-mail address: yuri.fedoriw@unchealth.unc.edu

surgpath.theclinics.com

MATURE B-LINEAGE NEOPLASMS

The great majority of systemic lymphomas and those involving the GI tract are of B-lineage origin, including mature B-cell and plasma cell neoplasms. The mature B-cell neoplasms commonly express B-cell antigens (ie, CD20, PAX5, CD19, CD79a, and CD22), whereas plasma cell tumors typically express CD138, CD38, MUM1, and cytoplasmic immunoglobulin (Ig). Although plasma cell neoplasms often express CD79a, they typically lack other B-cell antigens. B-cell neoplasms with a germinal center B-cell (GCB) phenotype express CD10 and BCL6, whereas those with a non-GCB phenotype lack these markers. Conversely, B-cell lymphomas may show extensive plasmacytic differentiation and show a more plasmacytic immunophenotype with the lack of B-cell antigens.[1] Most B-lineage neoplasms show clonal rearrangement of the Ig heavy (IgH) and/or kappa light chain (IgK) genes,[1] which can be demonstrated via polymerase chain reaction (PCR) analysis.

Table 1 reviews the morphologic and immunophenotypic characteristics useful in the differentiation of morphologically low-grade B-cell lymphomas of the GI tract.

B-CELL LYMPHOMAS

EXTRANODAL MARGINAL ZONE LYMPHOMA OF MUCOSA-ASSOCIATED LYMPHOID TISSUE

Mucosa-associated lymphoid tissue (MALT) lymphoma is a morphologically low-grade neoplasm that most commonly involves the stomach and far less frequently the small intestine. Small intestinal MALT lymphoma can present as a primary alpha heavy chain disease (AHCD). Many MALT lymphomas are associated with chronic inflammation due to infection or autoimmune disease. Gastric MALT lymphoma is associated with *Helicobacter pylori* infection, and AHCD may be associated with *Campylobacter* infection.[1]

Microscopic Features

MALT lymphoma is composed of small- to intermediate-sized mature lymphocytes with slightly irregular nuclei and inconspicuous nucleoli. Cells may show a monocytoid appearance with moderate to abundant pale cytoplasm. There may be plasmacytic differentiation, and an increase in plasma cells may be extensive (Fig. 1). The neoplastic lymphocytes infiltrate and disrupt residual germinal centers. Lymphoepithelial lesions (LELs) showing distortion or destruction of the epithelium by lymphoma cells are frequent.[1] Admixed large cells may be seen; however, if sheets of large cells are present, the neoplasm is best classified as diffuse large B-cell lymphoma (DLBCL).[1]

AHCD typically involves the small intestine and shows a prominent plasmacytic infiltrate with admixed small lymphocytes. LELs may be present.[1]

Ancillary Studies, Diagnostic

MALT lymphoma expresses B-cell antigens with or without CD43 and CD11c and is typically negative for CD5, CD10, BCL6, and CD23 (Fig. 2). The admixed plasma cells express plasma cell markers and frequently show Ig light chain restriction by kappa and lambda immunohistochemical or in situ hybridization (ISH) stains. The proliferation rate, demonstrated by Ki67 or MIB1, is low (<20%). *H pylori* organisms may be identified by routine or special stains in gastric lesions.

Associated Genetic Changes/Alterations

Table 1 includes the cytogenetic alterations associated with GI tract MALT lymphomas. There are no specific or diagnostic gene mutations associated with MALT lymphomas.

Prognosis

MALT lymphoma has an indolent clinical course. *H pylori*-associated tumors often respond to antibiotic therapy alone; therefore, gastric lesions should be evaluated for *H pylori*.

DUODENAL-TYPE FOLLICULAR LYMPHOMA

Duodenal-type follicular lymphoma (DFL) is an indolent mature B-cell lymphoma that involves the second portion of the duodenum but may involve other portions of the small intestine.[1,4–6]

Microscopic Features

DFL shows mucosal and submucosal neoplastic follicles. The neoplastic follicles are composed mostly of centrocytes, which are small mature lymphocytes with angulated nuclei, inconspicuous nucleoli, and scant cytoplasm, consistent with WHO grade 1–2 follicular lymphoma. Larger cells with open chromatin and conspicuous nucleoli (centroblasts) are infrequent. Lymphoma cells may extend into the lamina propria[1,4–6] (Fig. 3).

Ancillary Studies, Diagnostic

DFL expresses mature B-cell markers, GCB markers, and BCL2 (Fig. 4), they are negative for CD5, and it is usually low proliferation rate. Follicular dendritic cell meshworks are often present at the periphery of the neoplastic follicles.[1,4–6]

Table 1
Characteristics useful in the differentiation of morphologically low-grade B-cell lymphomas of the gastrointestinal tract

B-cell Lymphoma	Morphologic Characteristics	Immunophenotype	Genetic Characteristics	Clinical Course
Extranodal marginal zone lymphoma of mucosa-associated lymphoid tissue (MALT lymphoma)	• Small-to-intermediate-sized mature lymphocytes • Cells may contain moderate to abundant cytoplasm • Lymphoepithelial lesions • May show extensive plasmacytic differentiation • May be associated with *H pylori* (gastric) or *Campylobacter* (intestinal) infection	Neoplastic B cells • Positive for B-cell markers[a] and BCL2 • CD43 +/– • Negative for CD5, CD10, CD23, BCL6 Neoplastic plasma cells (if present) • Plasma cell markers[b] • Immunoglobulin light chain restriction or skew	• t(11;18) (q21;q21)[c,d,e] • t(14;18) (q32;q21)[c,f] • t(1;14) (p22;q32)[d] • Trisomy 3[c,d] • Trisomy 18[c,d] • Abnormalities of TNFAIP3 (chromosome 6q23)	• Generally indolent • May transform to diffuse large B-cell lymphoma
Duodenal-type follicular lymphoma	• Nodular proliferation of small mature lymphocytes with angulated nuclei (centrocytes) and occasional larger cells with conspicuous nucleoli (centroblasts)	• Positive for B-cell markers,[a] CD10, BCL6, and BCL2 • Negative for CD5 • Follicular dendritic cell meshworks (CD21, CD23, CD35) at the periphery of the neoplastic nodules	• t(14;18) (q32;q21) (*IGH::BCL2*) • Deletion 1p (*TNFRSF14*)	• Generally indolent

Mantle cell lymphoma	• Diffuse to vaguely nodular proliferation of small-to-intermediate-sized mature lymphocytes with irregular nuclei, inconspicuous nucleoli, and scant cytoplasm
	• Blastoid or pleomorphic morphology (associated with more aggressive disease)
		• Positive for B-cell markers,[a] BCL2, CD5, Cyclin D1, and SOX11
		• Negative for CD10
		• CD23 is usually negative but may be weakly positive
			• t(11;14) (q13;q23) (*IGH::CCND1*)
			• Rare variant CCND1 or CCND2 translocations
			• Often contain secondary chromosomal aberrations
			  ○ Gains of 3q26, 7p21, and 8q24
			  ○ Losses of 1p13–31, 6q23–27, 9p21, 11q22–
				• Generally an aggressive disease
				• Some features are associated with worse outcomes:
				  ○ High proliferation rate
				  ○ Blastoid/pleomorphic morphology
				  ○ Complex karyotype
				  ○ *TP53* or *CDNK2A* aberrations

(continued on next page)

Table 1
(continued)

B-cell Lymphoma	Morphologic Characteristics	Immunophenotype	Genetic Characteristics	Clinical Course
			23, 13q14–34, and 17p13 • Mutations in *CCND1, KMT2D, NOTCH1/2, CDKN2A/C*	

Chronic lymphocytic leukemia/small lymphocytic lymphoma	• Small mature lymphocytes with inconspicuous nucleoli and scant cytoplasm
	• Proliferations may be present in which neoplastic cells are slightly larger with open chromatin, conspicuous nucleoli, and more abundant cytoplasm
		• Positive for B-cell markers,[a] BCL2, CD5, CD23, LEF1
		• Negative for cyclin D1 and SOX11
			• Deletion 13q14.3
			• Trisomy 12
			• Deletion 11q22–23
			• Deletion 6q21
			• Mutations in *NOTCH1, SF3B1, TP53, ATM, BIRC3, POT1, MYD88*
				• Generally indolent
				• Some features are associated with worse outcomes:
				  ○ Expression of ZAP70, CD38
				  ○ Unmutated IGHV genes
				  ○ Deletion 11q or deletion 17p
				  ○ *TP53* abnormalities
				  ○ Complex karyotype
				  ○ Mutations in *ATM, NOTCH1, SF3B1, BIRC3*

[a] B-cell markers: CD20, PAX5, CD19, CD79a, CD22.
[b] Plasma cell markers: CD138, CD38, MUM1, and cytoplasmic immunoglobulin.
[c] Present in gastric MALT lymphoma.
[d] Present in intestinal MALT lymphoma.
[e] Resistant to *H pylori* eradication therapy.
[f] Indistinguishable from t(14;18) (q32;q21) (*IGH::BCL2*) seen in follicular lymphoma by FISH analysis.

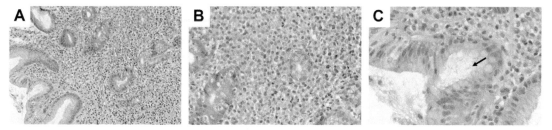

Fig. 1. Hematoxylin and eosin-stained sections of a gastric extranodal marginal zone lymphoma of mucosa-associated lymphoid tissue (MALT lymphoma). The neoplastic lymphocytes infiltrate the lamina propria (*A*, 200×), and they form lymphoepithelial lesions (*B*, 400×). They also show morphologic evidence of plasmacytic differentiation with many cells showing plasmacytic morphology. *H. pylori* organisms are identifiable (*C, arrow*).

Associated Genetic Changes/Alterations

DFL harbors the t(14;18) (q32;q21) (*IGH::BCL2*) translocation common to systemic follicular lymphoma (FL).[1] As such, evaluation for intestinal involvement by a systemic FL is recommended at primary diagnosis.

Prognosis

DFL has a very favorable prognosis and an indolent clinical course.[1,4–6]

MANTLE CELL LYMPHOMA

Mantle cell lymphoma (MCL) typically presents with nodal disease but may present with GI tract involvement as multiple lymphomatous polyposis.

Microscopic Features

The lesions of MCL are composed of a diffuse or vaguely nodular small- to intermediate-sized mature lymphocytes with irregular nuclear contours, inconspicuous nucleoli, and scant cytoplasm (**Fig. 5**). Increased hyalinized small vessels and admixed epithelioid histiocytes may be seen. Blastoid or pleomorphic morphology may be observed and should be reported as such as both have significant negative prognostic implications.[1,7]

Ancillary Studies, Diagnostic

MCL expresses mature B-cell markers and BCL2 and unsurprisingly expresses CD5, a marker of naïve B-cells populating the mantle zone. They are also

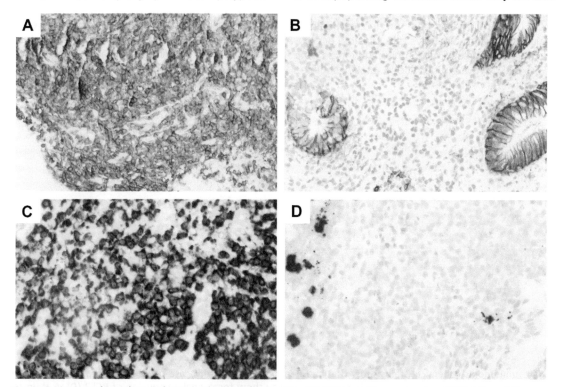

Fig. 2. By immunohistochemical stains, the neoplastic cells of MALT lymphoma express CD20 (*A*) and they are negative for CD138 (*B*). The neoplastic B cells show the evidence of plasmacytic differentiation with lambda light chain restriction by in situ hybridization (*C*), and they are negative for kappa light chain (*D*).

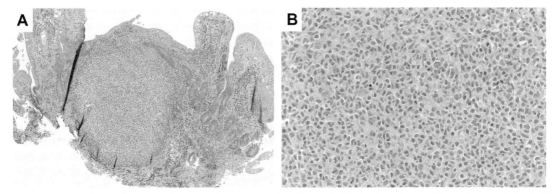

Fig. 3. Hematoxylin and eosin-stained sections of duodenal-type follicular lymphoma. There is a nodular infiltrate of neoplastic cells involving the lamina propria (A, 200×). The neoplastic cells are mostly small centrocytes and there are very few centroblasts (B, 400×).

usually positive for FMC7 and CD43 and typically show overexpression of cyclin-D1 (see Fig. 5) and SOX11. CD23 is negative or weakly positive.[1,7]

Associated Genetic Changes/Alterations

Most MCL demonstrate the t(11;14) (q13;q32) (*IGH::CCND1*) translocation. Rarely, variant *CCND1* translocations with the Ig light chain genes or *CCND2* translocations have been reported. Secondary chromosomal aberrations are frequent.[1,7]

Prognosis

MCL usually carries a poor prognosis. Features including a high proliferative rate, blastoid or pleomorphic morphology, a complex karyotype, and *TP53* or *CDKN2A* aberrations are associated with adverse outcomes.[1,7]

Differential Diagnosis

It is important to differentiate MCL from chronic lymphocytic leukemia/small lymphocytic lymphoma (CLL/SLL), which typically has a more indolent clinical course. In contrast to MCL, CLL/SLL is negative for cyclin D1 and SOX11, does not contain the *IGH::CCND1* translocation, and typically shows strong expression of CD23 (see Table 1). The proliferation centers of CLL/SLL may show partial expression of cyclin D1.

Oncogenic virus-associated B-lineage lymphoproliferative disorders involving the gastrointestinal tract

Some B-cell neoplasms of the GI tract are driven by oncogenic viruses, namely Epstein-Barr Virus (EBV) and Human Herpes Virus 8 (HHV8). These neoplasms usually occur in immunocompromised patients, including those with Human Immunodeficiency Virus

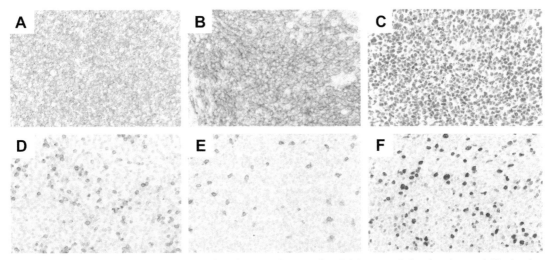

Fig. 4. Immunohistochemical stains show that the neoplastic cells of this case of duodenal-type follicular lymphoma express CD20 (A), CD10 (B), and BCL6 (C), and they show focal weak expression of BCL2 (D). A stain for CD3 (E) shows rare, admixed T cells. The Ki67 proliferation index is low (F).

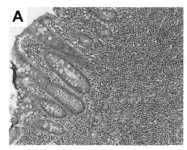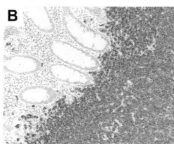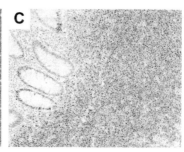

Fig. 5. Hematoxylin and eosin-stained sections of intestinal mantle cell lymphoma show a lamina propria infiltration by a monotonous proliferation of small-to-intermediate-sized lymphocytes (*A*). The neoplastic cells express CD20 (*B*) and cyclin D1 (*C*) by immunohistochemical analysis.

(HIV) infection, other immunodeficiency disorders, and elderly patients. The detection of EBV-encoded small RNA (EBER) via ISH is ideal for detection of EBV in tissue sections, as staining for EBV latent membrane protein-1 is less sensitive. Immunostaining for HHV8-associated latency-associated nuclear antigen-1 is useful in detecting the presence of HHV8.[1]

Table 2 lists the morphologic, immunophenotypic, and genetic features useful in the differentiation of the oncogenic virus-associated B-lineage LPDs of the GI tract.

BURKITT LYMPHOMA

Non-endemic Burkitt lymphoma (BL) is an aggressive mature B-cell lymphoma that commonly presents as a GI or abdominal mass. Patients often have advanced disease at diagnosis, and central nervous system involvement is frequent.[1,8]

Microscopic Features

BL contains monomorphic intermediate-sized cells with regular nuclei, finely clumped chromatin, conspicuous nucleoli, and basophilic cytoplasm. On touch preparations or cytology specimens, cytoplasmic vacuoles are often seen. Mitotic figures, apoptotic bodies, and tingible body macrophages imparting a "starry-sky" appearance are frequent.[1,8] (Fig. 6).

Ancillary Studies, Diagnostic

BL expresses mature B-cell markers and has a GCB phenotype. CD38 is usually positive. MYC protein is overexpressed and the proliferation rate approaches 100%. The cells are negative or show minimal expression of BCL2, and they lack CD5, CD23, TdT, and plasma cell markers (Fig. 7). EBV-EBER is positive in a subset of BL.[1,8]

Associated Genetic Changes/Alterations

BL is characterized by t(8;14) (q24;q32) (*MYC::IGH*). Less commonly, t(2;8) (*MYC::IGK*)or t(8;22) (*MYC::IGL*) translocations occur. Other chromosomal abnormalities may occur and mutations in *TCF3* and *ID3* are common.[1,8–10]

Prognosis

BL is aggressive but is highly curable with intensive chemotherapy.[1,8]

EXTRACAVITARY PRIMARY EFFUSION LYMPHOMA

Primary effusion lymphoma (PEL) is an uncommon and aggressive mature B-cell lymphoma that occasionally may present as an extracavitary PEL (ePEL) solid tumor mass involving the GI tract.[1,8,11]

Microscopic Features

ePEL contains sheets of large, atypical lymphocytes with prominent nucleoli, moderate-to-abundant basophilic cytoplasm, and occasional cytoplasmic vacuoles. Cells have immunoblastic, plasmablastic, or anaplastic morphology, resembling Hodgkin/Reed-Sternberg (HRS) cells. Tumors are mitotically active and lymphovascular involvement may be seen[8,11] (Fig. 8).

Ancillary Studies, Diagnostic

PEL is usually negative for mature B-cell markers and surface/cytoplasmic Ig; however, some ePEL may show expression of CD20 and CD79a. Plasma cell markers, CD30, and EMA are often positive. HHV8 is positive (see Fig. 8). EBV is usually positive in patients with HIV infection but is often negative in HIV-negative patients.[1,8,11]

Associated Genetic Changes/Alterations

PEL typically exhibits a complex karyotype with no specific or defining genetic alterations.[1,8,11]

Prognosis

PEL is aggressive with a median survival of less than 6 months.[1,8,11]

Table 2
Characteristics useful in the differentiation of the oncogenic virus-associated B-lineage lymphoproliferative disorders of the gastrointestinal tract

B-lineage Lymphoproliferative Disorders	Associated Virus(es)	Morphologic Characteristics	Immunophenotype	Genetic Characteristics	Clinical Course
Burkitt lymphoma	• EBV (+/−)	• Monomorphic intermediate-sized cells with conspicuous nucleoli and basophilic cytoplasm • "Starry-sky" pattern due to numerous tingible body macrophages • Frequent mitotic and apoptotic figures	• Positive for B-cell markers,[a] CD10, BCL6, CD38 • Overexpression of cMYC protein • Proliferation rate ~100% • Negative for BCL2, CD5, CD23, TdT	• t(8;14) (q24;q32) (MYC::IGH)[b] • Other chromosomal abnormalities may be identified • Mutations in TCF3 and ID3	• Aggressive disease • Highly curable with intensive chemotherapy

Extracavitary primary effusion lymphoma	• HHV8 +
	• EBV +/−
		• Large atypical cells with prominent nucleoli, basophilic cytoplasm, and occasional cytoplasmic vacuoles
		  ○ May resemble Hodgkin/Reed-Sternberg cells
		• Frequent mitotic figures
		• May show lymphovascular infiltration
			• Often positive for plasma cell markers,[c] CD30, EMA
			• Negative for B-cell markers[a]
			  ○ May express CD20 or CD79a
			• Negative for surface/cytoplasmic immunoglobulin
				• Complex karyotype
				• No specific or defining genetic alterations
					• Aggressive disease with a short median survival (<6 months)

Plasmablastic lymphoma	• EBV + • HHV8-negative	• Large immunoblastic cells with varying plasmacytic differentiation	• Positive for plasma cell markers[c] • Negative or weakly positive for B-cell markers[a]	• MYC rearrangements in >50% • Often has a complex karyotype	• Aggressive disease with a median survival of <1 year

		Morphology	Immunophenotype	Genetics	Clinical features
		• Frequent mitotic figures and apoptotic debris	• Often positive for CD30 and EMA • CD79a, CD10, and CD56 may be expressed • cMYC may be overexpressed	• No specific or defining genetic alterations	• Benign clinical course • Lesions often resolve with reduction of immunosuppressive therapy • May show local recurrence
EBV-positive mucocutaneous ulcer	EBV +	• Polymorphous inflammatory infiltrate containing plasma cells, histiocytes, eosinophils, intermediate-sized mature lymphocytes, and admixed large atypical Hodgkin/Reed-Sternberg (HRS)-like cells with prominent nucleoli • Band-like infiltrate of small mature lymphocytes present at the edge of the lesion	HRS-like cells • Positive for CD30, MUM1, PAX5, OCT2 • Variable CD20, CD79a, BOB1, CD15 • Negative for CD10 and BCL6 • EBV is positive in large, intermediate, and small neoplastic cells Admixed Small Lymphocytes • CD8-positive T-cells • EBV-negative		

a B-cell markers: CD20, PAX5, CD19, CD79a, CD22.
b Less commonly, t(2;8) (MYC::IGK) or t(8;22) (MYC::IGL) translocations may be identified.
c Plasma cell markers: CD138, CD38, MUM1, and cytoplasmic immunoglobulin.

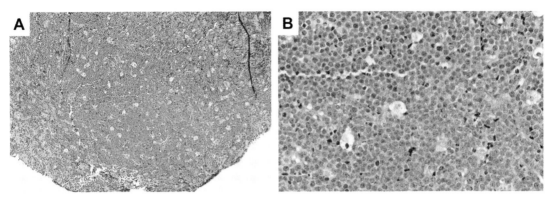

Fig. 6. Hematoxylin and eosin-stained sections of Burkitt lymphoma show effacement of the tissue architecture by a proliferation of neoplastic lymphocytes. On low power (A, 200×), tingible body macrophages impart a "starry-sky" appearance. The neoplastic cells are monomorphic with conspicuous nucleoli (B, 400×).

PLASMABLASTIC LYMPHOMA

Plasmablastic lymphoma (PBL) is a mature B-cell neoplasm with an aggressive clinical course. Outside of the head and neck, the GI tract is frequently involved.[1,8,12]

Microscopic Features

PBL contains sheets of large immunoblastic cells with varying plasmacytic differentiation. Mitoses and apoptotic debris are present (**Fig. 9**).[1,8,12]

Ancillary Studies, Diagnostic

PBL is positive for plasma cell markers and typically lacks or weakly expresses mature B-cell markers. CD30 and EMA are often expressed, and CD79a, CD10, and CD56 are expressed in a subset of cases. Most cases are EBV-EBER-positive and HHV8 is negative. MYC protein overexpression may be seen in association with *MYC* gene rearrangement.[1,8,12]

Associated Genetic Changes/Alterations

Approximately half of PBL harbor *MYC* rearrangements and many show a complex karyotype.[1,8,12]

Prognosis

PBL is an aggressive disease with a median survival of less than 1 year.[1,8,12]

Differential Diagnosis

It is important to differentiate PBL from anaplastic or plasmablastic plasma cell myeloma (PCM) (**Box 1**). Both diseases carry a poor prognosis; however, therapy differs between the two and anaplastic/plasmablastic PCM may have a longer overall survival with appropriate therapy.

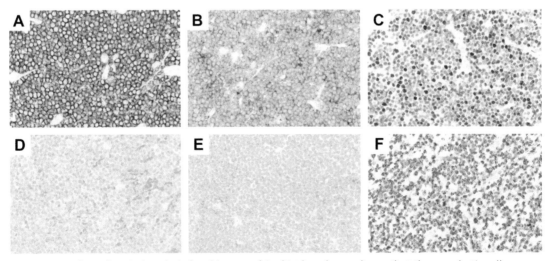

Fig. 7. Immunohistochemical analysis for this case of Burkitt lymphoma shows that the neoplastic cells are positive for CD20 (A), CD10 (B), and BCL6 (C), and they are negative for BCL2 (D), and TdT (E). The Ki67 proliferation index is >95% in the neoplastic cells (F).

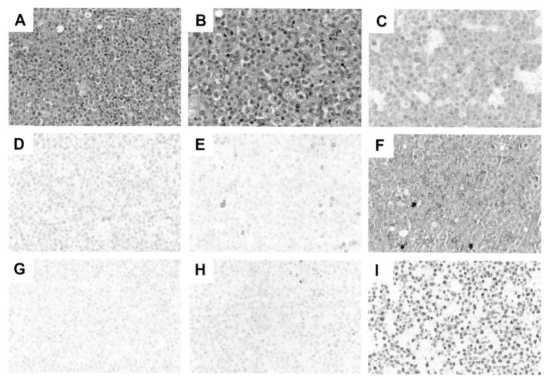

Fig. 8. Hematoxylin and eosin-stained sections of extracavitary primary effusion lymphoma at 400× (*A*) and 600× (*B*) involving an abdominal lymph node. The neoplastic cells are large in size with vesicular chromatin and prominent nucleoli, and they show evidence of plasmacytic differentiation. The neoplastic cells are positive for MUM1 (*C*) and HHV8 (*D*) and show focal expression of CD79a (*E*). They also show focal lambda light chain restriction (*F*). They are negative for CD30 (*G*) and PAX5 (*H*), and they have a high Ki67 proliferation index (*I*).

EBV-POSITIVE MUCOCUTANEOUS ULCER

EBV-positive mucocutaneous ulcer (EBV-MCU) may present in the oral cavity or throughout the GI tract and is associated with age-related or iatrogenic immunosuppression.[1,8]

Gross Features

EBV-MCU presents as a well-circumscribed ulcerated lesion with indurated, hyperemic borders.[1,8]

Microscopic Features

EBV-MCU contains a polymorphous inflammatory infiltrate with plasma cells, histiocytes, eosinophils, intermediate-sized mature lymphocytes, and admixed large, atypical lymphocytes with prominent nucleoli that may resemble HRS cells (**Fig. 10**). Lesions may resemble classic Hodgkin lymphoma (CHL) or DLBCL. A band-like infiltrate of mature lymphocytes is often present at the deep edge of the lesion.[1,8]

Ancillary Studies, Diagnostic

The HRS-like cells of EBV-MCU are positive for CD30, MUM1, PAX5, and OCT2 with variable expression of CD20, CD79a, BOB1, and CD15 and are negative for CD10 and BCL6. EBV-EBER is positive in both small and large/HRS-like B-lineage cells. The admixed lymphocytes and those at the edge of the lesion are CD8-positive, EBV-negative T-cells.

Prognosis

EBV-MCU has a benign clinical course and lesions often resolve with reduction of immunosuppressive therapy. Some cases show local recurrence, but distal involvement is rare.[1,13]

Differential Diagnosis

It is important to distinguish EBV-MCU from CHL and DLBCL to appropriately guide patient management (**Box 2**).

Plasma cell neoplasms and amyloidosis involving the GI tract

Plasma cell neoplasms and amyloidosis may present as GI lesions. These cases usually represent involvement by systemic disease; however, isolated GI involvement may be seen.

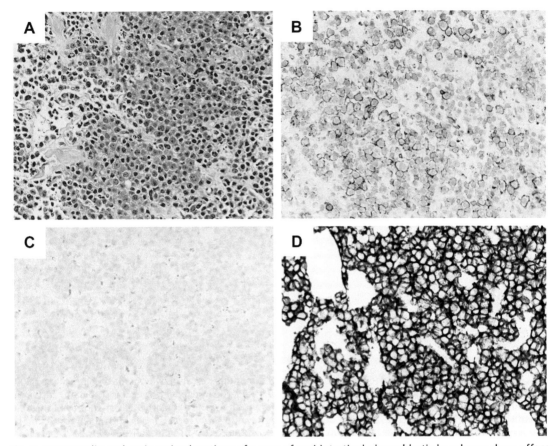

Fig. 9. Hematoxylin and eosin-stained sections of a case of peri-intestinal plasmablastic lymphoma show efface-ment of the tissue by a proliferation of large atypical lymphocytes with vesicular chromatin, prominent nucleoli, and amphophilic cytoplasm (*A*, 200×). The neoplastic cells show variable expression of CD138 (*B*) and they show lambda light chain restriction on in situ hybridization stains (*C*, kappa, and *D*, lambda).

PLASMA CELL NEOPLASMS

Microscopic Features

Plamsa cell neoplasm (PCN) are composed of neoplastic plasma cells, which are oval with an eccentrically placed round nucleus, "clock-face" chromatin, and inconspicuous nucleoli. Some cases may contain large atypical plasma cells with prominent nucleoli or multinucleation, and pleomorphic, plasmablastic, or anaplastic morphology can also be seen. Cytoplasmic inclu-sions such as multiple cytoplasmic grape-like ac-cumulations (Mott cells), cherry-red refractile inclusions (Russell bodies), prominent cyto-plasmic fibrils (pseudo-Gaucher cells), and crys-talline cytoplasmic rods may be seen.[1,14]

Ancillary Studies, Diagnostic

PCN express plasma cell markers with mono-clonal light chain restriction. CD56, CD117, and CD20 may be aberrantly expressed, though CD45 and CD19 are usually negative (**Fig. 11**). MYC protein may be overexpressed and cyclin-D1 may be positive, particularly in cases with t(11;14) (q13;q32) (*IGH::CCND1*).

Box 1
Differentiating PBL from PCM

Cases of EBV-negative PBL may be difficult to differentiate from anaplastic or plasmablastic PCM. PBL typically lacks features seen in PCM, such as lytic bone lesions, monoclonal serum Igs, bone marrow involvement, and PCM cytogenetics. If these features are present in the setting of a poorly differenti-ated neoplasm with plasmacytic differentiation, a diagnosis of anaplastic or plasmablastic PCM is favored.

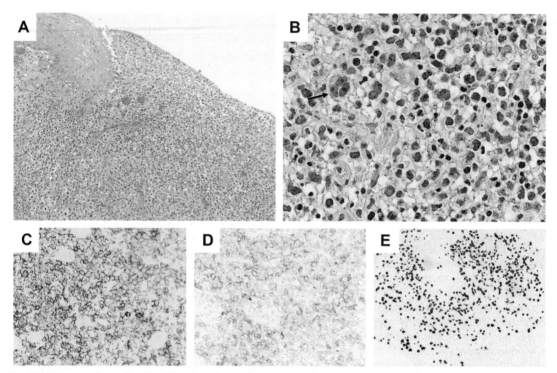

Fig. 10. Hematoxylin and eosin-stained sections of an EBV-positive mucocutaneous ulcer show mucosal ulceration with an associated mixed inflammatory infiltrate (*A*, 100×). The lesion shows scattered large Hodgkin/Reed-Sternberg-like cells (*arrow*), intermediate-sized atypical cells, and small lymphocytes with scattered mitotic and apoptotic bodies (*B*, 400×). Immunohistochemical stains show that the lesional cells exhibit variable expression of CD20 (*C*) and CD30 (*D*), and EBV is positive in the neoplastic small, intermediate, and large cells (*E*).

Associated Genetic Changes/Alterations

Clonal genetic abnormalities are present in approximately one-third of PCN (**Table 3**).[14–16]

Prognosis

PCN have a variable prognosis. Certain genetic features have been associated with less favorable outcomes (see **Table 3**).

Differential Diagnosis

In addition to differentiation from PBL, PCN must be differentiated from reactive plasma cell proliferations and B-cell lymphomas with plasmacytic differentiation. See **Box 3** for features useful in the differential diagnosis of a plasma cell neoplasm versus PBL.

Box 2
Differentiating EBV-MCU from CHL and DLBCL

It can be difficult to differentiate EBV-MCU from CHL and DLBCL. This is an important distinction, because EBV-MCU has a favorable prognosis and typically requires limited or non-intensive therapy. CHL and DLBCL are more aggressive diseases that require chemotherapy with or without radiation therapy for adequate treatment.

CHL consists of HRS cells with prominent nucleoli scattered in a mixed inflammatory background containing eosinophils, neutrophils, plasma cells, histiocytes, and small lymphocytes. The HRS cells express CD30, MUM1, weak PAX5, and variable CD15. HRS cells are negative or show partial weak expression of CD20 and CD79a, and they are negative for OCT2 and BOB1. EBV-EBER may be positive in the HRS cells. CHL rarely if ever presents as a mucocutaneous lesion, and a diagnosis of CHL in these sites should be made with extreme caution to prevent patient overtreatment.

DLBCL consists of sheets of large, atypical lymphocytes. B-cell markers are typically strongly expressed. Neoplastic cells show a GCB or non-GCB phenotype. CD30 and CD15 are usually negative, though a subset of cases may show expression of CD30. There are typically few background inflammatory cells, consisting primarily of small, mature-appearing T-cells.

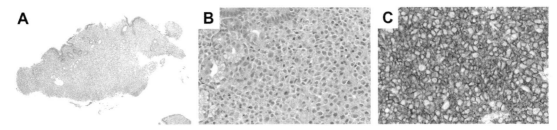

Fig. 11. Hematoxylin and eosin-stained section of a stomach biopsy with involvement by a plasma cell neoplasm (*A*, 40×, and *B*, 400×). The plasma cells are highlighted by a CD138 immunohistochemical stain (*C*), and they show kappa light chain restriction (not pictured).

IMMUNOGLOBULIN-RELATED (AL) AMYLOIDOSIS

Ig-related (AL) amyloidosis (WHO-HAEM5),[3] or Ig light chain amyloidosis (ICC),[2] is typically associated with a PCN or, rarely, a B-cell LPD with plasmacytic differentiation (lymphoplasmacytic lymphoma or MALT lymphoma). Lesions contain abnormally folded proteins, typically Ig light chains, secreted by the neoplastic plasma cells or lymphoplasmacytic cells. Mass spectrometry may be used to subtype amyloid protein when abundant amyloid is biopsied.[1,17–19] The diagnosis of amyloidosis is typically made on bone marrow or abdominal fat pad biopsy, but the GI tract and many other organs may be involved.[1,17,19]

Microscopic Features

Amyloid deposits consist of amorphous eosinophilic material within blood vessel walls, basement membranes, or the interstitium. An associated plasma cell infiltrate may be present.[1,17]

Ancillary Studies, Diagnostic

The Congo red stain is used to identify amyloid on tissue sections. Deposits stain salmon-pink-to-red with yellow-green or apple-green birefringence under polarized light[1,17] (**Fig. 12**). Associated plasma cells show monoclonal light chain restriction by immunohistochemical or ISH stains.[1]

Associated Genetic Changes/Alterations

IGH::CCND1 may be found in a significant portion of patients with amyloidosis. The deletion of chromosome 13q14 and gain of 1q21 are also frequently identified.[1]

Prognosis

Primary amyloidosis carries a variable prognosis. High-stage disease, PCM involving the bone marrow, and cardiac involvement portend worse outcomes.[1]

Table 3
Genetic abnormalities frequently identified in plasma cell neoplasms

Gene Rearrangements	Genetic Mutations	Other Frequent Cytogenetic Abnormalities
t(11;14) (q13;q32) (*CCND1::IGH*)[a]	*TP53*/deletion 17p[c]	
t(4;14) (p16;q32) (*FGFR3::IGH*)[b]	*KRAS*	Hyperdiploid[a]
t(14;16) (q32;q23) (*IGH::MAF*)[c]	*NRAS*	Non-hyperdiploid
t(6;14) (p25;q32) (*CCND3::IGH*)[a]	*BRA*	Hypodiploid[b]
t(14;20) (q32;q11) (*IGH::MAFB*)[c]	*FGFR3* (seen in cases with t(4;14))	Deletion 13q14
t(8;14) (q24;q32) (*IGH::MAFA*)[a]	*CDKN2C*	Gains in odd-numbered chromosomes (3,5,7,9,11,15,19,21)
t(12;14) (p13;q32) (*CCND2::IGH*)[a]	*RB1*	Gains of 1q and loss of 1p
	FAM46C	
	DIS3	

[a] Standard risk.
[b] Intermediate risk.
[c] High risk.

Box 3
PReactive vs. Neoplastic Plasma Cell Proliferations

Although plasma cell neoplasms may involve the GI tract, reactive plasma cell proliferations are also common in this region. A reactive plasma cell proliferation will show polytypic expression of kappa and lambda light chains by ISH or immunohistochemistry, whereas a plasma cell neoplasm will show monotypic expression of either kappa or lambda light chain.

B-cell lymphomas with extensive plasmacytic differentiation can be very difficult to differentiate from a plasma cell neoplasm. These typically are either classified as a marginal zone lymphoma or lymphoplasmacytic lymphoma. In these entities, a neoplastic B-cell component with light chain restriction identical to the plasma cell component (ie, both the B-cell and plasma cell components are kappa-restricted) can be identified. ISH and immunohistochemical stains for kappa and lambda are often not reliable in B cells. Flow cytometry is the ideal method for determination of B-cell clonality; however, IgH or IgK gene rearrangement studies may also be used to determine clonality.

T-CELL AND NK-CELL NEOPLASMS

T-cell and NK-cell neoplasms are less common than B-lineage neoplasms; however, there are several entities of this lineage that primarily involve the GI tract.

Mature T-cell neoplasms express pan-T-cell antigens (CD2, surface CD3, CD5, and CD7), with expression of either CD4 or CD8. CD4-positive T-cells are mainly regulatory or helper subclass. CD8-positive T-cells are mainly cytotoxic or suppressor subtype. Mature T-cells also contain either $\alpha\beta$ or $\gamma\delta$ T-cell receptors (TCR). $\gamma\delta-$T cells lack CD4 and CD5, and are CD4/CD8-double-negative or express CD8. $\gamma\delta-$T cells are found predominantly in the intestinal epithelium, splenic red pulp, and other epithelial sites.

NK-cells express cytoplasmic CD3-ε and -ζ chains, CD2, CD7, CD16, CD56, variable CD57, and cytotoxic granule proteins (ie, TIA-1, granzyme, and perforin) and are negative for surface CD3.

Clonal T-cell neoplasms typically show clonal TCR-β and/or TCR-γ gene rearrangements by PCR analysis. NK-cells do not show clonal TCR gene rearrangements, but killer-cell Ig-like receptor analysis may be used to evaluate for NK-cell clonality.

Table 4 reviews the morphologic features useful in the differential diagnosis of T-cell and NK-cell neoplasms involving the GI tract. Table 5 describes the immunophenotypic characteristics of the described T-cell and NK-cell neoplasms.

INDOLENT T-CELL LYMPHOMA OF THE GASTROINTESTINAL TRACT

Indolent T-cell lymphoma of the GI (ITCL-GI) tract (WHO-HAEM5),[3] also referred to as indolent T-cell LPD of the GI tract (ICC),[2] is a heterogeneous disorder.[1–3]

Microscopic Features

The lesions of ITCL-GI show the expansion of the lamina propria by small, round, mature lymphocytes. There may be admixed epithelioid granulomas resembling inflammatory bowel disease; however, lesions are typically nondestructive and do not show significant epitheliotropism.[1,20,21] Lesions may occasionally show superficial ulceration with an inflammatory background.[20]

Ancillary Studies, Diagnostic

ITCL-GI expresses pan-T-cell antigens with variable loss of CD7, either CD4 or CD8, with the latter predominating in the literature, and a minor subset

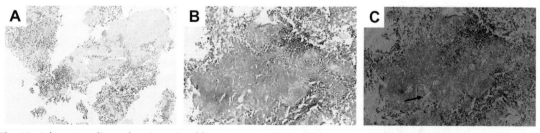

Fig. 12. A hematoxylin and eosin-stained bone marrow biopsy shows deposits of amorphous eosinophilic material (*A*, 40×). Congo red shows salmon-pink staining of the eosinophilic material (*B*) with apple-green birefringence under polarized light (*C, arrow*), consistent with amyloid.

Table 4
Morphologic, genetic, and clinical characteristics of T-cell and NK-cell lymphoproliferative disorders of the gastrointestinal tract

Lymphoproliferative Disorder	Morphologic Characteristics	Genetic Characteristics	Clinical Course
Indolent T-cell lymphoma of the GI tract	• Nondestructive expansion of the lamina propria • Small, round, mature lymphocytes • May contain epithelioid granulomas • No significant epitheliotropism	• STAT3::JAK2 • Mutations in TET2 and KMT2D	• Generally indolent • Rarely may progress to peripheral T-cell lymphoma
Enteropathy-associated T-cell lymphoma (EATL)	• Sheets of pleomorphic intermediate-to-large-sized cells with angulated nuclei, vesicular chromatin, prominent nucleoli, and pale cytoplasm • May have anaplastic morphology, angioinvasion, or necrosis • Mixed inflammatory background • Variable epitheliotropism	• Recurrent gains of chromosomes 9q34, 1q, or 5q • Deletion 16q12.1 or 17p12-p13.2 (TP53) • Loss of heterozygosity at 9p • Mutations in JAK1 and STAT3	• Aggressive disease with suboptimal response to conventional chemotherapy • Intensive chemotherapy and autologous stem cell transplant may improve survival
Monomorphic epitheliotropic intestinal T-cell lymphoma (MEITL)	• Sheets of monomorphic intermediate-sized lymphocytes with round nuclei, inconspicuous nucleoli, and limited cytoplasm • Prominent epitheliotropism May show more pleomorphism, necrosis, angiocentricity, or a "starry-sky" pattern	• Gains of chromosomes 9q34.3 or 8q24 (MYC) • Deletion 7p14.1 or 16q12.1 • Mutations in SETD2, STAT5B, JAK3, GNAI2 • Some genetic overlap with EATL	• Generally poor prognosis
Hepatosplenic T-cell lymphoma	• Intermediate-sized mature lymphocytes with inconspicuous nucleoli and scant cytoplasm • Splenic red pulp, hepatic sinusoids, and bone marrow involvement (intrasinusoidal pattern)	• Most cases contain isochromosome 7q • May contain trisomy 8 • Mutations in STAT5B, STAT3, SETD2, INO80, and ARID1B	• Generally an aggressive disease with frequent relapse

Indolent NK-cell lymphoproliferative disorder of the gastrointestinal tract	• Expansion of the lamina propria • Intermediate-to-large lymphocytes with variably conspicuous nucleoli and pale cytoplasm • Often contains eosinophilic cytoplasmic granules • May have a mixed inflammatory background • Locally destructive but *no* angiocentricity or necrosis	• Recurrent *JAK3* mutations	• Generally indolent but with frequent recurrence • Gastric lesions may show spontaneous regression
Extranodal NK/T-cell lymphoma	• Effacement of architecture with prominent angiocentricity and angiodestruction • Variably sized irregular lymphocytes with vesicular/granular chromatin, inconspicuous nucleoli, and pale cytoplasm • Frequent necrosis and apoptotic debris	• Deletion 6q21-q25 • Isochromosome 6p10 Mutations in *DDX3X*, JAK/STAT pathway constituents, tumor suppressors, RAS family oncogenes, *MYC*, epigenetic modifiers, and cell cycle and apoptosis regulators	• Generally poor prognosis • Limited response to therapy

Table 5
Immunophenotypic characteristics useful in the differentiation of T-cell and NK-cell lymphoproliferative disorders of the gastrointestinal tract

Lymphoproliferative Disorder	CD2	Surface CD3	Cytoplasmic CD3-ε	CD5	CD7	CD4	CD8	CD30	CD56	Cytotoxic Markers	EBV
Indolent T-cell lymphoma of the GI tract	+	+		+	-/+	-/+	+/-	-	-	-	-
Enteropathy-associated T-cell lymphoma (EATL)	+	+		-	+	-	-/+	+/-	-	+	-
Monomorphic epitheliotropic intestinal T-cell lymphoma (MEITL)	+	+		-	-/+	-	+	-	+	+	-
Hepatosplenic T-cell lymphoma	+	+		-	-/+	-	-/+	-	+/-	TIA1 + Granzyme M + Granzyme B – Perforin –	-
Indolent NK-cell lymphoproliferative disorder of the gastrointestinal tract	+	-	+	-	+	-	-	-	+	+	-
Extranodal NK/T-cell lymphoma	+	-	+	-/+	+/-	-	-/+	-/+	+	+	+

of reported cases are CD4/CD8 double-negative. CD30 and CD56 are negative and the proliferative index is low.[1,20,21]

Associated Genetic Changes/Alterations

STAT3::JAK2 fusions are common, especially CD4-positive lesions.[22] Mutations in *TET2* and *KMT2D* have also been reported.[3]

Prognosis

ITCL-GI typically follows a chronic clinical course with rare progression or evolution to peripheral T-cell lymphoma.[1,20,21,23]

ENTEROPATHY-ASSOCIATED T-CELL LYMPHOMA

Enteropathy-associated T-cell lymphoma (EATL) is associated with refractory celiac disease (CD) and the presence of the HLA-DQ2 or -DQ8 alleles. EATL is the most common primary intestinal T-cell lymphoma and typically involves the small intestine but is often multifocal.[1,24-28]

Gross Features

EATL may present as nodules, plaques, or strictures with associated ulceration, or uncommonly may form a large exophytic mass.[1,24]

Microscopic Features

EATL is composed of pleomorphic intermediate-to-large atypical lymphocytes with angulated nuclei, vesicular chromatin, prominent nucleoli, and moderate-to-abundant pale cytoplasm. Large-cell and/or anaplastic morphology, angioinvasion, and necrosis are common, as is a mixed inflammatory background (**Fig. 13**). Epitheliotropism is variable, although the adjacent uninvolved mucosa often shows changes consistent with CD.[1,24-28]

Ancillary Studies, Diagnostic

EATL expresses CD3, CD7, CD103, and cytotoxic markers, may show CD8-positivity, and is typically negative for CD5 and CD4. CD30 may be positive, particularly in cases with a large cell component (see **Fig. 13**).[1,24-28]

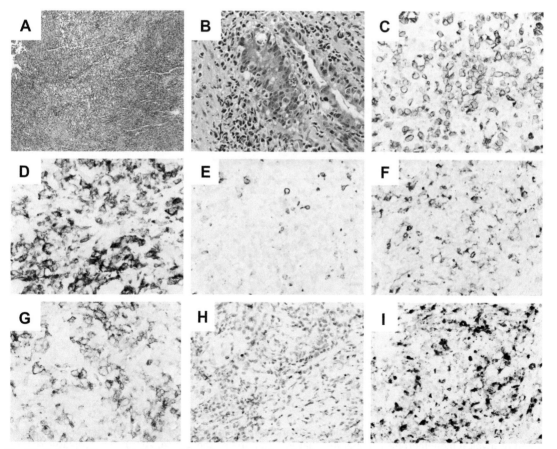

Fig. 13. Enteropathy-associated T-cell lymphoma involving the ileum. On hematoxylin and eosin-stained sections, the neoplastic cells are pleomorphic (*A*, 20×) and show some epitheliotropism (*B*, 40×). The neoplastic cells express CD3 (*C*) and CD7 (*D*), and they are largely negative for CD4 (*E*). They show partial loss of CD5 (*F*). CD30 (*G*) is also positive. The neoplastic cells show a cytotoxic phenotype with expression of TIA-1 (*H*) and Granzyme B (*I*).

Associated Genetic Changes/Alterations

EATL usually shows recurrent gains of chromosomes 9q34, 1q, or 5q, or deletions of chromosome 16q12.1. A subset also shows the loss of heterozygosity at chromosome 9p or loss of 17p12-p13.2 (*TP53*). Mutations in the JAK-STAT pathway, including *JAK1* and *STAT3* mutations, have also been reported.[1,27,29]

Prognosis

EATL generally has an unfavorable prognosis with suboptimal response to conventional chemotherapy.[1] Intensive chemotherapy and autologous stem cell transplant may improve outcomes.[1,24]

MONOMORPHIC EPITHELIOTROPIC INTESTINAL T-CELL LYMPHOMA

Monomorphic epitheliotropic intestinal T-cell lymphoma (MEITL) is a primary intestinal T-cell lymphoma. This entity was previously classified as type II EATL; however, MEITL shows no association with CD and is now classified as a unique entity.[1,30,31]

Microscopic Features

MEITL contains sheets of atypical intermediate-sized lymphocytes with round nuclei, mature chromatin, inconspicuous nucleoli, and limited cytoplasm. Cells are usually monomorphic with prominent epitheliotropism[1,30] (**Fig. 14**), though some cases may show more pleomorphism, necrosis, angiocentricity, or admixed tingible body macrophages imparting a starry-sky pattern.[30]

Ancillary Studies, Diagnostic

MEITL is positive for CD3, CD7, CD8, CD56, CD103, cytotoxic markers, and either αβ or γδ, with the latter being more common[1,30] (see **Fig. 13**).

Associated Genetic Changes/Alterations

MEITL commonly shows the gains of chromosome 9q34.3 or gains in 8q24 (*MYC*).[1,30] Other chromosomal gains and loss of 7p14.1 or 16q12.1 may be seen, and there is some genetic overlap with EATL.[1]

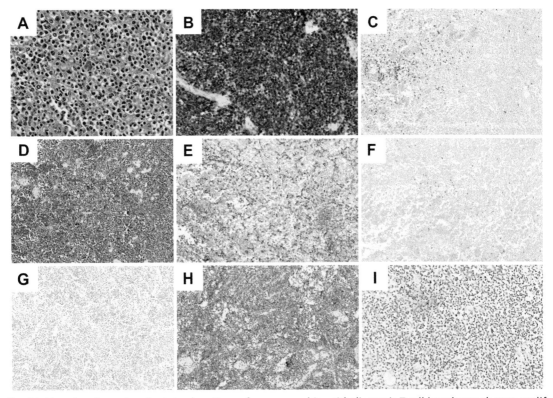

Fig. 14. Hematoxylin and eosin-stained sections of monomorphic epitheliotropic T-cell lymphoma show a proliferation of atypical monomorphic lymphocytes that infiltrate the epithelium (*A*, 200×). The neoplastic cells express CD3 (*B*), show loss of CD5 (*C*), and retain expression of CD7 (*D*). They are largely negative for CD4 (*E*) and CD8 (*F*). CD30 is also negative (*G*). The cells show a cytotoxic phenotype with TIA-1 expression (*H*), and they are negative for TCR-BF1 (*I*).

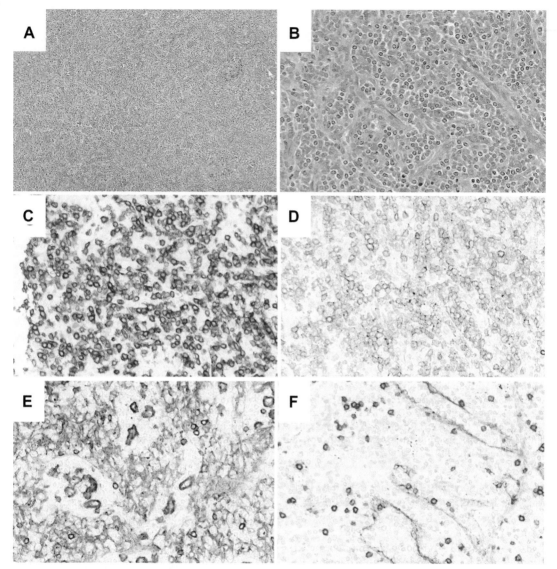

Fig. 15. Hematoxylin and eosin-stained sections of the spleen (*A*, 40×, and *B*, 400×) revealed expansion of the splenic red pulp by a predominantly sinusoidal proliferation of predominantly small mature lymphocytes. By immunohistochemistry, the neoplastic cells express CD3 (*C*) and CD56 (*D*). CD4 highlights numerous background histiocytes and is largely negative in the neoplastic cells (*E*). The tumor cells are negative for CD8 (*F*) as well as CD30, ALK1, TdT, TCR beta-F1, and EBV-EBER ISH (not pictured).

SETD2 and *STAT5B* mutations are common, and *JAK3* and *GNAI2* mutations have been reported.[1,30,31]

Prognosis

MEITL has a poor prognosis, with a median survival rate of approximately 7 months.[1]

HEPATOSPLENIC T-CELL LYMPHOMA

Hepatosplenic T-cell lymphoma (HSTL) is an aggressive entity that presents with involvement and enlargement of the liver and spleen without prominent nodal disease.[1,32]

Microscopic Features

HSTL contains a proliferation of intermediate-sized cells with mature chromatin, inconspicuous nucleoli, and scant cytoplasm. The neoplastic infiltrate is concentrated in the splenic red pulp and hepatic sinusoids and the bone marrow with an intrasinusoidal distribution. Progressive lesions may show prominent cytologic atypia[1] (**Figs. 15** and **16**).

Ancillary Studies, Diagnostic

HSTL expresses CD3, TCR-γδ, and cytotoxic markers TIA1 and granzyme M, often with expression of CD56.[1,32] CD8 may be positive. CD4, CD5,

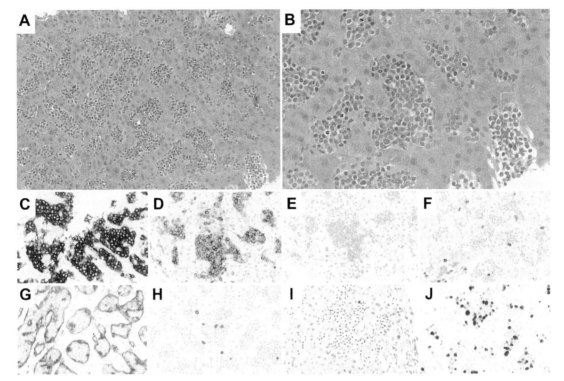

Fig. 16. Hematoxylin and eosin-stained sections of a liver biopsy involved by hepatosplenic T-cell lymphoma show a sinusoidal infiltrate of small to intermediate-sized mature lymphocytes (*A*, 200×, and *B*, 400×. The neoplastic lymphocytes are positive for CD3 (*C*), CD7 (*D*) and show weak expression of CD56 (*E*). The cells are negative for CD5 (*F*), CD4 (*G*), CD8 (*H*), TCR-betaF1 (*I*), and the Ki67 proliferation index is approximately 20-30% (*J*). Additional immunostains performed at the outside institution showed that the neoplastic cells were also positive for TCR-delta and negative for TIA-1, granzyme B, and perforin (not pictured).

and CD30 are negative. The tumor cells may lack granzyme B and perforin[1] (see **Figs. 15** and **16**).

Associated Genetic Changes/Alterations

Most cases of HSTL harbor isochromosome 7q. Trisomy 8 and ring chromosomes causing 7q amplification have been reported. Mutations in *STAT5B*, *STAT3*, *SETD2*, *INO80*, and *ARID1B* are also frequent.[1,32]

Prognosis

HSTL is generally clinically aggressive. Although patients may initially respond to chemotherapy, relapse is common. Median overall survival is less than 2 years, but high-dose chemotherapy and stem cell transplantation may lead to improved outcomes.[1,32]

INDOLENT NK-CELL LYMPHOPROLIFERATIVE DISORDER OF THE GASTROINTESTINAL TRACT

Indolent NK-cell LPD of the GI tract (INKLPD-GI) includes lesions formerly classified as lymphomatoid gastropathy and NK-cell enteropathy.[2,3]

Microscopic Features

INKLPD-GI shows expansion of the lamina propria by intermediate to large lymphocytes with round to irregular nuclei, mature chromatin, variably conspicuous nucleoli, and moderate pale cytoplasm, and occasional eosinophilic cytoplasmic granules.[3,20] Some cases may show a mixed inflammatory background. Lesions may be locally destructive, but do not show angiocentricity or necrosis.[20]

Ancillary Studies, Diagnostic

INKLPD-GI has a mature NK-cell immunophenotype with a low-to-moderate proliferation index. EBV-EBER is negative.[20]

Associated Genetic Changes/Alterations

Recurrent *JAK3* mutations have been identified in INKLPD-GI.[3]

Prognosis

INKLPD-GI has an indolent clinical course. Gastric lesions often showing spontaneous regression, but intestinal lesions may show a more protracted clinical course. Recurrence is frequent.[20]

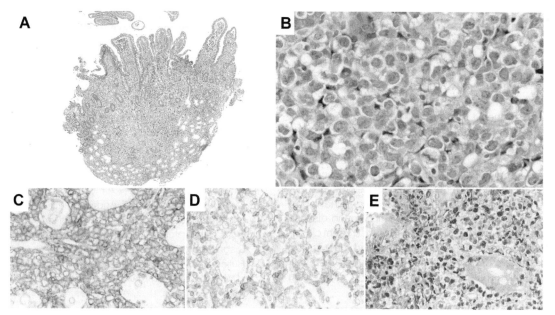

Fig. 17. Hematoxylin and eosin-stained sections show a duodenal biopsy involved by extranodal NK/T-cell lymphoma involving the lamina propria (*A*, 400×). The neoplastic cells are intermediate-to-large in size with conspicuous nucleoli and pale cytoplasm, and scattered mitotic figures and apoptotic bodies are identified (*B*, 600×). The neoplastic cells express CD2 (*C*) and weak CD3 (*D*), and they are EBV-EBER-positive (*E*).

Differential Diagnosis

It is important to differentiate INKLPD-GI from extranodal NK/T-cell lymphoma. In contrast to extranodal NK/T-cell lymphoma (ENKTL), INKLPD-GI is EBV-negative and the lesions do not show angiocentricity or prominent necrosis.[3,20]

EXTRANODAL NK/T-CELL LYMPHOMA

ENKTL most frequently presents in the upper aerodigestive tract; however, the GI tract may also be involved.[1,25,33]

Microscopic Features

ENKTL shows effacement of tissue architecture with prominent angiocentricity and angiodestruction. The malignant cells vary in size with irregular nuclei, granular or vesicular nuclei, variably conspicuous nucleoli, and moderate pale cytoplasm (**Fig. 17**). Necrosis and apoptotic debris are common.[1]

Ancillary Studies, Diagnostic

ENKTL has a variable immunophenotype. The neoplastic cells usually have an NK-cell phenotype with expression of CD2, CD56, and cytoplasmic CD3-ε, are negative for CD4, CD5, and surface CD3, and show variable expression of CD7. CD8, CD16, and CD57 are typically negative, though a subset of cases may show a CD8-positive cytotoxic T-cell phenotype with CD5 co-expression. EBV-EBER is positive.[1,25,33] (see **Fig. 17**).

Associated Genetic Changes/Alterations

Deletion 6q21q25 or isochromosome 6p10 are the most common cytogenetic aberrancies identified. Mutations in *DDX3X*, JAK/STAT pathway constituents, tumor suppressors, RAS family oncogenes, *MYC*, epigenetic modifiers, and cell cycle and apoptosis regulators are also common.[1,25,33]

Box 4
Differentiating INKLPD-GI and ENKTL

It can be very difficult to differentiate INKLPD-GI and ENKTL. Both entities may show an extensive infiltrate of intermediate to large neoplastic lymphocytes with an NK-cell phenotype. In contrast to INKLPD-GI, ENKTL usually shows prominent angiocentricity and angiodestruction and often has a higher proliferation index. ENKTL is also strongly associated with EBV, whereas INKLPD-GI is EBV-negative. This distinction is important, as INKLPD-GI follows an indolent clinical course and ENKTL is an aggressive disease with an overall poor prognosis.

Prognosis

Extranasal ENKTL has a generally poor prognosis with a limited response to therapy[1] **(Box 4)**.

SUMMARY

LPDs of the GI tract are a heterogeneous group of neoplasms ranging from indolent LPDs to aggressive lymphomas. Although there may be significant morphologic and immunophenotypic overlap, ever-increasing knowledge on the genetic landscape of this group of tumors provides new insights into disease classification and risk stratification. The importance of molecular and genetic findings in disease classification is highlighted by the most recent classification schema for hematolymphoid neoplasms. Nonetheless, morphologic and immunophenotypic evaluation remains a cornerstone in diagnosing these neoplasms.

CLINICS CARE POINTS

- The majority of LPDs of the GI tract are B-cell in origin.
- Patients with immunodeficiency may present with unique and aggressive oncogenic virus-associated LPDs.
- There are several indolent LPDs of the GI tract that mimic more aggressive diseases by morphology alone. Correlation with clinical, radiographic, and genetic findings is often useful in differentiating these disorders.

DISCLOSURE

The authors have nothing to disclose.

REFERENCES

1. Swerdlow S, Campo E, Harris NL, et al. WHO classification of Tumours of haematopoietic and lymphoid tissues. Revised 4th edition. Lyon, France: International Agency for Research on Cancer (IARC); 2017.
2. Campo E, Jaffe ES, Cook JR, et al. The international consensus classification of mature lymphoid neoplasms: a report from the clinical advisory committee. Blood 2022;140(11):1229–53.
3. Alaggio R, Amador C, Anagnostopoulos I, et al. The 5th edition of the World Health Organization classification of haematolymphoid tumours: lymphoid neoplasms. Leukemia 2022;36(7):1720–48.
4. Duffles Amarante G, Collins G, Rocha V. What do we know about duodenal-type follicular lymphoma? From pathological definition to treatment options. Br J Haematol 2020;188(6):831–7.
5. Marks E, Shi Y. Duodenal-type follicular lymphoma: a clinicopathologic review. Arch Pathol Lab Med 2018; 142(4):542–7.
6. Takata K, Miyata-Takata T, Sato Y, et al. Gastrointestinal follicular lymphoma: current knowledge and future challenges. Pathol Int 2018;68(1):1–6.
7. Nadeu F, Martin-Garcia D, Clot G, et al. Genomic and epigenomic insights into the origin, pathogenesis, and clinical behavior of mantle cell lymphoma subtypes. Blood 2020;136(12): 1419–32.
8. Grimm KE, O'Malley DP. Aggressive B cell lymphomas in the 2017 revised WHO classification of tumors of hematopoietic and lymphoid tissues. Ann Diagn Pathol 2019;38:6–10.
9. Hüllein J, Słabicki M, Rosolowski M, et al. MDM4 is targeted by 1q gain and drives disease in Burkitt lymphoma. Cancer Res 2019;79(12): 3125–38.
10. Panea RI, Love CL, Shingleton JR, et al. The whole-genome landscape of Burkitt lymphoma subtypes. Blood 2019;134(19):1598–607.
11. Shimada K, Hayakawa F, Kiyoi H. Biology and management of primary effusion lymphoma. Blood 2018; 132(18):1879–88.
12. Ambrosio MR, Mundo L, Gazaneo S, et al. MicroRNAs sequencing unveils distinct molecular subgroups of plasmablastic lymphoma. Oncotarget 2017;8(64):107356–73.
13. Maxfield CM, Thorpe MP, Desser TS, et al. Awareness of implicit bias mitigates discrimination in radiology resident selection. Med Educ 2020;54(7): 637–42.
14. Caers J, Garderet L, Kortüm KM, et al. European Myeloma Network recommendations on tools for the diagnosis and monitoring of multiple myeloma: what to use and when. Haematologica 2018; 103(11):1772–84.
15. Flores-Montero J, Sanoja-Flores L, Paiva B, et al. Next Generation Flow for highly sensitive and standardized detection of minimal residual disease in multiple myeloma. Leukemia 2017;31(10): 2094–103.
16. Furukawa Y, Kikuchi J. Molecular basis of clonal evolution in multiple myeloma. Int J Hematol 2020; 111(4):496–511.
17. Picken MM. The pathology of amyloidosis in classification: a review. Acta Haematol 2020;143(4): 322–34.
18. Wechalekar AD, Gillmore JD, Hawkins PN. Systemic amyloidosis. Lancet 2016;387(10038): 2641–54.
19. Wisniowski B, Wechalekar A. Confirming the diagnosis of amyloidosis. Acta Haematol 2020;143(4): 312–21.

20. Matnani R, Ganapathi KA, Lewis SK, et al. Indolent T- and NK-cell lymphoproliferative disorders of the gastrointestinal tract: a review and update. Hematol Oncol 2017;35(1):3–16.

21. Küçük C, Wei L, You H. Indolent T-Cell lymphoproliferative disease of the gi tract: insights for better diagnosis, prognosis, and appropriate therapy. Front Oncol 2020;10:1276.

22. Sharma A, Oishi N, Boddicker RL, et al. Recurrent. Blood 2018;131(20):2262–6.

23. Perry AM, Bailey NG, Bonnett M, et al. Disease progression in a patient with indolent T-cell lymphoproliferative disease of the gastrointestinal tract. Int J Surg Pathol 2019;27(1):102–7.

24. Al Somali Z, Hamadani M, Kharfan-Dabaja M, et al. Enteropathy-associated T cell lymphoma. Curr Hematol Malig Rep 2021;16(2):140–7.

25. Nishimura MF, Nishimura Y, Nishikori A, et al. Primary gastrointestinal T-cell lymphoma and indolent lymphoproliferative disorders: practical diagnostic and treatment approaches. Cancers 2021;13(22). https://doi.org/10.3390/cancers13225774.

26. Soderquist CR, Bhagat G. Gastrointestinal T- and NK-cell lymphomas and indolent lymphoproliferative disorders. Semin Diagn Pathol 2020;37(1):11–23.

27. Chander U, Leeman-Neill RJ, Bhagat G. Pathogenesis of enteropathy-associated T cell lymphoma. Curr Hematol Malig Rep 2018;13(4):308–17.

28. Ondrejka S, Jagadeesh D. Enteropathy-associated T-cell lymphoma. Curr Hematol Malig Rep 2016; 11(6):504–13.

29. Moffitt AB, Ondrejka SL, McKinney M, et al. Enteropathy-associated T cell lymphoma subtypes are characterized by loss of function of SETD2. J Exp Med 2017;214(5):1371–86.

30. Veloza L, Cavalieri D, Missiaglia E, et al. Monomorphic epitheliotropic intestinal T-cell lymphoma comprises morphologic and genomic heterogeneity impacting outcome. Haematologica 2023;108(1):181–95.

31. Tomita S, Kikuti YY, Carreras J, et al. Monomorphic Epitheliotropic Intestinal T-Cell Lymphoma in Asia Frequently Shows. Cancers 2020;12(12). https://doi.org/10.3390/cancers12123539.

32. Yabe M, Miranda RN, Medeiros LJ. Hepatosplenic T-cell Lymphoma: a review of clinicopathologic features, pathogenesis, and prognostic factors. Hum Pathol 2018;74:5–16.

33. de Mel S, Hue SS, Jeyasekharan AD, et al. Molecular pathogenic pathways in extranodal NK/T cell lymphoma. J Hematol Oncol 2019;12(1):33.

Gastrointestinal Biopsies in the Patient Post-Stem Cell Transplant
An Approach to Diagnosis

Tao Zhang, MD, Catherine E. Hagen, MD*

KEYWORDS

- Stem cell transplantation • Graft-versus-host disease • Gastrointestinal pathology • Apoptosis

---

Key points

- Gastrointestinal (GI) graft-versus-host disease (GVHD) is a pauci-inflammatory process histologically characterized by crypt apoptosis.
- Apoptosis in the GI tract is nonspecific and can also be seen with drug-induced injury and infection.
- Identifying significant inflammation (eosinophilic or neutrophilic) can be a histologic clue to underlying medication-related injury.
- GI biopsies from stem cell transplantation patients should be assessed for infectious organisms, particularly cytomegalovirus.
- Distinguishing GVHD for other entities in the differential diagnosis is important for clinical management.

ABSTRACT

Graft-versus-host disease (GVHD) is a major complication of hematopoietic stem cell transplantation (SCT), leading to a significant morbidity and mortality. Histologically, gastrointestinal GVHD is characterized by crypt apoptosis and dropout. However, similar histologic features can also be seen in drug-induced injury and opportunistic infection. Knowledge of the timing of biopsy, patient medications, evidence of infection, and presence of GVHD at other organ sites can aid in the correct diagnosis and subsequent management of these patients. This review focuses on the pathologic differential diagnosis of apoptosis in gastrointestinal biopsies obtained from SCT patients.

OVERVIEW

Hematopoietic stem cell transplantation (SCT) encompasses a series of procedures in which patients with various acquired or inherited malignant and nonmalignant disorders of the bone marrow are treated with chemotherapy and/or radiation therapy, followed by the infusion of hematopoietic stem/progenitor cells to reestablish marrow and immune function.[1] SCT can be lifesaving; unfortunately, it is also associated with substantial morbidity and mortality. Graft-versus-host disease (GVHD), a disease in which donor lymphocytes recognize host antigens as foreign resulting in tissue destruction, is considered one of the most severe and difficult to treat complications.[2]

Department of Laboratory Medicine and Pathology, Mayo Clinic, 200 1st Street Southwest, Rochester, MN 55905, USA
* Corresponding author.
E-mail address: hagen.catherine@mayo.edu

Surgical Pathology 16 (2023) 745–753
https://doi.org/10.1016/j.path.2023.05.009
1875-9181/23/

The gastrointestinal (GI) tract is one of the most common sites affected by GVHD, second only to the skin.[3] Histologic diagnosis of GI GVHD is challenging for many reasons including lack of consensus for the lower diagnostic threshold, nonspecific histologic features that raise a broad differential diagnosis, and lack of a gold standard for diagnosis. Furthermore, the diagnosis of GVHD comes with high clinical stakes, requiring increased immunosuppression for resolution, but increased immunosuppression is not without its own risks, namely infection. In this review, the authors present an overview of histopathologic evaluation of GI biopsies in patients status post SCT with a focus on GVHD and its differential diagnosis.

CLINICAL AND ENDOSCOPIC FEATURES

Acute GVHD is a consequence of alloreactive donor T cells and cytokine effectors leading to host tissue damage. In short, donor T cells recognize recipient human leukocyte antigen (HLA) complexes as foreign which leads to T-cell activation. The T-cell activation results in cytokine and inflammatory effectors which result in direct tissue damage and consequently the symptoms of GVHD. Within the GI tract, damage of the intestine results in translocation of microbial products such as lipopolysaccharide which creates a positive feedback loop that potentiates the tissue injury. Chronic GVHD is less well-understood but typically involves aberrant tissue repair with resulting fibrosis.[4,5]

Diagnosis of GI GVHD requires clinical, endoscopic, and histologic correlation. GVHD occurs primarily in allogeneic stem cell transplant patients but may rarely occur in autologous stem cell transplant patients or solid organ transplant recipients. GVHD has been historically divided into acute and chronic disease based on the time elapsed between the transplantation and symptom onset (<100 days vs >100 days, respectively).[6] Currently, patients with GVHD are subclassified into classic acute GVHD, persistent, recurrent, or late-onset acute GVHD, classic chronic GVHD, and overlap syndrome based on the timing of presentation and clinical features. Classification into these categories is based solely on clinical criteria as there are no histologic features specific for chronic GVHD in the GI tract.[7]

Symptoms of GI GVHD include anorexia, nausea, vomiting, diarrhea, weight loss, and failure to thrive.[8] Endoscopic findings are nonspecific and vary from subtle mucosal erythema and edema to frank ulceration and mucosal sloughing.[9,10] Commonly both the upper and lower GI tract are involved and therefore upper and lower endoscopy with biopsy may be indicated.[11,12] Not uncommonly endoscopic findings and histologic findings are discrepant, likely owing to biopsy sampling error, in which case diagnosis may be made based solely on the endoscopic and clinical features.[7]

MICROSCOPIC FEATURES AND HISTOLOGIC DIAGNOSIS

The histologic hallmark of GI GVHD is epithelial cell apoptosis, involving intestinal crypts in the small bowel and colon and gastric pits in the stomach. In the squamous-lined esophagus histologic features may include basal vacuolization, apoptosis, or dyskeratotic cells (**Fig. 1**).[13] In mild cases, biopsies may only show scattered apoptotic bodies, but in more severe cases, apoptotic microabscesses, hypereosinophilic crypts, crypt loss, and ulceration may be seen.[4,7] Only sparse inflammation is typically present. Grading of GVHD is not required, and utilization of grading systems usually varies based on institutional preferences. The Lerner system is the most widely used grading system but does not correlate well with patient outcome (particularly low-grade disease) and therefore provides limited clinical utility (**Table 1**).[7,14] Newer grading systems have been proposed that use quantification of apoptotic bodies or a combined grading system scoring apoptotic counts and crypt damage independently. However, these systems have not been widely adopted.[15,16]

The lower diagnostic threshold for GI GVHD remains debated. Rare crypt apoptosis may be seen in normal GI biopsies, and apoptosis is not specific for GVHD, most notably being seen in other diagnoses such as infection and drug-induced injury.[17] Varying thresholds have a tradeoff of sensitivity and specificity. The Lerner system considers the presence of a single apoptotic body sufficient for diagnosis of GVHD.[14] Although cases with rare apoptosis may represent GVHD, more recent studies have shown that patients with rare apoptosis on biopsy may symptomatically resolve without treatment, suggesting rare apoptosis is not sufficient for a diagnosis of GVHD. The 2014 National institutes of Health (NIH) consensus guidelines recommend ≥1 apoptosis per biopsy fragment.[7] Other authors have suggested using a cutoff of greater than 6 apoptotic bodies per 10 contiguous crypts with cases having ≤6 apoptotic bodies per 10 contiguous crypts being classified as "indeterminate for GVHD (iGVHD)." Utilization of this terminology alerts clinicians to the presence of minimal crypt apoptosis, allowing them to treat based on clinical judgment.[18–20] It is also worth

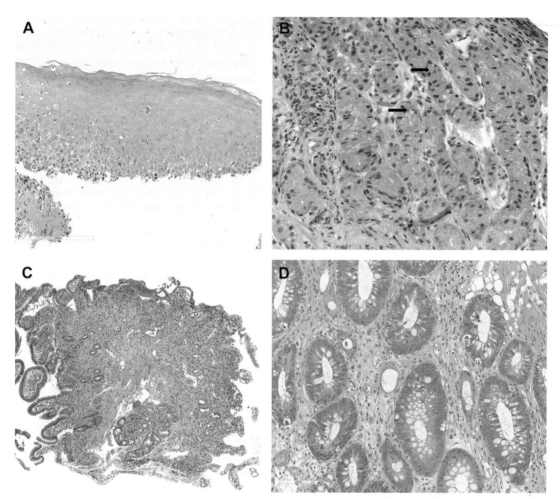

Fig. 1. GVHD involving different organ sites within the tubal GI tract. An esophageal biopsy showing basal lymphocytosis and scattered dyskeratotic cells (*A*). Gastric biopsy showing sparse inflammation and rare pit apoptosis (*arrows*) (*B*). Duodenal biopsy with contiguous crypt dropout and ulceration (Lerner grade 4) (*C*). Colonic biopsy with abundant crypt apoptosis and eosinophilic crypts with crypt dropout (*D*).

noting that the same diagnostic threshold may not be applicable to all sites within the GI tract. Most of the above criteria are based on colonic biopsies. Pit apoptosis in the stomach tends to be less conspicuous than in the small bowel or colon. At least one study has suggested a lower diagnostic threshold of ≥1 apoptotic body per biopsy fragment and at least one focus of ≥ 2 apoptotic bodies per 10 contiguous pits for the stomach.[21] Studies addressing the diagnostic threshold in the esophagus are largely lacking.

To help standardize the diagnosis of GI GVHD, the NIH consensus Project on Criteria for Clinical Trials in Chronic GHVD Pathology Working Group (2014) published guidelines for pathologic reporting of GVHD. The guidelines include three diagnostic categories: not GVHD, possible GVHD, and likely GVHD.[7] The Mount Sinai Acute GVHD International Consortium has also proposed pathologic reporting criteria for GI GVHD with categories including negative, equivocal, positive, and nondiagnostic.[22] The full definition of each

Table 1	
Modified grading system for acute graft-versus-host disease described by Lerner	
Grade 1	Isolated apoptotic epithelial cells, without crypt loss
Grade 2	Loss of isolated crypts, without loss of contiguous crypts
Grade 3	Loss of two or more contiguous crypts
Grade 4	Extensive crypt loss with mucosal denudation

category for of the above guidelines are listed in **Table 2.**

DIFFERENTIAL DIAGNOSIS

Apoptosis is a common pattern of injury within the GI tract of patients who have undergone SCT. The differential diagnosis is broad and includes drug-induced injury and opportunistic infections (**Table 3**). This can be problematic as SCT patients are often immunosuppressed, putting them at risk for infection, and are exposed to several medications for prophylaxis and treatment. Furthermore, some patients can have more than one coexisting diagnosis. A diagnostic algorithm for GI biopsies obtained to rule out GVHD is provided in **Fig. 2.**

CONDITIONING CHEMORADIATION THERAPY

It is well known that the cytotoxic effect of conditioning chemotherapy and total body irradiation can cause changes indistinguishable from GVHD. Typically, these findings are most prominent in the first 3 weeks following SCT and resolve by 21 days posttransplantation. Histologic changes include crypt apoptosis, increased mitotic activity, and regenerative eosinophilic crypts with nuclear atypia. Many authors advise against making a definitive diagnosis of GVHD on GI biopsies performed less than 21 days posttransplantation.

Exceptions to this rule would include autologous stem cell transplant patients and patients with biopsies showing abundant apoptosis close to the 21-day mark.[23] Compared with allogeneic SCT patients, autologous SCT are more likely to undergo early biopsy (median 20 days vs 87 days), and they lack the numerical T-cell attenuation that is usually seen in allogeneic patients early posttransplant. Therefore, diagnosis of early GVHD in allogeneic patients seems reasonable.[24] As noted above, the effects of chemoradiation tend to taper down by 21 days posttransplant, so presence of severe histologic injury at this timepoint likely indicates GVHD.[25]

MEDICATIONS

Mycophenolate is an immunosuppressive agent used predominantly in solid organ transplant patients but is also occasionally used as GVHD prophylaxis in a subset of SCT, particularly those that have undergone reduced intensity conditioning regimens.[26,27] Mycophenolate is well-known to cause GI toxicity which can manifest in various histologic patterns, including a GVHD-like pattern with increased apoptosis.[28] Although theoretically patients receiving mycophenolate as GVHD prophylaxis are at risk for developing both GVHD and mycophenolate toxicity, in reality, mycophenolate

Table 2
Comparison of NIH and Mount Sinai diagnostic categories

NIH Category	Definition	Mount Sinai Category	Definition
Not GVHD	No evidence for GVHD	Negative	Unequivocal evidence of diagnosis other than GVHD
Possible GVHD	Evidence of GVHD but other possible explanations	Equivocal	Findings are consistent with GVHD or other etiologies but pathologist cannot definitively confirm diagnosis of GVHD
Likely GVHD	Clear evidence of GVHD without a competing cause of injury OR clear evidence of GVHD with mitigating factors OR GVHD most likely diagnosis but relevant clinical information is limited OR GVHD is validated by sequential biopsy or by the absence of competing diagnosis	Positive	GVHD clearly identified on biopsy
		Nondiagnostic	Subtle changes that are insufficient to determine an etiology or insufficient tissue

Table 3
Distinguishing histologic features of the differential diagnosis

	Crypt Apoptosis	Eosinophilic or Neutrophilic Inflammation	Apoptotic Microabscesses	Lerner Grade 4 Disease with Neuroendocrine Aggregates	Viral Cytopathic Effect
GVHD	++	+/−	++	+	-
Drug-induced injury	+	++	+/−	-	-
Infection (CMV)	+	+/−	-	-	+

toxicity in SCT patients seems to be exceedingly rare. A search of our institutional archives yielded only one possible biopsy case of mycophenolate (MMF) toxicity in an SCT patient, and when pathologists at other large institutions were inquired, they likewise found rare or no cases (anecdotal evidence). Solid organ transplant patients are often on mycophenolate therapy indefinitely, whereas SCT patients often receive mycophenolate for a few months.[26,27] Although certainly mycophenolate toxicity can occur in SCT patients, GVHD is much more likely. Star and colleagues reported histologic features to distinguish GVHD from mycophenolate toxicity. Cases of mycophenolate toxicity are more likely to have increased lamina propria eosinophils, absence of neuroendocrine aggregates, and absence of apoptotic microabscesses (Fig. 3).[29] In our experience, lamina propria eosinophils are the

most important distinguishing histologic feature, but ultimately most cases require clinical correlation for distinction.[30]

Many medications not specifically used in the SCT setting can cause apoptosis within the GI tract. Proton-pump inhibitor (PPI) use is relatively ubiquitous both for treatment of gastroesophageal reflux and as a prophylactic agent for stress ulcers. PPI use has been shown to result in increased apoptosis within the gastric mucosa, particularly the antrum. However, the identification of apoptotic bodies within the gastric body or other sites along the GI tract would be in favor of GVHD.[31] Historically, oral sodium phosphate (NaP), an agent used in endoscopic preparatory regimens, was known to cause crypt apoptosis is some patients, possibly mimicking GVHD. However, NaP preparations are not currently available in the United States due to

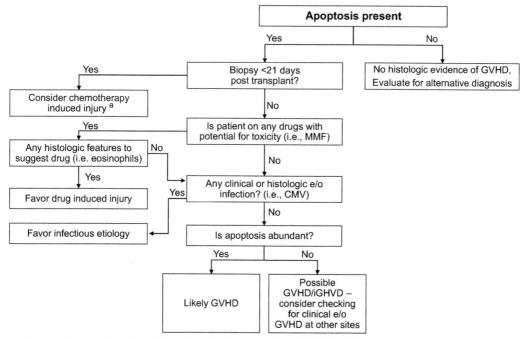

Fig. 2. Diagnostic algorithm for GI biopsies obtained to rule out GVHD. [a]Still consider GVHD, especially in autologous SCT patients or if abundant apoptosis & close to 21-day mark.

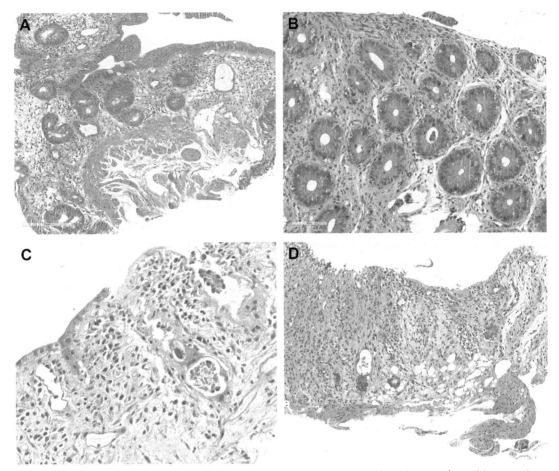

Fig. 3. Distinguishing features between GVHD and mycophenolate toxicity. The sole case of possible mycophenolate toxicity in an SCT patient from our archives. Crypt dropout is present, and eosinophils are prominent in the lamina propria (*A*). A case of GVHD with prominent eosinophilic inflammation, including an eosinophilic crypt abscess. The patient was not on mycophenolate and thus eosinophilic inflammation can sometimes be prominent in cases of GVHD (*B*). A case of GVHD with an apoptotic crypt abscess (*C*). A case of GVHD with Lerner grade 4 disease and residual neuroendocrine aggregates. This finding is likely a function of disease severity rather than a specific feature of GVHD (*D*).

reported renal complications and electrolyte abnormalities. Currently used bowel preparation agents (ie, polyethylene glycol [PEG] or magnesium citrate) may result in changes of the superficial epithelium (mucin loss and apoptosis) but do not lead to alterations of the crypts. Therefore, the histologic changes resulting from these agents usually do not complicate the diagnosis of GVHD.[32–34] Finally, several additional agents such as immune checkpoint inhibitors, tumor necrosis factor (TNF)-α inhibitors, and nonsteroidal anti-inflammatory drugs can result in increased crypt apoptosis. Noting significant acute inflammation or specific colitis patterns (ie, microscopic colitis pattern) can serve as histologic clues, and the review of the patient's medication list for known offending agents is prudent (Fig. 4).[35]

OPPORTUNISTIC INFECTIONS

Owing to their immunocompromised state, SCT patients are at risk for opportunistic infection. Cytomegalovirus (CMV) is the most common infection seen in this setting but other viral infections such as adenovirus can also occur. Histologically, viral infection can result in increased crypt apoptosis. The identification of viral inclusions, either on hematoxylin and eosinophil (H&E) stain or via immunohistochemistry, allows for definitive diagnosis. *Cryptosporidium* can also cause increased crypt apoptosis, mimicking GVHD. However, *cryptosporidium* infection is relatively uncommon in the SCT setting. Diagnosis can be made by identification of 2 to 5 μm basophilic spherules along the luminal GI tract border.[36–38]

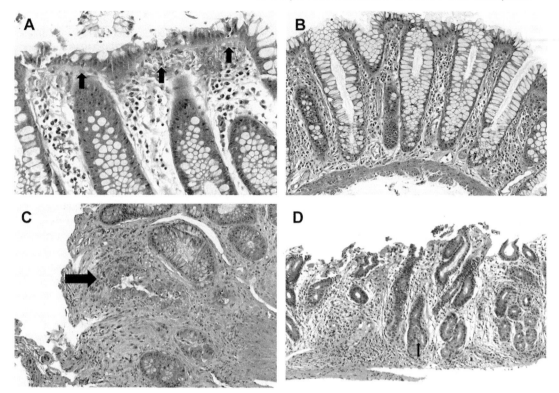

Fig. 4. Differential diagnosis of GVHD. Surface apoptosis (*arrows*) and regenerative changes in colonic mucosa are likely a result of colonoscopy preparatory agents and are not indicative of GVHD (*A*). A case of immune checkpoint inhibitor colitis showing abundant crypt apoptosis. Taken out of context, this could be interpreted as GVHD and thus knowing clinical history is essential (*B*). A case of CMV colitis. Crypt apoptosis is present but numerous endothelial viral inclusions (*arrow*) are present facilitating the correct diagnosis (*C*). Gastric biopsy showing active chronic gastritis and rare pit apoptosis (*arrow*). Although this may represent GVHD, the degree of inflammation is not typical and should raise consideration for infection or drug toxicity (*D*).

TREATMENT AND PROGNOSIS

Early mortality following SCT is most often related to underlying disease recurrence, whereas late mortality and morbidity are often related to GVHD. Up to 70% of SCT patients will develop acute GVHD. Those with severe disease have a poor overall survival (1 year overall survival approximately 30%) and those surviving the first year are likely to develop late comorbidities.[39] First-line therapy for GVHD consists of systemic corticosteroids. No standard guidelines exist for second-line therapy and several different agents can be used for steroid-refractory disease.[26,27] The distinction of GVHD from other diagnoses in the differential is crucial for clinical management. Drug toxicity often requires dose reduction or medication withdrawal, whereas infection requires antimicrobial therapy ± decreased immunosuppression.

SUMMARY

GVHD is a common complication in SCT patients histologically characterized by crypt apoptosis and

dropout. Common entities to consider in the differential diagnosis when assessing a GI biopsy for GVHD include chemotherapy-induced injury, medication effect, and infection. Biopsies containing abundant apoptosis with exclusion of other entities can confidently be diagnosed as GVHD. Biopsies containing rare apoptosis are not sufficient for a diagnosis of GVHD and are best classified as possible GVHD or iGVHD. Clinical knowledge of GVHD affecting other organ sites can be helpful when assessing biopsies with minimal histologic findings. Correctly diagnosing GVHD is imperative for clinical management and treatment.

CLINICS CARE POINTS

- Rare apoptosis in gastrointestinal biopsies may represent graft-versus-host disease (GVHD) but is not sufficient for a definitive diagnosis. Such cases are best signed out descriptively or classified as "indeterminate for GVHD."

- The timing of the biopsy posttransplantation is important to determine if histologic findings may be related to chemotherapy-induced injury.

- Eosinophilic or neutrophilic inflammation or specific patterns of colitis other than apoptosis can serve as clues to possible drug-induced injury.

- Infection, particularly CMV, should be excluded in biopsies from stem cell transplantation patients.

- Knowledge of GVHD affecting other organ sites can be helpful clinical information, especially in histologically subtle cases.

DISCLOSURE

The authors have nothing to disclose.

REFERENCES

1. Gratwohl A, Baldomero H, Aljurf M, et al. Hematopoietic stem cell transplantation: a global perspective. JAMA 2010;303(16):1617–24.

2. Wong NACS. Gastrointestinal pathology in transplant patients. Histopathology 2015;66(4):467–79.

3. Mastaglio S, Stanghellini MTL, Bordignon C, et al. Progress and prospects: graft-versus-host disease. Gene Ther 2010;17(11):1309–17.

4. Washington K, Jagasia M. Pathology of graft-versus-host disease in the gastrointestinal tract. Hum Pathol 2009;40(7):909–17.

5. Ferrara JL, Deeg HJ. Graft-versus-host disease. N Engl J Med 1991;324(10):667–74.

6. Shulman HM, Sullivan KM, Weiden PL, et al. Chronic graft-versus-host syndrome in man. A long-term clinicopathologic study of 20 Seattle patients. Am J Med 1980;69(2):204–17.

7. Shulman HM, Cardona DM, Greenson JK, et al. NIH Consensus development project on criteria for clinical trials in chronic graft-versus-host disease: II. The 2014 Pathology Working Group Report. Biol Blood Marrow Transplant 2015;21(4):589–603.

8. Jagasia MH, Greinix HT, Arora M, et al. National Institutes of Health Consensus Development Project on Criteria for Clinical Trials in Chronic Graft-versus-Host Disease: I. The 2014 Diagnosis and Staging Working Group report. Biol Blood Marrow Transplant 2015;21(3):389–401.e1.

9. Ponec RJ, Hackman RC, McDonald GB. Endoscopic and histologic diagnosis of intestinal graft-versus-host disease after marrow transplantation. Gastrointest Endosc 1999;49(5):612–21.

10. Altun R, Gökmen A, Tek İ, et al. Endoscopic evaluation of acute intestinal graft-versus-host disease after allogeneic hematopoietic cell transplantation. Turk J Gastroenterol 2016;27(4):312–6.

11. Daniel F, Hassoun L, Husni M, et al. Site specific diagnostic yield of endoscopic biopsies in Gastrointestinal Graft-versus-Host Disease: A tertiary care Center experience. Curr Res Transl Med 2019;67(1):16–9.

12. Ross WA, Ghosh S, Dekovich AA, et al. Endoscopic biopsy diagnosis of acute gastrointestinal graft-versus-host disease: rectosigmoid biopsies are more sensitive than upper gastrointestinal biopsies. Am J Gastroenterol 2008;103(4):982–9.

13. Kamboj AK, Agarwal S, Yarlagadda MK, et al. Clinical, Endoscopic, and Histopathology Features of Esophageal Graft-vs-Host Disease. Am J Gastroenterol 2022;117(7):1154–7.

14. Lerner KG, Kao GF, Storb R, et al. Histopathology of graft vs. host reaction (GvHR) in human recipients of marrow from HL A matched sibling donors. Transplant Proc 1974;6(4):367–71.

15. Farooq A, González IA, Byrnes K, et al. Multi-institutional development and validation of a novel histologic grading system for colonic graft-versus-host disease. Mod Pathol 2022;35(9):1254–61.

16. Myerson D, Steinbach G, Gooley TA, et al. Graft-versus-Host Disease of the Gut: A Histologic Activity Grading System and Validation. Biol Blood Marrow Transplant 2017;23(9):1573–9.

17. Nguyen T, Park JY, Scudiere JR, et al. Mycophenolic acid (cellcept and myofortic) induced injury of the upper GI tract. Am J Surg Pathol 2009;33(9):1355–63.

18. Lin J, Fan R, Zhao Z, et al. Is the presence of 6 or fewer crypt apoptotic bodies sufficient for diagnosis of graft versus host disease? A decade of experience at a single institution. Am J Surg Pathol 2013;37(4):539–47.

19. Rowan DJ, Hartley CP, Carrillo-Polanco LF, et al. Diagnostic phrasing is independently correlated with the decision to treat for graft-versus-host disease: retrospective review of colon biopsies with rare apoptosis. Histopathology 2016;69(5):802–11.

20. Gomez AJ, Arai S, Higgins JP, et al. Clinicopathologic Threshold of Acute Colorectal Graft-versus-Host Disease. Arch Pathol Lab Med 2016;140(6):570–7.

21. Mostafa M, Hartley CP, Hagen CE. Evaluation of the lower histologic threshold for gastric graft versus host disease. Mod Pathol 2020;33(5):962–70.

22. Harris AC, Young R, Devine S, et al. International, Multicenter Standardization of Acute Graft-versus-Host Disease Clinical Data Collection: A Report from the Mount Sinai Acute GVHD International Consortium. Biol Blood Marrow Transplant 2016;22(1):4–10.

23. Zubkova SM. [Mechanism of biological effect of helium-neon laser irradiation]. Nauchnye Dokl Vysshei Shkoly Biol Nauki 1978;7:30–7.

24. Hartley CP, Carrillo-Polanco LF, Rowan DJ, et al. Colonic graft-vs.-host disease in autologous versus allogeneic transplant patients: earlier onset, more apoptosis, and lack of regulatory T-cell attenuation. Mod Pathol 2018;31(10):1619–26.

25. Epstein RJ, McDonald GB, Sale GE, et al. The diagnostic accuracy of the rectal biopsy in acute graft-versus-host disease: a prospective study of thirteen patients. Gastroenterology 1980;78(4):764–71.

26. Penack O, Marchetti M, Ruutu T, et al. Prophylaxis and management of graft versus host disease after stem-cell transplantation for haematological malignancies: updated consensus recommendations of the European Society for Blood and Marrow Transplantation. Lancet Haematol 2020;7(2):e157–67.

27. Ruutu T, Gratwohl A, de Witte T, et al. Prophylaxis and treatment of GVHD: EBMT-ELN working group recommendations for a standardized practice. Bone Marrow Transplant 2014;49(2):168–73.

28. Selbst MK, Ahrens WA, Robert ME, et al. Spectrum of histologic changes in colonic biopsies in patients treated with mycophenolate mofetil. Mod Pathol 2009;22(6):737–43.

29. Star KV, Ho VT, Wang HH, et al. Histologic features in colon biopsies can discriminate mycophenolate from GVHD-induced colitis. Am J Surg Pathol 2013;37(9):1319–28.

30. Abstracts from USCAP 2021: Gastrointestinal Pathology (311-404). Mod Pathol 2021;34(2):501–620.

31. Welch DC, Wirth PS, Goldenring JR, et al. Gastric Graft-Versus-Host Disease Revisited: Does Proton Pump Inhibitor Therapy Affect Endoscopic Gastric Biopsy Interpretation? Am J Surg Pathol 2006; 30(4):444–9.

32. Driman DK, Preiksaitis HG. Colorectal inflammation and increased cell proliferation associated with oral sodium phosphate bowel preparation solution. Hum Pathol 1998;29(9):972–8.

33. ASGE Standards of Practice Committee, Saltzman JR, Cash BD, et al. Bowel preparation before colonoscopy. Gastrointest Endosc 2015; 81(4):781–94.

34. Pockros PJ, Foroozan P. Golytely lavage versus a standard colonoscopy preparation. Effect on normal colonic mucosal histology. Gastroenterology 1985; 88(2):545–8.

35. Marginean EC. The Ever-Changing Landscape of Drug-Induced Injury of the Lower Gastrointestinal Tract. Arch Pathol Lab Med 2016;140(8):748–58.

36. Weidner AS, Panarelli NC, Rennert H, et al. Immunohistochemistry Improves the Detection of Adenovirus in Gastrointestinal Biopsy Specimens From Hematopoietic Stem Cell Transplant Recipients. Am J Clin Pathol 2016;146(5):627–31.

37. Baniak N, Kanthan R. Cytomegalovirus Colitis: An Uncommon Mimicker of Common Colitides. Arch Pathol Lab Med 2016;140(8):854–8.

38. Lumadue JA, Manabe YC, Moore RD, et al. A clinicopathologic analysis of AIDS-related cryptosporidiosis. AIDS Lond Engl 1998;12(18):2459–66.

39. Rashid N, Krakow EF, Yeh AC, et al. Late Effects of Severe Acute Graft-versus-Host Disease on Quality of Life, Medical Comorbidities, and Survival. Transplant Cell Ther 2022;28(12):844.e1–8.

Mast Cell Disorders of the Gastrointestinal Tract
Clarity out of Chaos

Nicole C. Panarelli, MD

KEYWORDS

- Mast cells • Systemic mastocytosis • Irritable bowel syndrome • Mast cell enterocolitis
- Mast cell activation syndrome

Key points

- KIT and CD25 immunostains can aid evaluation of patients with suspected gastrointestinal involvement by systemic mastocytosis.

- Mast cells are likely involved in the pathogenesis of irritable bowel syndrome, but mast cell counts and immunostains for their evaluation have no proven utility in this setting.

- Idiopathic mast cell activation syndrome is caused by aberrant release of mediators by morphologically and immunophenotypically normal mast cells.

- Aggregates of mast cells may be seen in gastrointestinal mucosae of patients with hereditary alpha-tryptasemia.

ABSTRACT

Pathologists are increasingly asked to evaluate mast cell infiltrates in the gastrointestinal tract when there is clinical concern for systemic mastocytosis or a variety of functional disorders, including irritable bowel syndrome and mast cell activation syndrome. Neoplastic mast cells have established quantitative, morphologic, and immunohistochemical features that facilitate their identification in gastrointestinal mucosal biopsies. Specific qualitative and quantitative findings are lacking for inflammatory mast cell–mediated disorders. This review covers histopathologic features of mast cell disorders that affect the gastrointestinal tract and offers practical guidance for their assessment in mucosal biopsies.

OVERVIEW

Release of mast cell mediators causes gastrointestinal symptoms, such as abdominal pain, nausea, vomiting, and diarrhea, in patients with neoplastic and nonneoplastic mast cell disorders. Criteria for the diagnosis of mast cell neoplasia, namely systemic mastocytosis and mast cell leukemia, include mast cell quantification, aberrant immunohistochemical profiles, and molecular features that are established by the World Health Organization.[1] Most other mast cell–mediated disorders feature phenotypically normal mast cells and lack other morphologic hallmarks. Although many groups report increased numbers of mucosal mast cells in samples from patients who experience gastrointestinal symptoms, there are no universally accepted ranges for baseline numbers of mucosal mast cells nor are there validated thresholds for abnormally high mast cell counts at gastrointestinal sites. A recent report from the American Academy of Allergy, Asthma, and Immunology Allergic Skin Diseases Community Work Group acknowledged that there is broad variability in reported mast cell densities in the published literature and extensive overlap between mast cell–mediated disorders and physiologic and reactive states.[2] Thus, establishment of meaningful diagnostic thresholds is not possible on the basis of available data. Pathologists may nonetheless be asked to perform mast cell counts and immunohistochemical stains for

---

Albert Einstein College of Medicine, 1300 Morris Park Avenue, Bronx, NY 10461, USA

Surgical Pathology 16 (2023) 755–764
https://doi.org/10.1016/j.path.2023.05.010

patients with suspected inflammatory disorders despite a lack of evidence supporting these practices.[2] This review covers the role of mast cells in neoplastic and nonneoplastic mast cell–related disorders that affect the gastrointestinal tract and provides practical guidance for their histologic and immunohistochemical evaluation.

MAST CELLS IN NORMAL GASTROINTESTINAL MUCOSAE

Mast cells are key to intestinal hemostasis and immunity. They release histamine and prostaglandins that regulate peristalsis and nociception. They also regulate epithelial and vascular permeability through release of proteases and proinflammatory cytokines.[3–5] Finally, they contain antimicrobial and antiparasitic proteins that help maintain the mucosal barrier. Submucosal and serosal mast cells produce tryptase, chymase, and carboxypeptidase, whereas mucosal mast cells only elaborate tryptase.[6]

Mast cells are oval with central hyperchromatic nuclei and faintly basophilic to clear cytoplasm in hematoxylin and eosin stains (Fig. 1A).[7] They are singly dispersed in the lamina propria and muscularis mucosae and inconspicuously admixed with other resident inflammatory cells. They label with immunohistochemical stains for tryptase, a protease component of their secretory granules, and show membranous and cytoplasmic staining for the transmembrane tyrosine kinase receptor, KIT (CD117) (Fig. 1B). KIT is positive in all mast cells, whereas tryptase stains may be negative in degranulated mast cells and show absent or faint staining in up to 5% of mastocytosis cases.[1,8] Neither stain is entirely mast cell–specific because tryptase labels some basophils, and both tryptase and CD117 stain immature myeloid leukemic cells.[9–11] Mast cells reportedly comprise 2% to 3% of resident lamina propria immune cells, but reported "normal" ranges are broad and highly discrepant in various studies.[2,12]

SYSTEMIC MASTOCYTOSIS IN THE GASTROINTESTINAL TRACT

Mastocytosis is a clonal mast cell proliferation that involves one or more organ systems. Cutaneous mastocytosis causes urticaria pigmentosa, telangiectasia macularis eruptiva perstans, or solitary mastocytomas. Systemic disease frequently involves the bone marrow, liver, and gastrointestinal tract and has indolent and aggressive forms. Patients with indolent disease develop skin lesions, symptoms related to mast cell degranulation, and hepatosplenomegaly. High tumor burden may produce malabsorption, portal hypertension, ascites, and hypersplenism in the aggressive form.[1] Systemic mastocytosis is diagnosed in the presence of one major and one minor or three minor criteria. The major criterion is the presence of aggregates of ≥15 mast cells at extracutaneous sites. Minor criteria include the following: coexpression of CD25 and/or CD2 by neoplastic mast cells, morphologic atypia of 25% of mast cells, activating point mutations in c-KIT codon D816V, and serum tryptase greater than 20 ng/mL. Of note, CD25 is preferred because CD2 immunostains also label T and natural killer cells and thus may be challenging to interpret.[13] Mast cell leukemia features neoplastic mast cell burden in the bone marrow of greater than 20%. Patients with concurrent hematologic neoplasms are designated to have systemic mastocytosis associated with hematologic non–mast cell lineage disease.

Patients with mastocytosis often experience gastrointestinal symptoms even in the absence

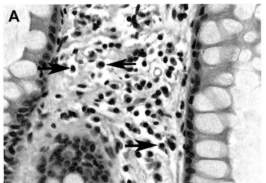
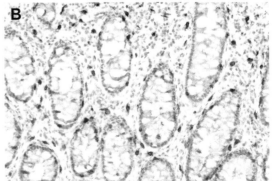

Fig. 1. Mast cells (*arrows*) are singly dispersed in the lamina propria and have hyperchromatic oval nuclei and granular cytoplasm (*A*). A KIT immunostain highlights their normal distribution throughout the lamina propria (*B*). (Original magnifications: 400x [*A*], 100x [*B*]; hematoxlin and eosin [*A*]; CD117 immunostain [*B*]).

of direct gastrointestinal involvement.[14] The true prevalence of gastrointestinal involvement is unknown because patients with established systemic disease rarely undergo endoscopy. Extramedullary mast cells in systemic mastocytosis are arranged in sheets or bandlike subepithelial aggregates and are often associated with numerous eosinophils (Fig. 2A). They have atypical morphology, including spindled contours and irregular or bilobed nuclei (Fig. 2B). Architectural changes, including villous blunting and irregular crypts, are often present in the small intestine.[15,16] Doyle and colleagues[17] reported that upper gastrointestinal biopsies from patients with systemic mastocytosis may show only scattered mast cell aggregates or singly dispersed mast cells with fewer eosinophils. In light of the fact that mast cell aggregates from patients with systemic mastocytosis may be subtle, obscured by eosinophils, or scant, it is reasonable to perform KIT (Fig. 2C) and CD25 (Fig. 2D) immunohistochemical stains to identify and characterize mast cell aggregates in patients with documented or suspected systemic mastocytosis. However, there

are very few indications to do so outside of this setting, as discussed subsequently.

Mast cell aggregates that meet criteria for systemic mastocytosis are occasionally detected incidentally in gastrointestinal mucosae of otherwise healthy patients. Shih and colleagues[16] encountered 2 such patients in a series of systemic mastocytosis, neither of whom developed symptoms during the follow-up interval of their study (2–3 years). Doyle and colleagues[17] reported that systemic mastocytosis was first diagnosed on the basis of gastrointestinal biopsies in 16 (67%) cases. The disease was aggressive for some patients with concurrent skin and/or bone marrow involvement, but those without extragastrointestinal disease experienced an indolent or asymptomatic course (follow-up: 12–312 months). Johncilla and colleagues[18] described 16 asymptomatic patients with colonic or duodenal mast cell aggregates, all of which showed diffuse aberrant expression of CD25, thus fulfilling criteria for systemic mastocytosis. Bone marrow biopsies, when performed, were normal, and all patients either remained asymptomatic or symptoms spontaneously

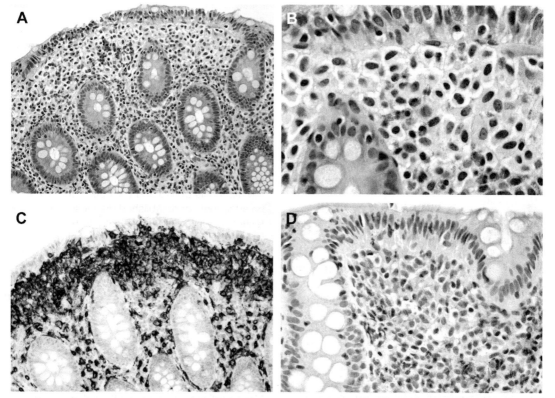

Fig. 2. In systemic mastocytosis, neoplastic mast cells display a bandlike distribution in the superficial lamina propria (*A*). The tumor cells show cytologic atypia, including spindled contours and binucleation (*B*). A KIT immunostain highlights dense mast cell aggregates (*C*). A proportion of the neoplastic mast cells aberrantly express CD25 (*D*). (Original magnifications: 100x [*A*], 200x [*B*], 400x [*B, D*]; hematoxylin and eosin [*A, B*], CD117 immunostain [*C*], CD25 immunostain [*D*]).

resolved during follow-up (range: 3–104 months). Although these patients meet existing criteria for indolent systemic mastocytosis, the collective findings of these studies imply that abnormal enterocolic mast cell aggregates may be clinically inconsequential in asymptomatic patients. Pathologists may consider more descriptive terms, such as "atypical mast cell aggregate," in order to prompt clinical follow-up, but avoid labeling otherwise healthy patients with malignant disease.

IRRITABLE BOWEL SYNDROME

Irritable bowel syndrome (IBS) is a functional disorder that causes recurrent abdominal pain and bowel habit disturbances (diarrhea and/or constipation) in the absence of structural or biochemical abnormalities.[19] The Rome IV criteria are clinical features used to identify patients with potential IBS. These include recurrent abdominal pain on average at least 1 d/wk for 3 months associated with at least two of the following: pain related to defecation, change in stool frequency, or change in stool form.[20] Patients may experience diarrhea-predominant, constipation-predominant, or alternating/mixed symptoms.[21] The pathogenesis of IBS is incompletely understood, but likely involves dysregulation of the enteric nervous system and mucosal immunity, as well as dysbiosis, psychosocial factors, and genetic susceptibility.[19] Most cases have no known cause, but association with prior infectious enterocolitis is reported in some. IBS is a substantial source of morbidity and health care cost in the United States.[22] Identification of diagnostic markers and therapeutic targets would be an important step toward improving quality of life for these patients.

MAST CELLS IN IRRITABLE BOWEL SYNDROME

Low-grade mucosal inflammation likely contributes to IBS development. In particular, aberrant release of mast cell mediators is implicated in increased intestinal permeability, visceral hypersensitivity, and smooth muscle contraction.[23] Spatial analyses reveal that mast cells may aggregate around nerves and plasma cells in IBS, whereas ultrastructural studies indicate that degranulated mast cells are more abundant in samples from patients with IBS.[24,25] Numerous studies purport to demonstrate elevated numbers of mast cells in small intestinal and colonic biopsies obtained from patients with IBS. A recent meta-analysis reported that mast cells in duodenal and jejunal mucosa do not differ significantly from controls, but mast cells are increased in the terminal ileum of patients with IBS.[26] For example, Di Nardo and colleagues[27] demonstrated

a marginally significant increase in mast cells/mm^2 in ileal mucosa of patients with IBS compared with controls using digital image analysis. On the other hand, mean ileal mast cell counts per 400× field (10–49) overlap substantially with controls (6–47) in other studies.[28–30] Another recent meta-analysis, including pooled data from 332 patients, showed that mean mast cell counts in the rectosigmoid colon were higher in IBS compared with controls, but ranges for the former (4–48/400× field) also overlapped with the latter (6–37/400× field).[28,31–35] On the other hand, several recent studies report similar numbers of colonic mucosal mast cells among patients with IBS and controls.[15,17,35–37]

MAST CELL COUNTS IN THE DIAGNOSIS OF IRRITABLE BOWEL SYNDROME

Numbers of mucosal mast cells vary widely among the aforementioned studies, despite the fact that most report an average derived from counting in multiple 400× fields. Possible explanations for these discrepancies include the use of different immunohistochemical stains to identify mast cells (tryptase vs KIT/CD117), reporting of peak versus mean mast cell counts, technical differences among laboratories, differences in the field dimensions of 400× objectives, and interobserver variability for manual mast cell counts. The extensive overlap among study patients and controls, both within cohorts and across different studies, implies that baseline mast cell counts may differ among individuals owing to environmental and genetic variables. This may partially explain why the prospective value of performing mast cell counts in individual patients has not yet been demonstrated. All studies reviewed here have included study patients who already met Rome criteria for the diagnosis of IBS and controls who have either no symptoms or established diagnoses of other intestinal disorders. Mast cell counts have not been used as a diagnostic tool to prospectively identify IBS. Although mast cells and their products likely contribute to the pathogenesis of IBS, the use of mast cell counts to diagnose and monitor disease likely oversimplifies complex relationships between mast cell mediators and other cell types.[24,27]

CORRELATION BETWEEN MAST CELL COUNTS AND SYMPTOMS IN PATIENTS WITH IRRITABLE BOWEL SYNDROME

Most studies that examined the link between mast cell numbers and IBS symptoms fail to support a correlation. For example, Ahn and colleagues[32] counted mast cells in colonic biopsy samples from 83 patients with diarrhea-predominant inflammatory bowel syndrome (IBS-D), 49 with ulcerative colitis (UC), and 25 healthy controls. Mast cell numbers were highest in the UC group (mean: 34/400× field), followed by patients with IBS-D (mean: 19/400× field) compared with controls (mean: 7/400× field). Numbers of mast cells did not correlate with self-reported gastrointestinal symptoms, stool form and frequency, or quality of life in the IBS-D group. Sohn and colleagues[33] used digital image analysis to quantify tryptase-positive mast cells in IBS-D patients (10/400× field) versus controls (6/400× field) and also reported no association between these counts and symptoms of abdominal pain, bloating, flatulence, or stool frequency. Park and colleagues[28] also found a lack of correlation between mast cell counts and IBS symptoms or rectal hypersensitivity measured by barostat tests in a series of 18 patients.

CORRELATION BETWEEN MAST CELLS AND THERAPEUTIC RESPONSE

Potential therapies for IBS include mast cell stabilizers, antihistamines, anti-inflammatory agents, and opioid receptor agonists. Relatively few studies have correlated the efficacy of therapies with histopathology. Lobo and colleagues[38] examined mast cell counts, small bowel fluid tryptase levels, ultrastructural evidence of mast cell degranulation, and expression of proinflammatory genes in IBS-D patients who were (n = 18) and were not (n = 25) treated with the mast cell stabilizer, disodium cromoglycate compared with controls (n = 16). In biopsy samples taken after therapy or placebo, mast cell counts and degranulation did not differ across these 3 groups. On the other hand, tryptase levels and expression of some proinflammatory molecules (eg, TLR4, Ly96) were reduced to levels similar to controls in the treatment arm. Patients in the treated group also experienced reduced abdominal pain and decreased bowel movements. Klooker and colleagues[39] treated 29 patients with IBS and 22 healthy volunteers with the mast cell stabilizer, ketotifen. Although 20% of study patients reported symptom relief, baseline numbers of mast cells, histamine, or tryptase levels in gut biopsy supernatant were not predictive of treatment response. Corinaldesi and colleagues[40] reported that mesalazine therapy reduced numbers of mast cells in colonic mucosa of patients with IBS compared with placebo, and improved overall well-being of treated patients; however, there was no significant effect on stool frequency, bloating, or abdominal pain. A follow-up randomized control trial of mesalazine therapy failed to show superiority to placebo, further suggesting that reduction in mucosal mast cell numbers is not a meaningful indicator of therapeutic response and has limited utility for disease monitoring.[41]

MASTOCYTIC ENTEROCOLITIS

Some investigators consider intractable diarrhea with increased mucosal mast cells to represent a separate, but related subtype of IBS-D termed "mastocytic enterocolitis." Only 2 papers have described its pathologic features. Jakate and colleagues[42] used mast cell tryptase stains to quantify duodenal and colonic mucosal mast cells in 47 patients with intractable diarrhea of unknown cause, 50 healthy controls, and 63 patients with established diagnoses of microscopic colitis, inflammatory bowel disease, and gluten sensitivity. They reported that normal mucosae contained a mean of 13 mast cells per 400× field, whereas 33 study patients had greater than 20 mast cells per 400× field, representing an increase of greater than 2 standard deviations above the mean in controls. Twenty-two of these patients who received histamine receptor antagonists and/or mast cell stabilizers experienced reduced diarrhea. Akhavein and colleagues[43] performed KIT stains on samples from 24 patients with diarrhea, constipation, and delayed gastric emptying using 20 mast cells per 400× field as a threshold for abnormal levels. They report increased mast cells in gastric, small intestinal, and colonic mucosae, as well as elevated whole blood histamine levels in this cohort. Of note, the study did not include a control group or provide follow-up data on any patients. Limited available data suggest that mastocytic enterocolitis does not represent a distinct disorder, but likely a heterogeneous group of patients with IBS and other medication, infectious, and immune-related diarrhea, all of which may feature mildly increased mucosal mast cells.

MAST CELL ACTIVATION SYNDROME

Idiopathic mast cell activation syndrome (MCAS) describes patients who (1) experience symptoms related to mast cell activation (urticaria, flushing, pruritus, headache, abdominal cramping, diarrhea, vomiting, respiratory symptoms, and hypotension); (2) have elevated serum tryptase, histamine, and/or prostaglandin D_2; and (3) respond to therapy with histamine receptor blockers in the absence of other clonal (ie, mastocytosis) or nonclonal (ie, allergic or autoimmune) mast cell disorders.[44] Alvarez-Twose and colleagues[45] described 29 patients who met criteria for idiopathic MCAS. Although respiratory and cardiovascular symptoms dominated the clinical picture in that cohort, patients did reportedly experience nausea, vomiting, and diarrhea,

Table 1
Features of mast cell disorders in the gastrointestinal tract

Disorder	Diagnostic Criteria	Morphology and Distribution of Mast Cells in Gastrointestinal Mucosae	Recommended Pathology Workup for Gastrointestinal Biopsy Samples
Systemic mastocytosis	Major and one minor criterion or 3 minor criteria should be met Major criterion: extracutaneous aggregates of ≥15 mast cells Minor criteria: coexpression of CD2 and/or CD25, *c-KIT* D816V mutation, serum tryptase ≥20 ng/mL	Superficial or bandlike distribution of spindle or ovoid mast cells, some with bilobed nuclei or irregular nuclei Often numerous eosinophils	KIT, CD25, and CD2 immunostains indicated in the setting of clinically confirmed or suspected systemic mastocytosis
Irritable bowel syndrome	Rome IV criteria: Recurrent abdominal pain on average at least 1 d/wk for 3 mo associated with at least two of the following: pain related to defecation, change in stool frequency, or change in stool form	Normal	None
Mastocytic enterocolitis	Controversial entity, criteria not established	Normal	None
Idiopathic mast cell activation syndrome	Symptoms related to mast cell activation (urticaria, flushing, pruritus, headache, abdominal cramping, diarrhea, vomiting, respiratory symptoms, and hypotension), elevated serum tryptase, histamine, and/or prostaglandin D_2, respond to therapy with histamine receptor blockers in the absence of other clonal or nonclonal mast cell disorders	Normal	None
Monoclonal mast cell activation syndrome	Bone marrow mast cells with *c-KIT* D816V mutations ± aberrant expression of CD25, but failure to meet criteria for the diagnosis of systemic mastocytosis	Unknown	None

(continued on next page)

		Morphology and Distribution of Mast Cells in Gastrointestinal	Recommended Pathology Workup for Gastrointestinal Biopsy
Disorder	Diagnostic Criteria	Mucosae	Samples
Hereditary alpha-tryptasemia (HαT)	Increased *TPSAB1* copy number	Increased numbers of mast cells in clusters in the superficial lamina propria and submucosa	KIT stains for mast cell aggregates may be appropriate if clinical suspicion or genetic testing is positive for HαT

Table 1 (continued)

supporting the notion that aberrant release of mast cell mediators can cause intestinal dysfunction. Hamilton and colleagues[46] described 18 patients with idiopathic MCAS treated with anti–mast cell mediator therapy, all of whom experienced some degree of symptom regression. The mean numbers of mast cells in 10 patients who underwent endoscopic biopsies of the stomach (n = 7), duodenum (n = 7), left (n = 5) and right (n = 4) colon were similar to their previously published reference standards, as was their morphology and distribution.[15] Similarly, Doyle and colleagues[17] reported that peak mast cell counts in patients with MCAS (mean: 28; range: 14–48 per 400× field) were similar to controls (mean: 26; range: 11–55 per 400× field). Patients with MCAS who have abnormalities on complete blood count, unexplained osteoporosis, hepatomegaly, or splenomegaly may undergo bone marrow biopsy to evaluate for systemic mastocytosis.[47] Monoclonal mast cell activation syndrome (MMAS) is diagnosed when mast cell clonality is found in bone marrow biopsy specimens on the basis of *c-KIT* D816V mutations ± aberrant expression of CD25, in the absence of other criteria for systemic mastocytosis. MMAS is rare, and its diagnosis relies on bone marrow mast cell–enrichment techniques.[48] There is currently no role for gastrointestinal biopsy in the evaluation of idiopathic MCAS or MMAS.

HEREDITARY ALPHA-TRYPTASEMIA

TPSAB1 encodes serum tryptase-alpha/beta-1, which is highly expressed on mast cells. Patients with increased copy number of *TPSAB1* have a condition known as hereditary alpha-tryptasemia (HαT).[49] Some patients with HαT experience symptoms similar to MCAS; however, a recent survey indicated that a substantial proportion are asymptomatic.[50] The same group found an association between HαT and mastocytosis. Mucosal biopsy specimens from symptomatic patients

with HαT appear to have some morphologic hallmarks. Hamilton and colleagues[51] reported that duodenal biopsy samples from this group show significantly higher numbers of mast cells (median: 30/400× field) compared with idiopathic MCAS (median: 15/400× field) and controls (median: 15/400× field). Mast cells were also more likely to form clusters and be present in the superficial lamina propria and submucosa in the HαT group. These findings raise the possibility that increased mast cells or clusters of mast cells may help to identify patients with HαT and prompt appropriate genetic testing. On the other hand, all patients in this study were symptomatic and had documented increased *TPSAB1* copy number; thus, it is not clear whether these features would be helpful in prospectively identifying patients with HαT.

MAST CELLS IN OTHER DISORDERS

Increased mast cells are found in a variety of other inflammatory gastrointestinal disorders, such as eosinophilic esophagitis and eosinophilic gastroenteritis, but diagnostic features of those disease are well-established and do not rely on mast cell evaluation.[6,52] Mast cells are also involved in antibacterial, antifungal, and antiparasitic immunity.[53] Some evidence suggests that stress-induced mast cell degranulation contributes to IBD flares.[54] Mast cells also elaborate tryptases that promote fibroblast proliferation and collagen deposition.[55] Their accumulation in Crohn disease–related strictures may contribute to mural fibrosis in some cases.[56] Finally, some investigators suggest that mast cells contribute to IBS-like symptoms in patients with quiescent IBD, but there is minimal evidence for this claim.[57] Vivinus-Nebot and colleagues[57] reported similar mast cell counts in patients with quiescent Crohn disease and UC (12/400× field) and those with IBS (12/400× field), both significantly higher than in controls (6/400× field). On the other hand, mast cell counts did not differ among patients with IBD with and without IBS-like symptoms. A study by Fan and colleagues[58] also showed no difference in mast cell counts when patients with quiescent IBD were compared with those with IBS and controls. There is presently no role for enumerating mast cells in mucosal biopsy samples from patients with IBD nor is there any indication to use ancillary techniques for their detection.

SUMMARY

It is well-established that aberrant release of mast cell contents causes gastrointestinal symptoms in patients with neoplastic and nonneoplastic mast cell disorders (Table 1). Unfortunately, the role of gastrointestinal biopsy samples in their evaluation is quite narrow. Mast cell aggregates in patients with systemic mastocytosis are morphologically and immunophenotypically abnormal; thus, KIT and CD25 immunostains are indicated when systemic mastocytosis is established or suspected. Abnormal mast cell morphology and distribution may help to identify patients with HαT, but these features have not yet been prospectively evaluated in this rare situation. Conversely, there is currently no sound evidence to indicate that mast cell counts are useful in the diagnosis or monitoring of IBS. Similarly, MCAS features phenotypically normal mast cells in quantities that overlap substantially with controls. In the current era of resource-conscious and evidence-based medicine, pathologists should discourage the use of immunostains and mucosal mast cell counts to diagnose or monitor patients suspected to have IBS/mast cell enterocolitis or MCAS. The role of mucosal biopsies in these settings is limited to excluding other treatable disorders.

CLINICS CARE POINTS

- Abnormal-appearing mast cell aggregates with abberant immunophenotype may herald gastrointestinal involvement by systemic mastocystosis in the appropriate clinical context.

- There is no robust evidence for the use of mast cell counts in the gastroinestinal mucosae for the diagnosis or monitoring of patients with irritable bowel syndrome or mast cell activation syndrome.

- Mast cells in gastrointestinal biopsy specimens from some patients with hereditary alpha-tryptasemia have characteristic morphology and distribution, but the prospective value of these features has not been studied.

DISCLOSURE

The author has no relevant financial interests.

REFERENCES

1. Horny HP, Akin C, Arber DA, et al. Mastocytosis. In: Swerdlow SH, Campo E, Harris NL, et al, editors. WHO classification of tumours of haematopoietic and lymphoid tissues. Lyon (France): IARC Press; 2017. p. 61–9.
2. Zimmermann N, Abonia JP, Dreskin SC, et al. Developing a standardized approach for assessing mast cells and eosinophils on tissue biopsies: A Work Group Report of the AAAAI Allergic Skin Diseases Committee. J Allergy Clin Immunol 2021;148(4): 964–83.
3. Heib V, Becker M, Taube C, et al. Advances in the understanding of mast cell function. Br J Haematol 2008;142(5):683–94.
4. Krystel-Whittemore M, Dileepan KN, Wood JG, et al. A Multi-Functional Master Cell. Front Immunol 2015; 6:620.
5. Wouters MM, Vicario M, Santos J. The role of mast cells in functional GI disorders. Gut 2016;65(1): 155–68.
6. Hamilton MJ, Frei SM, Stevens RL. The multifaceted mast cell in inflammatory bowel disease. Inflamm Bowel Dis 2014;20(12):2364–78.
7. Ribatti D. The Staining of Mast Cells: A Historical Overview. Int Arch Allergy Immunol 2018;176(1):55–60.
8. Horny HP, Sotlar K, Valent P. Mastocytosis: immunophenotypical features of the transformed mast cells are unique among hematopoietic cells. Immunol Allergy Clin North Am 2014;34(2):315–21.
9. Sperr WR, Hauswirth AW, Valent P. Tryptase a novel biochemical marker of acute myeloid leukemia. Leuk Lymphoma 2002;43(12):2257–61.
10. Khafateh Y, Aqil B. Tryptase Positivity in Chronic Myeloid Leukemia With Marked Basophilia. Cureus 2020;12(8):e9577.
11. Ahmadi A, Poorfathollah AA, Aghaiipour M, et al. Diagnostic value of CD117 in differential diagnosis of acute leukemias. Tumour Biol 2014;35(7):6763–8.
12. Bischoff SC. Physiological and pathophysiological functions of intestinal mast cells. Semin Immunopathol 2009;31(2):185–205.
13. Reichard KK, Chen D, Pardanani A, et al. Morphologically occult systemic mastocytosis in bone marrow: clinicopathologic features and an algorithmic approach to diagnosis. Am J Clin Pathol 2015;144(3):493–502.
14. Jensen RT. Gastrointestinal abnormalities and involvement in systemic mastocytosis. Hematol Oncol Clin North Am 2000;14(3):579–623.
15. Hahn HP, Hornick JL. Immunoreactivity for CD25 in gastrointestinal mucosal mast cells is specific for

systemic mastocytosis. Am J Surg Pathol 2007; 31(11):1669–76.

16. Shih AR, Deshpande V, Ferry JA, et al. Clinicopathological characteristics of systemic mastocytosis in the intestine. Histopathology 2016;69(6):1021–7.

17. Doyle LA, Sepehr GJ, Hamilton MJ, et al. A clinicopathologic study of 24 cases of systemic mastocytosis involving the gastrointestinal tract and assessment of mucosal mast cell density in irritable bowel syndrome and asymptomatic patients. Am J Surg Pathol 2014;38(6):832–43.

18. Johncilla M, Jessurun J, Brown I, et al. Are Enterocolic Mucosal Mast Cell Aggregates Clinically Relevant in Patients Without Suspected or Established Systemic Mastocytosis? Am J Surg Pathol 2018; 42(10):1390–5.

19. Lacy BE, Pimentel M, Brenner DM, et al. ACG Clinical Guideline: Management of Irritable Bowel Syndrome. Am J Gastroentero 2021;116(1):17–44.

20. Mearin F, Lacy BE, Chang L, et al. Bowel Disorders. Gastroenterology 2016. https://doi.org/10.1053/j.gastro.2016.02.031.

21. Chadwick VS, Chen W, Shu D, et al. Activation of the mucosal immune system in irritable bowel syndrome. Gastroenterology 2002;122(7):1778–83.

22. Nyrop KA, Palsson OS, Levy RL, et al. Costs of health care for irritable bowel syndrome, chronic constipation, functional diarrhoea and functional abdominal pain. Aliment Pharmacol Ther 2007; 26(2):237–48.

23. Boeckxstaens GE. The Emerging Role of Mast Cells in Irritable Bowel Syndrome. Gastroenterol Hepatol (N Y) 2018;14(4):250–2.

24. Vicario M, Gonzalez-Castro AM, Martinez C, et al. Increased humoral immunity in the jejunum of diarrhoea-predominant irritable bowel syndrome associated with clinical manifestations. Gut 2015; 64(9):1379–88.

25. Barbara G, Stanghellini V, De Giorgio R, et al. Activated mast cells in proximity to colonic nerves correlate with abdominal pain in irritable bowel syndrome. Gastroenterology 2004;126(3):693–702.

26. Robles A, Perez Ingles D, Myneedu K, et al. Mast cells are increased in the small intestinal mucosa of patients with irritable bowel syndrome: A systematic review and meta-analysis. Neuro Gastroenterol Motil 2019;31(12):e13718.

27. Di Nardo G, Barbara G, Cucchiara S, et al. Neuroimmune interactions at different intestinal sites are related to abdominal pain symptoms in children with IBS. Neurogastroenterol Motil 2014;26(2):196–204.

28. Park JH, Rhee PL, Kim HS, et al. Mucosal mast cell counts correlate with visceral hypersensitivity in patients with diarrhea predominant irritable bowel syndrome. J Gastroenterol Hepatol 2006;21(1 Pt 1):71–8.

29. Wang SH, Dong L, Luo JY, et al. Decreased expression of serotonin in the jejunum and increased numbers of mast cells in the terminal ileum in patients with irritable bowel syndrome. World J Gastroenterol 2007;13(45):6041–7.

30. Wang LH, Fang XC, Pan GZ. Bacillary dysentery as a causative factor of irritable bowel syndrome and its pathogenesis. Gut 2004;53(8):1096–101.

31. Bashashati M, Moossavi S, Cremon C, et al. Colonic immune cells in irritable bowel syndrome: A systematic review and meta-analysis. Neurogastroenterol Motil 2018;30(1).

32. Ahn JY, Lee KH, Choi CH, et al. Colonic mucosal immune activity in irritable bowel syndrome: comparison with healthy controls and patients with ulcerative colitis. Dig Dis Sci 2014;59(5):1001–11.

33. Sohn W, Lee OY, Lee SP, et al. Mast cell number, substance P and vasoactive intestinal peptide in irritable bowel syndrome with diarrhea. Scand J Gastroenterol 2014;49(1):43–51.

34. Cenac N, Andrews CN, Holzhausen M, et al. Role for protease activity in visceral pain in irritable bowel syndrome. J Clin Investr 2007;117(3):636–47.

35. Lee H, Park JH, Park DI, et al. Mucosal mast cell count is associated with intestinal permeability in patients with diarrhea predominant irritable bowel syndrome. J Neurogastroenterol Motil 2013;19(2):244–50.

36. Chang L, Adeyemo M, Karagiannides I, et al. Serum and colonic mucosal immune markers in irritable bowel syndrome. Am J Gastroenterol 2012;107(2): 262–72.

37. El-Salhy M, Gundersen D, Hatlebakk JG, et al. Low-grade inflammation in the rectum of patients with sporadic irritable bowel syndrome. Mol Med Rep 2013;7(4):1081–5.

38. Lobo B, Ramos L, Martinez C, et al. Downregulation of mucosal mast cell activation and immune response in diarrhoea-irritable bowel syndrome by oral disodium cromoglycate: A pilot study. United European Gastroenterol J 2017;5(6):887–97.

39. Klooker TK, Braak B, Koopman KE, et al. The mast cell stabiliser ketotifen decreases visceral hypersensitivity and improves intestinal symptoms in patients with irritable bowel syndrome. Gut 2010;59(9): 1213–21.

40. Corinaldesi R, Stanghellini V, Cremon C, et al. Effect of mesalazine on mucosal immune biomarkers in irritable bowel syndrome: a randomized controlled proof-of-concept study. Aliment Pharmacol Ther 2009;30(3):245–52.

41. Barbara G, Cremon C, Annese V, et al. Randomised controlled trial of mesalazine in IBS. Gut 2016;65(1): 82–90.

42. Jakate S, Demeo M, John R, et al. Mastocytic enterocolitis: increased mucosal mast cells in chronic intractable diarrhea. Arch Pathol Lab Med 2006;130(3):362–7.

43. Akhavein MA, Patel NR, Muniyappa PK, et al. Allergic mastocytic gastroenteritis and colitis: an

unexplained etiology in chronic abdominal pain and gastrointestinal dysmotility. Gastroenterol Res Pract 2012;2012:950582.

44. Valent P, Akin C, Arock M, et al. Definitions, criteria and global classification of mast cell disorders with special reference to mast cell activation syndromes: a consensus proposal. Int Arch Allergy Immunol 2012;157(3):215–25.

45. Alvarez-Twose I, Gonzalez de Olano D, Sanchez-Munoz L, et al. Clinical, biological, and molecular characteristics of clonal mast cell disorders presenting with systemic mast cell activation symptoms. J Allergy Clin Immunol 2010;125(6):1269–1278 e2.

46. Hamilton MJ, Hornick JL, Akin C, et al. Mast cell activation syndrome: a newly recognized disorder with systemic clinical manifestations. J Allergy Clin Immunol 2011;128(1):147–152 e2.

47. Valent P, Akin C, Escribano L, et al. Standards and standardization in mastocytosis: consensus statements on diagnostics, treatment recommendations and response criteria. Eur J Clin Invest 2007;37(6):435–53.

48. Picard M, Giavina-Bianchi P, Mezzano V, et al. Expanding spectrum of mast cell activation disorders: monoclonal and idiopathic mast cell activation syndromes. Clin Ther 2013;35(5):548–62.

49. Lyons JJ, Chovanec J, O'Connell MP, et al. Heritable risk for severe anaphylaxis associated with increased alpha-tryptase-encoding germline copy number at TPSAB1. J Allergy Clin Immunol 2021;147(2):622–32.

50. Chollet MB, Akin C. Hereditary alpha tryptasemia is not associated with specific clinical phenotypes. J Allergy Clin Immunol 2022;149(2):728–735 e2.

51. Hamilton MJ, Zhao M, Giannetti MP, et al. Distinct Small Intestine Mast Cell Histologic Changes in Patients With Hereditary Alpha-tryptasemia and Mast Cell Activation Syndrome. Am J Surg Pathol 2021;45(7):997–1004.

52. Bolton SM, Kagalwalla AF, Arva NC, et al. Mast Cell Infiltration Is Associated With Persistent Symptoms and Endoscopic Abnormalities Despite Resolution of Eosinophilia in Pediatric Eosinophilic Esophagitis. Am J Gastroenterol 2020;115(2):224–33.

53. Jimenez M, Cervantes-Garcia D, Cordova-Davalos LE, et al. Responses of Mast Cells to Pathogens: Beneficial and Detrimental Roles. Front Immunol 2021;12:685865.

54. Boeckxstaens G. Mast cells and inflammatory bowel disease. Curr Opin Pharmacol 2015;25:45–9.

55. Douaiher J, Succar J, Lancerotto L, et al. Development of mast cells and importance of their tryptase and chymase serine proteases in inflammation and wound healing. Adv Immunol 2014;122:211–52.

56. Gelbmann CM, Mestermann S, Gross V, et al. Strictures in Crohn's disease are characterised by an accumulation of mast cells colocalised with laminin but not with fibronectin or vitronectin. Gut 1999;45(2):210–7.

57. Vivinus-Nebot M, Frin-Mathy G, Bzioueche H, et al. Functional bowel symptoms in quiescent inflammatory bowel diseases: role of epithelial barrier disruption and low-grade inflammation. Gut 2014;63(5):744–52.

58. Fan L, Wong M, Fan XS, et al. Quantitative Analysis of Intramucosal Mast Cells in Irritable Bowel Syndrome: A Comparison With Inflammatory Bowel Disease in Remission. J Clin Gastroenterol 2021;55(3):244–9.

A Practical Approach to Small Round Cell Tumors Involving the Gastrointestinal Tract and Abdomen

Khin Thway, MD, FRCPath[a,b,*],
Cyril Fisher, MD, DSc, FRCPath[b,c]

KEYWORDS

- *EWSR1* • *FUS* • *CIC* • *BCOR* • Sarcoma • Desmoplastic small round cell tumor • Ewing sarcoma
- Rhabdomyosarcoma

Key points

- Small round cell tumors are rare in the abdomen and gastrointestinal tract but include a range of sarcomas as well as carcinomas, lymphoma, and melanoma.

- Molecular investigation is increasingly required, so each core needle biopsy should be placed in a separate cassette to maximize the use of material.

- Desmoplastic small round cell tumor predilects for intra-abdominal locations and has a characteristic *EWSR1::WT1* fusion.

- Ewing sarcoma is the most common small round cell sarcoma.

- Many small round cell sarcomas have a polyphenotypic immunoprofile, with variable expression of CD99, keratins, and myoid and neuroendocrine markers, overlapping with other sarcomas and with small cell carcinomas and other non-mesenchymal tumors.

- Diagnosis requires awareness of the immunohistochemical spectra and expression patterns for these entities.

ABSTRACT

Small round cell neoplasms are diagnostically challenging owing to their clinical and pathologic overlap, necessitating use of large immunopanels and molecular analysis. Ewing sarcomas (ES) are the most common, but *EWSR1* is translocated in several diverse neoplasms, some with round cell morphology. Molecular advances enable classification of many tumors previously termed 'atypical ES'. The current WHO Classification includes two new undifferentiated round cell sarcomas (with *CIC* or *BCOR* alterations), and a group of sarcomas in which *EWSR1* partners with non-Ewing family transcription factor genes. This article reviews the spectrum of small round cell sarcomas within the gastrointestinal tract and abdomen.

OVERVIEW

Small round cell neoplasms are a group of genetically diverse, typically high-grade tumors

---

[a] Sarcoma Unit, Royal Marsden Hospital, London SW3 6JJ, UK; [b] Division of Molecular Pathology, The Institute of Cancer Research, London SW3 6JB, UK; [c] Department of Pathology, University Hospitals Birmingham NHS Foundation Trust, Birmingham B15 2GW, UK
* Corresponding author. Sarcoma Unit, The Royal Marsden NHS Foundation Trust, 203 Fulham Road, London SW3 6JJ, UK.
E-mail address: khin.thway@rmh.nhs.uk

Surgical Pathology 16 (2023) 765–778
https://doi.org/10.1016/j.path.2023.05.012
1875-9181/23/© 2023 Elsevier Inc. All rights reserved.

comprising small- to medium-sized cells with rounded nuclei and high nuclear:cytoplasmic ratios, generally in minimal stroma. Most small cell variants of epithelial, melanocytic, and hematolymphoid neoplasms can be discerned by clinical, histologic, and immunohistochemical correlation, but many small round cell tumors are undifferentiated without specific immunoprofiles, and are categorized as sarcomas, for which the prototype and commonest member of this group is Ewing sarcoma (ES). These tumors, frequently driven by defining pathogenic gene fusions, are becoming increasing well-defined. The current WHO Classification of Soft Tissue and Bone Tumors includes new entities of round cell sarcomas with capicua transcriptional repressor (CIC) rearrangements and BCOR-associated genetic alterations and also round cell sarcomas with EWSR1 fusions involving fusion partners that are not part of the erythroblast transformation specific (ETS) gene family (eg, PATZ1 and NFATC2). EWSR1 (the ES breakpoint region 1 gene) can fuse with many different genes to generate numerous clinically and histologically distinct neoplasms, or partner with the same gene to generate behaviorally and morphologically different tumors, with additional poorly understood molecular mechanisms of tumorigenesis.[1–3] Given the overlap in clinical presentation and morphologic and immunohistochemical findings between small round cell neoplasms, their diagnosis requires (1) clinicoradiologic correlation, including age group (pediatric, young adults, older adults); (2) use of a selected immunohistochemical panel; and (3) ancillary molecular investigation (eg, fluorescence in situ hybridization [FISH], reverse transcription-polymerase chain reaction [RT-PCR], next-generation sequencing [NGS]). This review discusses selected small round cell neoplasms that surgical pathologists can encounter within the gastrointestinal (GI) tract and abdomen, focusing on sarcomas.

SMALL ROUND CELL SARCOMAS WELL-DOCUMENTED TO OCCUR AS PRIMARY NEOPLASMS WITHIN ABDOMEN OR GASTROINTESTINAL TRACT

Desmoplastic Small Round Cell Tumor

This is a highly aggressive small round cell neoplasm characteristically occurring in the abdominal cavity (including retroperitoneum, pelvis, mesentery, and omentum,[4]) of adolescents and young adults, particularly males. Rarely, they occur in older adults or other sites,[5] including paratesticular and intrathoracic locations,[6] bowel, kidney, ovary,[7–11] and head and neck. Desmoplastic small round cell tumor (DSRCT) comprises

demarcated, angulated islands and nests of small cells with rounded nuclei, indiscernible nucleoli, and minimal cytoplasm (Fig. 1A–C), with mitotic activity and necrosis, within cellular desmoplastic stroma. Immunohistochemically, DSRCT is polyphenotypic, variably coexpressing desmin (see Fig. 1D, E) and markers of epithelial differentiation (epithelial membrane antigen [EMA] and keratins [see Fig. 1F]),[12] and neural markers (eg, neuron-specific enolase [NSE]). Approximately 65% to 90% show immunoreactivity to antibodies recognizing the Wilms tumor (WT1) protein carboxy terminus. Actin or S100 protein are variably expressed,[4,12] whereas CD99 is negative. Myogenin and MyoD1 are negative unlike in rhabdomyosarcoma (RMS). Antigen expression is variable and can be incomplete.

DSRCT is defined by a characteristic EWSR1::WT1 fusion,[13] of the WT1 gene with EWSR1, with the resultant chimeric transcription factor leading to gene dysregulation. The fusion is not wholly specific and is described in two pediatric intra-abdominal spindle cell tumors resembling leiomyosarcomas, but demonstrating favorable outcomes,[14] as well as in an indolent cauda equina low-grade small round cell tumor[15] expressing smooth muscle antigens and focal CD99.[15] Given the incipient lack of specificity of the EWSR1::WT1 fusion, it is mandatory to correlate this finding with the clinical and histopathologic picture. DSRCT may be solid with little stroma (see Fig. 1C), mimicking ES especially in biopsies. Because ES can arise intra-abdominally and show desmoplasia, RT-PCR or NGS to confirm EWSR1::WT1 fusion is required.

Ewing Sarcoma

This is an aggressive neoplasm of bone or soft tissues predominating in children and young adults.[16] Extraskeletal ES occurs in approximately 12% of patients,[17] favoring older patients (>30 years), with a wide anatomic distribution.[18] Primary ES is well-documented within the abdominopelvic cavity and retroperitoneum. Within the GI tract, there are greater than 30 cases arising in small intestine, most commonly ileum,[19,20] often involving the full bowel wall thickness and smaller numbers in the stomach (favoring antrum, lesser curvature, and posterior wall).[21,22] They present with pain, hemorrhage, or obstructive symptoms.[21] Rare visceral primary sites include liver, pancreas,[23] and genitourinary tract, especially kidney, and including bladder, ovary, and cervix.[24] As ES can show strong pankeratin expression, it can be mistaken for small cell or poorly differentiated carcinomas at these sites.

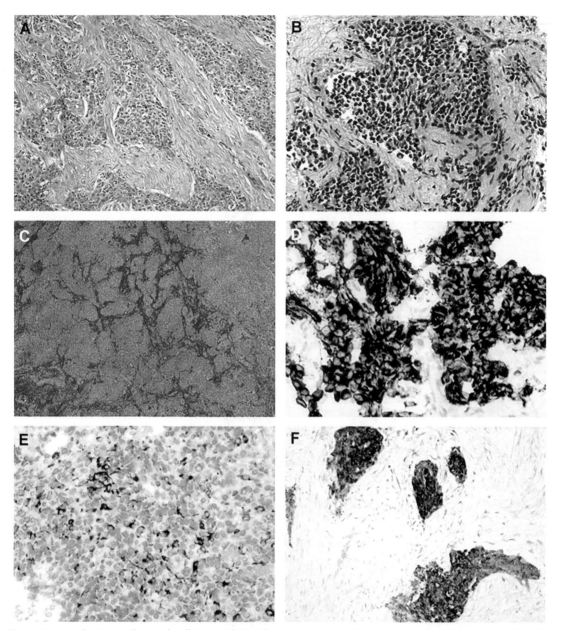

Fig. 1. Desmoplastic small round cell tumor (DSRCT) comprises angulated islands of uniform small cells with rounded nuclei (*A–C*), surrounded by desmoplastic collagenous stroma. It can show solid architecture (*C*), mimicking Ewing sarcoma. DSRCT coexpresses desmin (*D, E*) (often dot-like [*E*]) and markers of epithelial differentiation (AE1/AE3; *F*).

ES is defined by balanced translocations between *EWSR1* and genes encoding *ETS* family transcription factors (predominantly *FLI1* and *ERG*). Neural/neuroectodermal differentiation is not correlated with behavior. ES comprises sheets and nests of uniform small cells with rounded vesicular nuclei, sometimes small nucleoli, scanty amphophilic to clear (due to glycogen) cytoplasm, and minimal stroma

(Fig. 2A, B). There can be variable neural differentiation, with Homer Wright rosettes. Variants include large cell (atypical), clear cell, spindle cell, sclerosing, and adamantinoma-like (cytokeratin positive) ES. Greater than 90% show diffuse, strong membranous CD99 expression (see Fig. 2C), with ~65% displaying nuclear FLI1. Neural/neuroendocrine markers NSE, neurofilament, chromogranin, and synaptophysin are

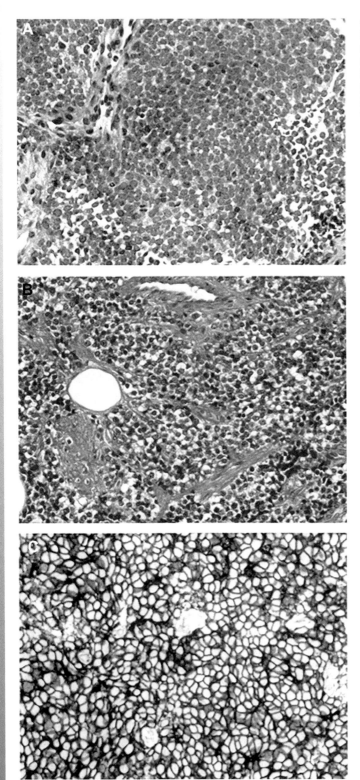

Fig. 2. Ewing sarcoma (ES). Sheets and nests of uniform small cells with rounded nuclei and scanty amphophilic (A) or clear (B) (due to glycogen) cytoplasm. Note the homogeneous morphology, with no atypia, and minimal intervening stroma. Diffuse strong membranous CD99 (C) is typical of ES (>90%).

variably positive. NKX2.2, a downstream target of EWSR1-ETS fusions, is a sensitive, not wholly specific marker.[25] ES associated with *ERG* rearrangement shows immunohistochemical nuclear ERG. There is variable positivity for S100 protein, cytokeratins (CK20 is negative), and CD117. Desmin expression is rare and myogenin always negative. *PAX7*, one of the most differentially expressed genes in ES compared with other small round cell sarcomas,[26,27] is expressed immunohistochemically in *EWSR1*-rearranged neoplasms with *FLI1*, *ERG,* and *NFATC2* partner genes.[28] CD56 and TLE1 are typically negative.

ESs are defined by translocations leading to EWSR1-ETS family fusion oncoproteins[29] (~85% *EWSR1::FLI1*[30]; 5%–10% *EWSR1::ERG*[31]). *EWSR1* is a member of the TET (translocated in liposarcoma [TLS]/fused in sarcoma [FUS], EWSR1, TATA-binding protein-associated factor 15 [TAF15]) (encompassing fused in sarcoma [FUS], EWSR1, and TAF15) family, a group of genes driving many translocation-associated neoplasms, with *FUS* and *EWSR1* functioning as alternative binding partners due to high homology. Oncogenesis involves numerous target genes, including *ERG*,[32] *cyclin D1,* and *NKX2.2.* Less than 1% contain non-*EWSR1::FLI1* or *EWSR1::ERG* fusions, harboring other TET-ETS fusions *EWSR1::ETV1/ETV4/FEV*,[33,34] or *FUS::ERG/FEV*[35] These usually display similar clinical, histologic, and immunohistochemical features. Round cell sarcomas in the differential diagnosis, discussed below, include *CIC*- and *BCOR*-associated undifferentiated round cell sarcomas (although the latter are extremely rare in the abdomen).[36] In contrast to the uniform features of ES, these show a range of appearances often containing myxoid foci and a spindle (or epithelioid) cell component. *CIC::DUX4* fusions are the most frequent genetic alterations in small round cell tumors lacking *EWSR1* fusions in pediatric and young adult populations,[37–40] whereas *BCOR*-associated tumors are rarer, accounting for ~5%.[41,42]

CIC-Rearranged Sarcomas

These are aggressive neoplasms with round and ovoid cell morphology, predilecting for young adults (median 25–35 years), with a wide age range (including <25% in the pediatric population).[43,44] Most arise within deep soft tissues of limbs or trunk, but can arise in retroperitoneum and pelvis. Approximately 10% present in viscera, including GI tract and kidney.[43,44] A minority (<5%) have primary osseous presentations, in contrast to ES.[44] *CIC*-rearranged sarcomas are markedly

aggressive with high metastatic potential, most frequently to lungs, and poor response to ES chemotherapeutic regimens,[44] with significantly worse overall survivals than ES.[43,44] They harbor *CIC* rearrangements, most frequently with *DUX4,* or *FOXO4, LEUTX, NUTM2A,* and *NUTM1,* with no described histologic differences between these.[45]

Histologically, these comprise monotonous sheets of predominantly rounded, small- to medium-sized cells, and often a smaller component of epithelioid to spindled cells, within fibromyxoid stroma (Fig. 3). In contrast to ES, *CIC*-rearranged sarcomas show at least focal mild atypia (see Fig. 3C) and small nucleoli, with small amounts of amphophilic or clear cytoplasm, mitoses, and necrosis. The stroma is sometimes focally myxoid (see Fig. 3C), unlike in ES. CD99 is frequently focally positive (see Fig. 3E), with a minority showing diffuse membranous expression.[44] The majority express ETV4 and WT1. ERG (see Fig. 3F), CD31, and calretinin are variably expressed,[43,46,47] and rarely there is positivity for cytokeratins, S100 protein, and myoid/myogenic markers. NKX2.2 is typically negative.[43] NUT protein is expressed by *CIC::NUTM1* sarcomas.[45] *CIC* rearrangement can be detected by FISH, RT-PCR, or NGS, although no technique has high sensitivity.

Poorly Differentiated Synovial Sarcoma

This rarer variant of synovial sarcoma (SS), occurs more frequently in older adults,[48] with a worse prognosis.[49] Subsets are described in the abdomen, pelvic cavity and retroperitoneum,[50] presenting as a mass or hemorrhage, in kidney, and sporadically in the GI tract and liver. Poorly differentiated synovial sarcoma (PDSS) typically comprises hypercellular sheets of cells with rounded hyperchromatic nuclei and small amounts of basophilic cytoplasm, mitoses, and necrosis (Fig. 4). Up to one-third of conventional SS may harbor poorly differentiated areas.[49] PDSS resembles other round cell neoplasms, though rarely demonstrating large cell epithelioid, and high-grade spindle cell morphology.[49] SS is defined by fusions of *SS18* (chromosome 18) with one of several *SSX* genes (usually *SSX1* or *SSX2*) (X chromosome). *SS18::SSX1/SSX2* are present in greater than 90%, generating *SS18-SSX* fusion oncogenes.

PDSS can closely mimic ES (see Fig. 4A, B). Greater than 90% of all SS focally express epithelial markers (keratin in ~40% of PDSS, most frequently AE1/AE3 or MNF116,[51] as well as CAM5.2, and sometimes high molecular weight

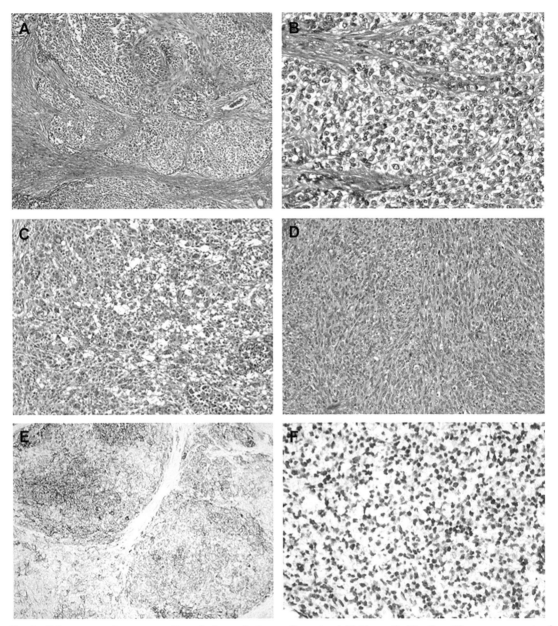

Fig. 3. *CIC*-rearranged sarcomas. Rounded, small- to medium-sized ES-like cells (*A*, *B*), with a component of epithelioid cells with focal atypia and myxoid stroma (*C*) or spindled cells (*D*). CD99 is often focal (*E*). The immunoprofile is nonspecific; this tumor shows diffuse nuclear ERG (*F*) (also seen in some ES).

keratins, and EMA up to 95%.[49]) (see **Fig. 4**D). EMA is sometimes the sole epithelial differentiation marker. Most express bcl-2, with variable CD99 (usually cytoplasmic) in ~60%, focal S100 protein (~40%), and rarely desmin, smooth muscle actin, and h-caldesmon.[52,53] TLE1 typically shows diffuse nuclear expression in greater than 90%[54–56] but has limited diagnostic specificity and is positive in spindle cell tumors in the differential diagnosis. CD34 is virtually always negative. AE1/AE3 is expressed in one-third of

ES, but these are negative for CK7 (positive in 50% of PDSS).[57] Nuclear FLI1, noted in ~70% of ES, is absent in PDSS.[58] Small round cell tumors are usually negative for TLE1, unlike PDSS. In the abdominal setting, it should be noted that focal cytoplasmic CD117 is seen in 11% of monophasic SS and 8% of PDSS,[53] and rarely weak or focal DOG1 expression is seen in SS. Recently, an *SSX18-SSX* fusion-specific antibody (E9X9V) showed positivity in 95% of SS; mimics were negative.[59]

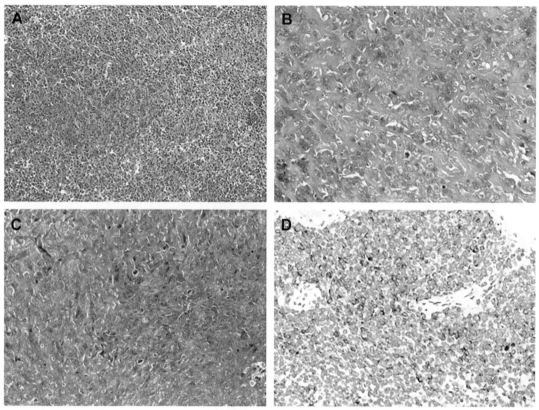

Fig. 4. Poorly differentiated synovial sarcoma (PDSS). Hypercellular sheets of cells with rounded nuclei and scanty cytoplasm (*A, B*), and frequently at least small areas of conventional SS (*C*). Greater than 90% of SS show variable epithelial marker expression (AE1/AE3 shown; *D*).

Rhabdomyosarcoma

Within the abdominopelvic cavity, embryonal RMS (ERMS) predominates, with ~50% occurring within the genitourinary tract (including bladder, prostate, vagina/vulva, cervix, and paratesticular soft tissues).[60,61] Rarer sites include abdomen, retroperitoneum, biliary tract, liver, and kidney. ERMS is the commonest RMS (~one-third arising in patients aged <5 years). The morphology is heterogeneous, frequently of fascicles of mildly and moderately atypical primitive ovoid to spindle cells (**Fig. 5**), in myxocollagenous stroma, with variable rhabdomyoblastic differentiation. ERMS shows variable desmin, and more focal myogenin and MyoD1. There is no specific molecular test; ERMS is not associated with specific fusions, generally showing aneuploidy, with multiple copy number (or whole chromosome) gains/losses. It is frequently associated with *RAS* family genes alterations (*HRAS, NRAS, KRAS*), and *NF1, FGFR4,* and *PIK3CA*.[62,63] Solid alveolar RMS (ARMS) arises in deep soft tissue. Primary intra-abdominal presentation is unusual; rare pelvic or pararectal neoplasms can cause bowel obstruction.[64] They comprise solid sheets of centrally discohesive cells with rounded nuclei. Most ARMS are associated with *PAX3* or *PAX7::FOXO1* fusions.

OTHER SMALL ROUND CELL SARCOMAS THAT ARE RARELY PRIMARY IN THE ABDOMEN OR GASTROINTESTINAL TRACT

Sarcomas with BCOR genetic alterations have hybrid spindle and round cell morphology, with either *BCOR*-associated fusions or *BCOR* internal tandem duplications (*BCOR*-ITDs). This group includes undifferentiated round cell sarcomas or primitive myxoid mesenchymal tumors of infancy (PMMTI) and clear cell renal sarcomas.[65,66] Sarcomas with *BCOR::CCNB3* fusions occur more frequently within bone than soft tissues (1.5:1), predisposing for extremities, pelvis and paraspinal areas,[41,42] with rarer sites including kidney, lungs, and head and neck.[67–69] *BCOR*-ITD sarcomas (including PMMTI) predominantly arise within soft tissues of trunk, retroperitoneum, and head and neck.[66] *Round cell sarcomas with EWSR1-non-*

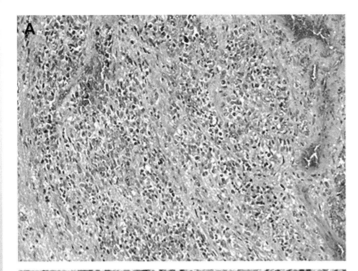

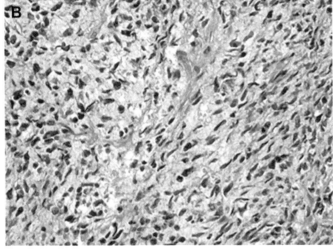

Fig. 5. Embryonal rhabdomyosarcoma (ERMS) shows fascicles of mildly and moderately atypical primitive ovoid to spindle cells in myxocollagenous stroma. When tightly packed rounded cells predominate, ERMS can resemble other small round cell sarcomas (*A*). Areas of more conventional ERMS with spindling and myxoid stroma can aid diagnosis (*B*).

ETS fusions are round and spindle cell sarcomas with *EWSR1/FUS* fusions with partners (principally *NFATC2* or *PATZ1*) that are non-ETS gene family members. These have heterogeneous morphologies and are rare intra-abdominally, typically arising in bones with extra-osseous extension (*NFATC2*) or in soft tissues including retroperitoneum (*PATZ1*).[70] *Sclerosing epithelioid fibrosarcoma (SEF)* can occur as a primary neoplasm within abdomen, stomach, small intestine, cecum, pelvis, or retroperitoneum,[71-73] comprising nests and cords of epithelioid cells within sclerotic stroma. SEF shows overlapping pathologic and molecular findings with low-grade fibromyxoid sarcoma, a fibroblastic neoplasm of bland spindle/ovoid cells in myxocollagenous matrix; tumors can have pure SEF morphology, or be hybrid. Most pure SEF contain *EWSR1* rearrangements with *CREB3L1/CREB3L2,* with occasional *FUS* rearrangements. Eighty percent to ninety percent show diffuse MUC4 expression[74]; MUC4-

negative SEF has more varied appearances, with other fusions, including of *YAP1* and *KMT2A*, or *KMT2A* and *PRRX1*.[75,76]

OTHER SMALL ROUND CELL NEOPLASMS TO CONSIDER IN THE ABDOMINOPELVIC CAVITY/GASTROINTESTINAL TRACT

Round cell epithelioid gastrointestinal stromal tumor: Epithelioid morphology is seen in up to 25% of gastrointestinal stromal tumors (GISTs). SDH-deficient GISTs are characteristically epithelioid and multinodular/plexiform.[77,78] Epithelioid GISTs have varied appearances, from large polygonal cells with eosinophilic cytoplasm to medium and even small cells with high nuclear:cytoplasmic ratios, rarely mimicking a small round cell neoplasm.[79] *PDGFRA*-mutated GISTs are usually epithelioid and arise predominantly in the stomach, with PDGFRA immunohistochemistry recently shown to be highly sensitive and moderately specific for these among GISTs.[80] *High-grade (formerly round cell) myxoid liposarcoma (MLPS)*, characterized by *FUS* or *EWSR1::DDIT3* fusions, arises within proximal extremity tissues, but can metastasize to abdomen and retroperitoneum. Round cell morphology can resemble other round cell sarcomas such as ES. When MLPS presents within the abdominal cavity or retroperitoneum, metastasis from typical sites should be first excluded. *Cytokeratin-positive malignant tumor in the abdomen with EWSR1/FUS::CREB fusion* represents an emerging group of neoplasms predilecting for the peritoneal cavity with cytokeratin expression, and *EWSR1/FUS::CREB* fusions.[81] These comprise multinodular distributions of monomorphic epithelioid cells with partly overlapping phenotypes with malignant mesothelioma, including diffuse strong AE1/AE3 and WT1 (and focal CD34), but negative calretinin.[81] Rarely, they comprise small ovoid cells

with nuclear molding, superficially resembling small cell carcinoma.[81] *EWSR1/FUS::ATF1* or *EWSR1::YY1* fusions are described in a group of *epithelioid mesotheliomas* in young to middle-aged adults, lacking histories of asbestos exposure, occurring in peritoneum or thorax. These show conventional epithelioid morphology (often solid nests/sheets with variable papillary or trabecular foci, within collagenous stroma, without mitotic activity or necrosis) with retained BAP1 expression, suggesting a novel subtype.[82,83] As the epithelioid cells are monomorphic within collagenous matrix, they may be mistaken for a small round cell sarcoma.[83] The abdominopelvic region is a well-documented site for MPNST, but the *small cell variant* is rare, comprising sheets or nests of rounded cells showing primitive neuroepithelial differentiation[84] and sometimes abortive rosettes.[84] Small cell MPNST can be distinguished from ES by its absence of CD99 expression[85]

Fig. 6. Low-grade endometrial stromal sarcoma (LGESS). This shows cellular sheets of small, uniform cells with ovoid/rounded nuclei without atypia and scant cytoplasm, with relatively minimal fibrous stroma and a delicate small arteriolar network (*A, B*).

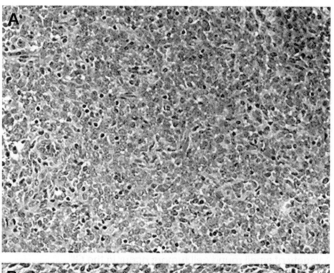

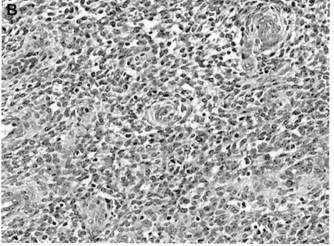

and foci of more typical MPNST (including alternating hypercellular and less cellular areas and at least focal atypia).

Endometrial stromal sarcoma (ESS) may recur in the abdominopelvic cavity, sometimes after a long interval, and can be diagnostically difficult on core biopsy. Low-grade ESS (LGESS) displays sheets of small, uniform cells with ovoid/rounded nuclei without atypia and scanty cytoplasm with minimal stroma (Fig. 6A, B). This can be mistaken for small round cell neoplasms such as ES, and it is important to be aware of this possibility in middle-aged to older adults and to correlate with the clinical history, including for histories of hysterectomy or endometriosis. LGESS often has a small arteriolar network (see Fig. 6B). ESS may express desmin, SMA, h-caldesmon, pankeratins, WT1, and CD99, but LGESS is typically diffusely strongly positive for CD10, estrogen receptor (ER), and progesterone receptor (PgR), and may show focal cyclin D1. LGESS is typically associated with a number of fusions, most commonly *JAZF1::SUZ12*. *Neuroblastoma* and pure or predominant blastemal *nephroblastoma* (Wilms tumor) typically occur in very young patients (neuroblastoma: <6 years; nephroblastoma: <10 years). These lack diffuse, membranous CD99. *Malignant rhabdoid tumor* can occasionally show predominant small round cell morphology, with minimal typical rhabdoid cells.[86,87] Most occur in infants and children younger than 3 years, although extrarenal and extracranial forms occur in adults.[88] Intact nuclear SMARCB1 (INI1) labeling aids distinction from other tumors in the differential diagnosis.[88]

SUMMARY

A variety of small round cell tumors occur in the GI tract and abdominal cavity. In these locations, small cell variants of more common lineage (particularly small cell carcinomas) might prevail, but small round cell sarcomas present as metastases or rarely as primary neoplasms. Given their heterogeneous morphology, immunohistochemical overlap, and often polyphenotypic immunoprofiles, diagnosis requires clinical correlation, awareness of the immunohistochemical and molecular spectra of each neoplasm, and the limitations of available ancillary molecular tests. The use of more newly available antibodies directed to protein changes of characteristic genetic alterations and the increasing availability of NGS techniques will further facilitate diagnosis, prognostic subtyping, and stratification of patients for targeted therapies.

CLINICS CARE POINTS

- Small round cell sarcomas are rare. When a small round cell neoplasm is encountered in the abdomen or gastrointestinal tract, carcinoma, lymphoma and melanoma should be first excluded.

- Diagnosis requires careful correlation with the clinical and radiologic picture, including for any previous history of a primary (eg, viscerally-based) neoplasm, and correlation with/review of any previous histology.

- The morphologic spectra of specific entities needs appreciation, as various mesenchymal or non-mesenchymal neoplasms may manifest, at least focally, with small round cell histology.

- Immunohistochemical evaluation should include sensitive, broad spectrum markers of lineages that need exclusion (eg, a broad spectrum pankeratin such as AE1/AE3, a broad spectrum neural marker such as SOX10, and broad spectrum hematolymphoid markers which should include TdT to assess for acute lymphoblastic leukemia).

- Due to the frequent polyphenotypic immunoprofiles of many small round cell sarcomas, the complete immunophenotype (including assessment of focality of positive markers and negative findings) needs careful consideration, and correlation with the histologic features and clinical picture.

- Pathologists should be aware of the limitations of ancillary molecular techniques used, including the non-specificity of the finding of particular gene rearrangements (eg, of EWSR1) or gene fusions.

DISCLOSURES

The authors have no conflicts of interest or funding to disclose.

REFERENCES

1. Mitelman F, Johansson B, Mertens F. The impact of translocations and gene fusions on cancer causation. Nat Rev Cancer 2007;7(4):233–45.
2. Thway K, Fisher C. Tumors with *EWSR1-CREB1* and *EWSR1-ATF1* fusions: the current status. Am J Surg Pathol 2012;36(7):e1–11.
3. Thway K, Fisher C. Mesenchymal Tumors with *EWSR1* Gene Rearrangements. Surg Pathol Clin 2019;12(1):165–90.

4. Ordonez NG. Desmoplastic small round cell tumor: I: a histopathologic study of 39 cases with emphasis on unusual histological patterns. Am J Surg Pathol 1998;22(11):1303–13.

5. Heikkila AJ, Prebtani AP. Desmoplastic small round cell tumour in a 74 year old man: an uncommon cause of ascites (case report). Diagn Pathol 2011; 6:55.

6. Gerald WL, Ladanyi M, de Alava E, et al. Clinical, pathologic, and molecular spectrum of tumors associated with t(11;22)(p13;q12): desmoplastic small round-cell tumor and its variants. J Clin Oncol 1998;16(9):3028–36.

7. Yaren A, Degirmencioglu S, Calli Demirkan N, et al. Primary mesenchymal tumors of the colon: a report of three cases. Turk J Gastroenterol 2014;25(3): 314–8.

8. Liu Q, Liu N, Chen D. Primary desmoplastic small round cell tumor of the duodenum. Eur J Med Res 2014;19:38.

9. Thway K. Primitive Round Cell Neoplasms. Surg Pathol Clin 2011;4(3):799–818.

10. da Silva RC, Medeiros Filho P, Chioato L, et al. Desmoplastic small round cell tumor of the kidney mimicking Wilms tumor: a case report and review of the literature. Appl Immunohistochem Mol Morphol 2009;17(6):557–62.

11. Rao P, Tamboli P, Fillman EP, et al. Primary intra-renal desmoplastic small round cell tumor: expanding the histologic spectrum, with special emphasis on the differential diagnostic considerations. Pathol Res Pract 2014;210(12):1130–3.

12. Ordonez NG. Desmoplastic small round cell tumor: II: an ultrastructural and immunohistochemical study with emphasis on new immunohistochemical markers. Am J Surg Pathol 1998;22(11):1314–27.

13. Sawyer JR, Tryka AF, Lewis JM. A novel reciprocal chromosome translocation t(11;22)(p13;q12) in an intraabdominal desmoplastic small round-cell tumor. Am J Surg Pathol 1992;16(4):411–6.

14. Alaggio R, Rosolen A, Sartori F, et al. Spindle cell tumor with EWS-WT1 transcript and a favorable clinical course: a variant of DSCT, a variant of leiomyosarcoma, or a new entity? Report of 2 pediatric cases. Am J Surg Pathol 2007;31(3):454–9.

15. Ud Din N, Pekmezci M, Javed G, et al. Low-grade small round cell tumor of the cauda equina with EWSR1-WT1 fusion and indolent clinical course. Hum Pathol 2015;46(1):153–8.

16. Gurney JG, Davis S, Severson RK, et al. Trends in cancer incidence among children in the. U.S. Cancer 1996;78(3):532–41.

17. Grunewald TGP, Cidre-Aranaz F, Surdez D, et al. Ewing sarcoma. Nat Rev Dis Primers 2018;4(1):5.

18. de Alava E, Lessnick SL, Stamenkovic I. Ewing Sarcoma. In: WHO classification of Tumours editorial board eds World Health organization classification of soft tissue and bone Tumours. 5th edition. Lyon: IARC Press; 2020.

19. Milione M, Gasparini P, Sozzi G, et al. Ewing sarcoma of the small bowel: a study of seven cases, including one with the uncommonly reported EWSR1-FEV translocation. Histopathology 2014; 64(7):1014–26.

20. Kolosov A, Dulskas A, Pauza K, et al. Primary Ewing's sarcoma in a small intestine - a case report and review of the literature. BMC Surg 2020;20(1): 113.

21. Shu Q, Luo JN, Liu XL, et al. Extraskeletal Ewing sarcoma of the stomach: A rare case report. World J Clin Cases 2023;11(1):201–9.

22. Czekalla R, Fuchs M, Stolzle A, et al. Peripheral primitive neuroectodermal tumor of the stomach in a 14-year-old boy: a case report. Eur J Gastroenterol Hepatol 2004;16(12):1391–400.

23. Wallace MW, Niec JA, Ghani MOA, et al. Distribution and surgical management of visceral Ewing sarcoma among children and adolescents. J Pediatr Surg 2023;S0022-S3468(23):00008.

24. Murthy SS, Challa S, Raju K, et al. Ewing Sarcoma With Emphasis on Extra-skeletal Ewing Sarcoma: A Decade's Experience From a Single Centre in India. Clin Pathol 2020;13, 2632010X20970210.

25. Yoshida A, Sekine S, Tsuta K, et al. NKX2.2 is a Useful Immunohistochemical Marker for Ewing Sarcoma. Am J Surg Pathol 2012;36(7):993–9.

26. Watson S, Perrin V, Guillemot D, et al. Transcriptomic definition of molecular subgroups of small round cell sarcomas. J Pathol 2018;245(1):29–40.

27. Charville GW, Wang WL, Ingram DR, et al. PAX7 expression in sarcomas bearing the EWSR1-NFATC2 translocation. Mod Pathol 2019;32(1):154–6.

28. Charville GW, Wang WL, Ingram DR, et al. EWSR1 fusion proteins mediate PAX7 expression in Ewing sarcoma. Mod Pathol 2017;30(9):1312–20.

29. Ordonez JL, Osuna D, Herrero D, et al. Advances in Ewing's sarcoma research: where are we now and what lies ahead? Cancer Res 2009;69(18):7140–50.

30. Delattre O, Zucman J, Plougastel B, et al. Gene fusion with ETS DNA-binding domain caused by chromosome translocation in human tumours. Nature 1992;359:162–5.

31. Sorensen PH, Lessnick SL, Lopez-Terrada D, et al. A second Ewing's sarcoma translocation, t(21;22), fuses the EWS gene to another ETS-family transcription factor, ERG. Nat Genet 1994;6(2):146–51.

32. Camoes MJ, Paulo P, Ribeiro FR, et al. Potential Downstream Target Genes of Aberrant ETS Transcription Factors Are Differentially Affected in Ewing's Sarcoma and Prostate Carcinoma. PLoS One 2012;7(11):e49819.

33. Jeon IS, Davis JN, Braun BS, et al. A variant Ewing's sarcoma translocation (7;22) fuses the EWS gene to the ETS gene ETV1. Oncogene 1995;10(6):1229–34.

34. Kaneko Y, Yoshida K, Handa M, et al. Fusion of an ETS-family gene, EIAF, to EWS by t(17;22)(q12;q12) chromosome translocation in an undifferentiated sarcoma of infancy. Genes Chromosomes Cancer 1996;15(2):115–21.

35. Ichikawa H, Shimizu K, Hayashi Y, et al. An RNA-binding protein gene, TLS/FUS, is fused to ERG in human myeloid leukemia with t(16;21) chromosomal translocation. Cancer Res 1994;54(11):2865–8.

36. Yamada Y, Kuda M, Kohashi K, et al. Histological and immunohistochemical characteristics of undifferentiated small round cell sarcomas associated with CIC-DUX4 and BCOR-CCNB3 fusion genes. Virchows Arch 2017;470(4):373–80.

37. Italiano A, Sung YS, Zhang L, et al. High prevalence of CIC fusion with double-homeobox (DUX4) transcription factors in EWSR1-negative undifferentiated small blue round cell sarcomas. Genes Chromosomes Cancer 2012;51(3):207–18.

38. Graham C, Chilton-MacNeill S, Zielenska M, et al. The CIC-DUX4 fusion transcript is present in a subgroup of pediatric primitive round cell sarcomas. Hum Pathol 2012;43(2):180–9.

39. Kawamura-Saito M, Yamazaki Y, Kaneko K, et al. Fusion between CIC and DUX4 up-regulates PEA3 family genes in Ewing-like sarcomas with t(4;19)(q35;q13) translocation. Hum Mol Genet 2006;15(13):2125–37.

40. Yoshimoto M, Graham C, Chilton-MacNeill S, et al. Detailed cytogenetic and array analysis of pediatric primitive sarcomas reveals a recurrent CIC-DUX4 fusion gene event. Cancer Genet Cytogenet 2009; 195(1):1–11.

41. Pierron G, Tirode F, Lucchesi C, et al. A new subtype of bone sarcoma defined by BCOR-CCNB3 gene fusion. Nat Genet 2012;44(4):461–6.

42. Puls F, Niblett A, Marland G, et al. BCOR-CCNB3 (Ewing-like) sarcoma: a clinicopathologic analysis of 10 cases, in comparison with conventional Ewing sarcoma. Am J Surg Pathol 2014;38(10):1307–18.

43. Yoshida A, Goto K, Kodaira M, et al. CIC-rearranged Sarcomas: A Study of 20 Cases and Comparisons With Ewing Sarcomas. Am J Surg Pathol 2016; 40(3):313–23.

44. Antonescu CR, Owosho AA, Zhang L, et al. Sarcomas With CIC-rearrangements Are a Distinct Pathologic Entity With Aggressive Outcome: A Clinicopathologic and Molecular Study of 115 Cases. Am J Surg Pathol 2017;41(7):941–9.

45. Le Loarer F, Pissaloux D, Watson S, et al. Clinicopathologic Features of CIC-NUTM1 Sarcomas, a New Molecular Variant of the Family of CIC-Fused Sarcomas. Am J Surg Pathol 2019;43(2):268–76.

46. Smith SC, Buehler D, Choi EY, et al. CIC-DUX sarcomas demonstrate frequent MYC amplification and ETS-family transcription factor expression. Mod Pathol 2015;28(1):57–68.

47. Specht K, Sung YS, Zhang L, et al. Distinct transcriptional signature and immunoprofile of CIC-DUX4 fusion-positive round cell tumors compared to EWSR1-rearranged Ewing sarcomas: further evidence toward distinct pathologic entities. Genes Chromosomes Cancer 2014;53(7):622–33.

48. Chan JA, McMenamin ME, Fletcher CD. Synovial sarcoma in older patients: clinicopathological analysis of 32 cases with emphasis on unusual histological features. Histopathology 2003;43(1):72–83.

49. van de Rijn M, Barr FG, Xiong QB, et al. Poorly differentiated synovial sarcoma: an analysis of clinical, pathologic, and molecular genetic features. Am J Surg Pathol 1999;23(1):106–12.

50. Fisher C, Folpe AL, Hashimoto H, et al. Intra-abdominal synovial sarcoma: a clinicopathological study. Histopathology 2004;45(3):245–53.

51. Hornick JL, Fletcher CD. Myoepithelial tumors of soft tissue: a clinicopathologic and immunohistochemical study of 101 cases with evaluation of prognostic parameters. Am J Surg Pathol 2003;27(9):1183–96.

52. Fisher C. Synovial sarcoma: ultrastructural and immunohistochemical features of epithelial differentiation in monophasic and biphasic tumors. Hum Pathol 1986;17(10):996–1008.

53. Pelmus M, Guillou L, Hostein I, et al. Monophasic fibrous and poorly differentiated synovial sarcoma: immunohistochemical reassessment of 60 t(X;18)(SYT-SSX)-positive cases. Am J Surg Pathol 2002;26(11):1434–40.

54. Terry J, Saito T, Subramanian S, et al. TLE1 as a diagnostic immunohistochemical marker for synovial sarcoma emerging from gene expression profiling studies. Am J Surg Pathol 2007;31(2):240–6.

55. Chuang HC, Hsu SC, Huang CG, et al. Reappraisal of TLE-1 immunohistochemical staining and molecular detection of SS18-SSX fusion transcripts for synovial sarcoma. Pathol Int 2013;63(12):573–80.

56. Jagdis A, Rubin BP, Tubbs RR, et al. Prospective evaluation of TLE1 as a diagnostic immunohistochemical marker in synovial sarcoma. Am J Surg Pathol 2009;33(12):1743–51.

57. Machen SK, Fisher C, Gautam RS, et al. Utility of cytokeratin subsets for distinguishing poorly differentiated synovial sarcoma from peripheral primitive neuroectodermal tumour. Histopathology 1998; 33(6):501–7.

58. Folpe AL, Hill CE, Parham DM, et al. Immunohistochemical detection of FLI-1 protein expression: a study of 132 round cell tumors with emphasis on CD99-positive mimics of Ewing's sarcoma/primitive neuroectodermal tumor. Am J Surg Pathol 2000; 24(12):1657–62.

59. Baranov E, McBride MJ, Bellizzi AM, et al. A Novel SS18-SSX Fusion-specific Antibody for the Diagnosis of Synovial Sarcoma. Am J Surg Pathol 2020; 44(7):922–33.

60. Hawkins DS, Chi YY, Anderson JR, et al. Addition of Vincristine and Irinotecan to Vincristine, Dactinomycin, and Cyclophosphamide Does Not Improve Outcome for Intermediate-Risk Rhabdomyosarcoma: A Report From the Children's Oncology Group. J Clin Oncol 2018;36(27):2770–7.

61. Walterhouse DO, Pappo AS, Meza JL, et al. Shorter-duration therapy using vincristine, dactinomycin, and lower-dose cyclophosphamide with or without radiotherapy for patients with newly diagnosed low-risk rhabdomyosarcoma: a report from the Soft Tissue Sarcoma Committee of the Children's Oncology Group. J Clin Oncol 2014;32(31): 3547–52.

62. Agaram NP. Evolving classification of rhabdomyosarcoma. Histopathology 2022;80(1):98–108.

63. Weber-Hall S, Anderson J, McManus A, et al. Gains, losses, and amplification of genomic material in rhabdomyosarcoma analyzed by comparative genomic hybridization. Cancer Res 1996;56(14): 3220–4.

64. Fuchs J, Dantonello TM, Blumenstock G, et al. Treatment and outcome of patients suffering from perineal/perianal rhabdomyosarcoma: results from the CWS trials–retrospective clinical study. Ann Surg 2014;259(6):1166–72.

65. Alaggio R, Ninfo V, Rosolen A, et al. Primitive myxoid mesenchymal tumor of infancy: a clinicopathologic report of 6 cases. Am J Surg Pathol 2006;30(3): 388–94.

66. Kao YC, Sung YS, Zhang L, et al. Recurrent BCOR Internal Tandem Duplication and YWHAE-NUTM2B Fusions in Soft Tissue Undifferentiated Round Cell Sarcoma of Infancy: Overlapping Genetic Features With Clear Cell Sarcoma of Kidney. Am J Surg Pathol 2016;40(8):1009–20.

67. Kao YC, Owosho AA, Sung YS, et al. BCOR-CCNB3 Fusion Positive Sarcomas: A Clinicopathologic and Molecular Analysis of 36 Cases With Comparison to Morphologic Spectrum and Clinical Behavior of Other Round Cell Sarcomas. Am J Surg Pathol 2018;42(5):604–15.

68. Argani P, Kao YC, Zhang L, et al. Primary Renal Sarcomas With BCOR-CCNB3 Gene Fusion: A Report of 2 Cases Showing Histologic Overlap With Clear Cell Sarcoma of Kidney, Suggesting Further Link Between BCOR-related Sarcomas of the Kidney and Soft Tissues. Am J Surg Pathol 2017;41(12):1702–12.

69. Matsuyama A, Shiba E, Umekita Y, et al. Clinicopathologic Diversity of Undifferentiated Sarcoma With BCOR-CCNB3 Fusion: Analysis of 11 Cases With a Reappraisal of the Utility of Immunohistochemistry for BCOR and CCNB3. Am J Surg Pathol 2017; 41(12):1713–21.

70. Mastrangelo T, Modena P, Tornielli S, et al. A novel zinc finger gene is fused to EWS in small round cell tumor. Oncogene 2000;19(33):3799–804.

71. Argani P, Lewin JR, Edmonds P, et al. Primary renal sclerosing epithelioid fibrosarcoma: report of 2 cases with EWSR1-CREB3L1 gene fusion. Am J Surg Pathol 2015;39(3):365–73.

72. Peng Y, Zhang D, Lei T, et al. The clinicopathological spectrum of sclerosing epithelioid fibrosarcoma: report of an additional series with review of the literature. Pathology 2023;55(3):355–61.

73. Dewaele B, Libbrecht L, Levy G, et al. A novel EWS-CREB3L3 gene fusion in a mesenteric sclerosing epithelioid fibrosarcoma. Genes Chromosomes Cancer 2017;56(9):695–9.

74. Doyle LA, Moller E, Dal Cin P, et al. MUC4 is a highly sensitive and specific marker for low-grade fibromyxoid sarcoma. American journal of surgical pathology 2011;35(5):733–41.

75. Puls F, Agaimy A, Flucke U, et al. Recurrent Fusions Between YAP1 and KMT2A in Morphologically Distinct Neoplasms Within the Spectrum of Low-grade Fibromyxoid Sarcoma and Sclerosing Epithelioid Fibrosarcoma. Am J Surg Pathol 2020;44(5): 594–606.

76. Kao YC, Lee JC, Zhang L, et al. Recurrent YAP1 and KMT2A Gene Rearrangements in a Subset of MUC4-negative Sclerosing Epithelioid Fibrosarcoma. Am J Surg Pathol 2020;44(3):368–77.

77. Miettinen M, Wang ZF, Sarlomo-Rikala M, et al. Succinate dehydrogenase-deficient GISTs: a clinicopathologic, immunohistochemical, and molecular genetic study of 66 gastric GISTs with predilection to young age. Am J Surg Pathol 2011;35(11): 1712–21.

78. Doyle LA, Nelson D, Heinrich MC, et al. Loss of succinate dehydrogenase subunit B (SDHB) expression is limited to a distinctive subset of gastric wild-type gastrointestinal stromal tumours: a comprehensive genotype-phenotype correlation study. Histopathology 2012;61(5):801–9.

79. Abrari A, Mukherjee U, Tandon R, et al. Round cell epithelioid GIST (gastrointestinal stromal tumour) in an endoscopic biopsy is a diagnostic confounder. BMJ Case Rep 2011;2011, bcr1020114996.

80. Papke DJ Jr, Forgo E, Charville GW, et al. PDGFRA Immunohistochemistry Predicts PDGFRA Mutations in Gastrointestinal Stromal Tumors. Am J Surg Pathol 2022;46(1):3–10.

81. Shibayama T, Shimoi T, Mori T, et al. Cytokeratin-positive Malignant Tumor in the Abdomen With EWSR1/FUS-CREB Fusion: A Clinicopathologic Study of 8 Cases. Am J Surg Pathol 2022;46(1): 134–46.

82. Desmeules P, Joubert P, Zhang L, et al. A Subset of Malignant Mesotheliomas in Young Adults Are Associated With Recurrent EWSR1/FUS-ATF1 Fusions. Am J Surg Pathol 2017;41(7):980–8.

83. Dermawan JK, Torrence D, Lee CH, et al. EWSR1::YY1 fusion positive peritoneal epithelioid

mesothelioma harbors mesothelioma epigenetic signature: Report of 3 cases in support of an emerging entity. Genes Chromosomes Cancer 2022;61(10):592–602.

84. Abe S, Imamura T, Park P, et al. Small round-cell type of malignant peripheral nerve sheath tumor. Mod Pathol 1998;11(8):747–53.

85. Shintaku M, Nakade M, Hirose T. Malignant peripheral nerve sheath tumor of small round cell type with pleomorphic spindle cell sarcomatous areas. Pathol Int 2003;53(7):478–82.

86. Kohashi K, Tanaka Y, Kishimoto H, et al. Reclassification of rhabdoid tumor and pediatric undifferentiated/unclassified sarcoma with complete loss of SMARCB1/INI1 protein expression: three subtypes of rhabdoid tumor according to their histological features. Mod Pathol 2016;29(10):1232–42.

87. Vokuhl C, Oyen F, Haberle B, et al. Small cell undifferentiated (SCUD) hepatoblastomas: All malignant rhabdoid tumors? Genes Chromosomes Cancer 2016;55(12):925–31.

88. Oda Y, Biegel JA, Pfister SM. Extrarenal rhabdoid tumour. In: WHO classification of Tumours editorial board eds World Health organization classification of soft tissue and bone Tumours. 5th edition. Lyon: IARC Press; 2020.

Infectious Disease Pathology of the Gastrointestinal Tract
Diagnosing the Challenging Cases

Laura W. Lamps, MD

KEYWORDS

- Gastrointestinal • Infection • Inflammatory bowel disease mimics • Fungus • Bacteria • Virus

Key points

- Many gastrointestinal infections mimic other diseases of the GI tract.
- Distinguishing between gastrointestinal infections and other disease processes is important because it significantly affects therapy.
- Immunohistochemistry, microbial culture, and molecular techniques are valuable diagnostic aids.

ABSTRACT

Infectious diseases of the GI tract mimic a variety of other GI diseases, including chronic idiopathic inflammatory bowel disease and ischemia. It can be challenging to identify pathogens in tissue sections as well, as many trainees are not exposed to infectious disease pathology other than in the context of microbiology. Our ability to diagnose infections in formalin fixed, paraffin embedded material has grown exponentially with the advent of new histochemical and immunohistochemical stains, as well as more options for molecular testing. Correlating these diagnostic techniques with morphology has led to increasing understanding of the histologic patterns that are associated with specific pathogens.

OVERVIEW

Infectious diseases of the gastrointestinal tract (GIT) can mimic a large number of other commonly encountered gastrointestinal (GI) diseases, including chronic idiopathic inflammatory bowel disease (CIIBD) and ischemia.[1–3] Broadly, GI infections are associated with neutrophilic inflammation and a lack of changes of chronicity (Fig. 1), but we have learned that many infections can cause changes of chronicity as well as a wide variety of other features that may mimic other GI diseases. The ability to diagnose infections in formalin-fixed, paraffin-embedded material has grown exponentially with the advent of new histochemical and immunohistochemical stains as well as enhanced options for molecular testing. As these techniques have emerged and evolved, our knowledge of morphologic patterns of inflammation associated with specific pathogens has also expanded.

INFECTIONS THAT MIMIC COMMONLY ENCOUNTERED GASTROINTESTINAL DISEASES

CHRONIC IDIOPATHIC INFLAMMATORY BOWEL DISEASE

Many infections that mimic CIIBD are caused by pathogens transmitted through contaminated

Department of Pathology, University of Michigan, NCRC Building 35, 2800 Plymouth Road, Ann Arbor, MI 48109, USA

E-mail address: lwlamps@med.umich.edu

Surgical Pathology 16 (2023) 779–804
https://doi.org/10.1016/j.path.2023.05.011
1875-9181/23/© 2023 Elsevier Inc. All rights reserved.

surgpath.theclinics.com

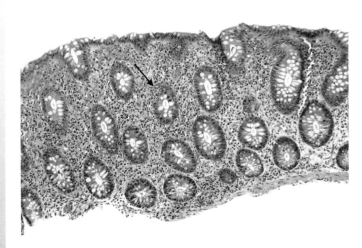

Fig. 1. This biopsy from a patient with bacterial enterocolitis shows neutrophilic cryptitis (*arrow*) and a mixed inflammatory infiltrate in the lamina propria. There is no significant architectural distortion (H&E, original magnification 20x).

food and water, such as *Salmonella, Shigella, Yersinia, Campylobacter*, and *Aeromonas* species, among others (**Table 1**).

Salmonella Species

The majority of clinically important *Salmonella* are in the species *Shigella enterica*. It is an important cause of both traveler's diarrhea and food-borne illness, as it can be found in dairy products, water, eggs, meat, and occasionally vegetables and fruits. *Salmonella* are differentiated by serotyping, and are often segregated into typhoid and non-typhoid serovars.[4,5] Typhoid serovars cause enteric (typhoid) fever; the most common are *S.* Typhi and *S.* Paratyphi. Non-typhoid serovars that cause clinically important infections include

Table 1
Summary of food and water-associated bacterial infections that mimic ulcerative colitis or Crohn's disease

	Aeromonas spp	Campylobacter spp	Salmonella spp	Shigella spp	Yersinia spp
Transmittal	Water, especially pond water; food	Food/water, especially undercooked meat	Food/water, often in the context of poor sanitation	Food/water, often in the context of poor sanitation	Meat/water, especially undercooked pork; dairy
Macroscopic features that mimic CIIBD	Segmental ulceration	Erythema, ulcers, friability	Ileocecal inflammation, apthous ulcers, thickened wall	Pancolitis or left-sided colitis	Ileocecal inflammation, thickened wall, aphthous ulcers
Key Histologic Features	Usually infectious type colitis pattern; sometimes architectural distortion	Usually infectious type colitis pattern; sometimes architectural distortion	Architectural distortion, basal plasmacytosis (especially typhoidal serovars)	Marked architectural distortion, especially later in course	Transmural inflammation, granulomas, mural fibrosis

Fig. 2. Ileal resection from a patient with typhoid fever shows ulceration overlying a Peyer patch, forming an aphthous ulcer, and significant architectural distortion. These features can mimic Crohn's disease (*A*, H&E, original magnification, 8x). Biopsy from a patient with infection by a nontyphoid serovar shows mild architectural distortion, basal plasmacytosis, and Paneth cell metaplasia (*B*, H&E, original magnificent 20x).

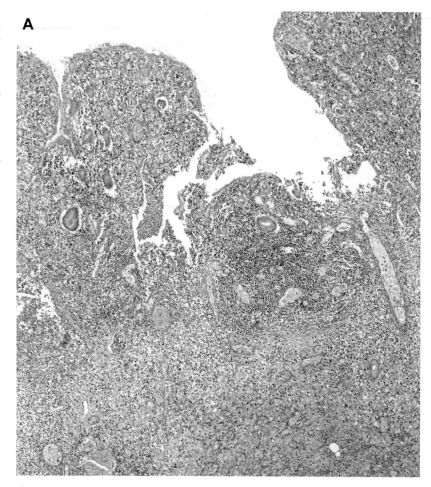

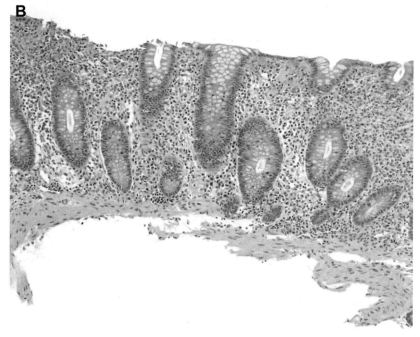

S. Enteritidis, S. Typhimurium, and S. Muenchen. Both typhoid and non-typhoid serovars may cause severe illness and pathologic features that mimic CIIBD.[6]

The ileum, right colon, and appendix are preferentially affected in typhoid fever due to the abundant lymphoid tissue at these sites. Common macroscopic features include aphthous ulcers overlying lymphoid follicles and deep or linear ulcers, mimicking Crohn's disease.[4–9] Architectural distortion is common, and basal plasmacytosis may be present (Fig. 2).

Shigellae species are virulent, invasive bacteria that are a major cause of infectious diarrhea worldwide. Populations at greatest risk include children under the age of six, homosexual males and chronically debilitated patients. Shigella typically involves the colon, and often the left colon is most severely affected. The inflammation may be contiguous, leading to confusion with ulcerative colitis.[10,11] Early infection is more likely to have an acute infectious-type colitis pattern, but later in the course mucosal destruction with architectural distortion and an expanded lamina propria may occur[12,13] (Fig. 3).

Yersinia is a common cause of bacterial enteritis in Western and Northern Europe, North America, and Australia. Yersinia enterocolitica and Yersinia pseudotuberculosis are the two species that cause human gastrointestinal disease. Yersiniosis may feature lymphoid hyperplasia, transmural lymphoid aggregates, granulomas, architectural distortion, and mural fibrosis, and thus it may be extremely difficult to distinguish from Crohn's disease[14–16] (Fig. 4). Features that favor Crohn's disease include cobblestoning of mucosa and fat wrapping grossly, involvement of multiple sites in the GI tract, and a more chronic clinical presentation.

Aeromonas and Campylobacter species occasionally cause severe illness with focal architectural distortion that can mimic CIIBD both clinically and pathologically.[17–20]

Stool cultures and/or stool PCR, ideally performed on samples obtained before antibiotics are started, are invaluable tools for the diagnosis of many food and water-born infections. A number of FDA-cleared multiplex PCR assays are available. These assays can detect a number of bacteria, viruses, and parasites, including many

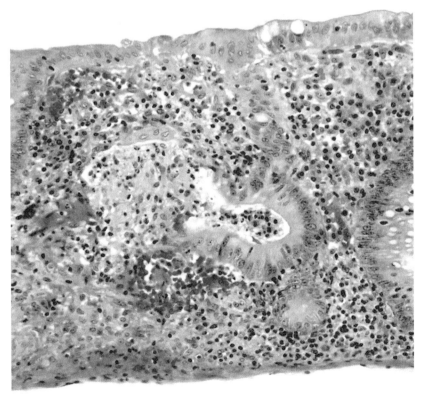

Fig. 3. Biopsy from a patient with S. sonnei shows a crypt abscess with associated mild architectural distortion and a granuloma associated with the damaged crypt (H&E, original magnification 40x).

Fig. 4. This patient had isolated granulomatous appendicitis due to *Yersinia enterocolitica* infection. The appendiceal wall contains granulomas with prominent lymphoid cuffs. There is overlying ulceration, neural hyperplasia, and transmural lymphoid aggregates, mimicking Crohn's disease (H&E, original magnification 4x).

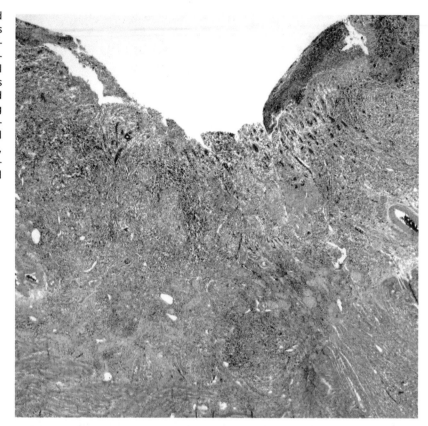

common causes of acute gastroenteritis, such as *Salmonella*, *Shigella*, *Campylobacter*, *Giardia*, *Cryptosporidum*, and Norovirus. The required specimen is liquid stool.

Enteric infections often (but not always) have a more acute clinical presentation than CIIBD, and there may be a history of exposure to possibly contaminated food or water. However, many patients with infectious colitis do not present for endoscopy until several weeks after the onset of symptoms, and the typical histologic features of acute infectious enterocolitis may no longer be present. In the resolving phase of infection mononuclear cells often predominate, with only occasional foci of neutrophilic cryptitis and a patchy increase in lamina propria inflammation. In addition, there may be abundant plasma cells and increased intra-epithelial lymphocytes (**Fig. 5**). Since these features are also seen in entities such as Crohn's disease and lymphocytic colitis, it is important to be aware of the duration of the patient's symptoms, and, ideally, the culture or PCR results, because a specific diagnosis may be difficult to determine on histologic grounds alone.

Sexually Transmitted Proctocolitides

The sexually acquired pathogens that most often mimic CIIBD are syphilis, caused by *Treponema pallidum,* and lymphogranuloma venereum (LGV), caused by *Chlamydia trachomatis*. These infections mimic CIIBD histologically because they cause architectural distortion, basal plasmacytosis, prominent lymphoid follicles, and/or granulomas, and endoscopically because they cause proctitis with mucosal changes similar to ulcerative colitis.[21,22]

The incidence of syphilis is increasing, especially among men who practice anal receptive intercourse and/or are HIV positive. Syphilitic proctitis often presents with pain at defecation, tenesmus, bleeding, and bloody or mucoid anal discharge. Endoscopic findings include ulcers, fissures, and inflammatory polypoid lesions, which may mimic IBD macroscopically. The most common histologic feature is a dense lymphoplasmacytic infiltrate[21] (**Fig. 6**). Neutrophilic inflammation and crypt architectural distortion are usually less prominent, although they may be variably present, and granulomas can be

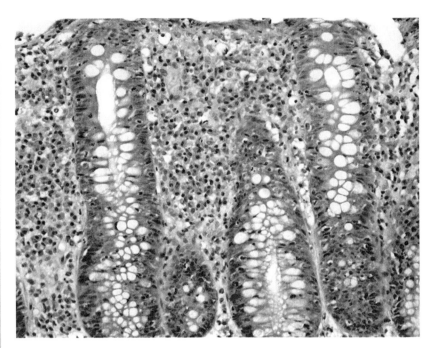

Fig. 5. Resolving bacterial infection may only have a few neutrophils, but increased intraepithelial lymphocytes and a mononuclear cell infiltrate in the lamina propria (H&E, original magnification 40x).

present as well. Small vessels with prominent endothelial cells may be noted, and the lamina propria may have prominent stromal reactive changes. Silver impregnation stains (Warthin–Starry, Steiner, and Dieterle) were historically been used for diagnosis, but have poor sensitivity, and immunohistochemistry for *T pallidum* is significantly more sensitive.

LGV is also most common among the MSM population. The primary stage of infection is characterized by anorectal pain, bleeding, mucopurulent discharge, and tenesmus. Lymphadenopathy develops during the second stage, followed by the tertiary stage during which fistulae and strictures may form. Some patients with anorectal LGV have evidence of urethral infection, but many do not. The macroscopic appearance of LGV proctitis features mucosal hyperemia, friability, ulcers, purulent exudate, or stricture. Similar to syphilis, the inflammatory infiltrate consists of a lymphoplasmacytic infiltrate with variably present neutrophils and lymphoid follicles[21,23] (**Fig. 7**). Granulomatous inflammation is occasionally present.

Laboratory testing is very helpful in distinguishing these infections from CIIBD.[21,22] In the case of syphilis, treponemal serologic tests that detect antibodies against the pathogen itself are highly sensitive at all stages of infection but can remain positive after treatment. Nontreponemal serologic tests (RPR and VDRL) are best used to track serologic response to therapy. LGV infection may be confirmed by molecular testing and nucleic acid amplification tests (NAATs) performed on swabs.[24]

ISCHEMIC COLITIS

Several different pathogens can mimic or cause ischemic colitis, as shown in **Box 1**.

The Shiga-toxin producing (formerly known as enterohemorrhagic) *Escherichia coli* (STEC or EHEC) are the bacteria that most frequently mimic ischemia. Bacteria adhere to intestinal epithelial cells and produce a cytotoxin similar to that produced by *S dysenteriae,* hence the name; however, unlike *S dysenteriae*, there is no tissue invasion. The most common strain is *E coli* 0157:H7. Contaminated meat is a frequent mode of transmission, but infection also occurs through water, milk, produce, and person-to-person contact. Bloody diarrhea and severe abdominal cramps are common; fever is mild or absent. Only one-third of patients have fecal leukocytes, which can confuse the clinical picture along with a predilection for the right side of the colon, which is unusual for ischemic colitis. The histologic features include marked edema and hemorrhage in the lamina propria and submucosa, with associated mucosal neutrophils, crypt withering, and necrosis[25,26] (**Fig. 8**). These features closely resemble

Fig. 6. Rectal biopsy from a patient with syphilitic proctitis shows a dense lymphoplasmacytic infiltrate within the lamina propria. Neutrophilic activity is sparse (*A*, H&E, original magnification 20x). Immunohistochemistry shows innumerable spirochetes in the lamina propria (*B*, *Treponema pallidum* IHC, original magnification 80x).

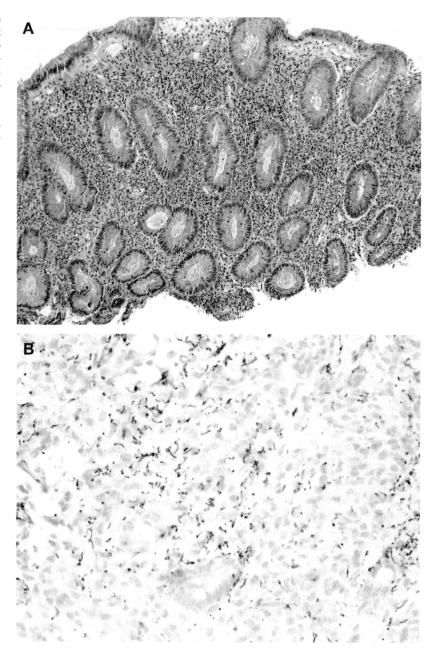

ischemic colitis, because the cytotoxin is believed to induce an ischemic insult. Microthrombi and pseudomembranes are occasionally present. Many multiplex PCR assays detect STEC. Microbial culture using selective Sorbital-MacConkey agar can be used to detect *E.coli* 0157:H7, but it will not detect other STEC serotypes.

Clostridium difficile may also mimic ischemia,[27] but pseudomembrane formation is more common in *C difficile* infection, as are dilated crypts with an "exploding" or "volcanic" exudate, intercrypt necrosis, and a lack of lamina propria hyalinization. A history of antibiotic use is also helpful. Viral and fungal pathogens that may cause ischemia are discussed later in discussion.

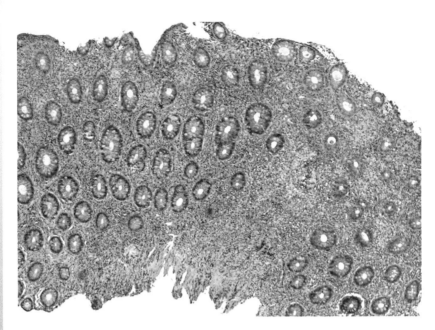

Fig. 7. Rectal biopsy from a patient with LGV proctitis shows lamina propria expansion by a lymphohistiocytic infiltrate and scattered loosely formed granulomas. (H&E, original magnification 20x. Courtesy Dr. Rhonda Yantiss).

MEDICALLY IMPORTANT FUNGI IN THE GASTROINTESTINAL TRACT

The incidence of invasive fungal infections, including those affecting the GI tract, has increased significantly over the past 2 to 3 decades as the number of patients with organ transplants, immunodeficiency states, and on long-term immunosuppression has risen.[28–31] Although GI fungal infections are most common in immunocompromised patients, many fungi also cause infection in immunocompetent people.

Accurate speciation of fungal infections is critical because it affects therapy. For this reason, tissue biopsy can be a very important diagnostic tool, as fungal cultures may require days to weeks for adequate growth and analysis (if culture material is even obtained), and

molecular studies may take a week or more as well. Fungal infections of the GIT are often part of a disseminated disease process, but GI findings may be the first sign of infection. Inflammatory reaction to fungi in immunosuppressed patients may be negligible. Organisms are often identifiable on H&E sections, particularly when numerous, but GMS and PAS stains are extremely useful. Fungi can often be correctly classified in tissue sections based on morphology, but it is important to note that fungi exposed to antifungal therapy or ambient air may produce bizarre and unusual forms. Fungi that may be encountered in the GIT are summarized in Table 2.

Mucor can be distinguished from other filamentous fungi by its broad, ribbon-like pauciseptate hyphae that branch randomly at various angles[32,33] (Fig. 9). When cut at cross-section, they have optically clear centers. *Mucor* are angioinvasive and frequently associated with necrosis. *B ranarum* is a more recently described gastrointestinal fungal pathogen related to *Mucor*.[34] It has an almost pathognomonic tissue reaction, featuring numerous eosinophils, necrosis, granulomas, and a Splendore-Hoeppli protein reaction to the organism (Fig. 10). There are generally fewer organisms than typically seen in mucormycosis, and a "crinkled cellophane ball" appearance is common on GMS.

Aspergillus and similar fungi, in contrast, have septate hyphae of uniform width that branch at

Box 1
Infections that cause or mimic ischemic colitis
Shiga-toxin producing *E. coli*
Clostridium difficile
Clostridium perfringens
CMV
Vasotrophic fungi (*Aspergillus* spp and *Mucor*)

Fig. 8. This biopsy from a patient with STEC shows features typical of ischemia, including lamina propria hyalinization, crypt withering, and ulceration. Numerous fibrin thrombi are also present (H&E, original magnification 20x).

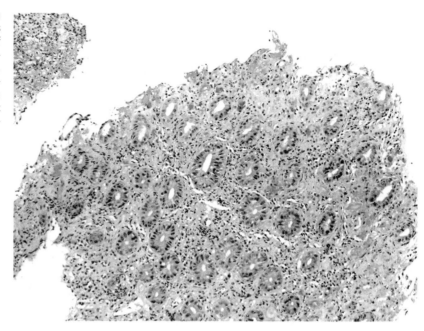

Table 2
Morphologic features of fungi that may be encountered in the gastrointestinal tract

Organism	Primary Geographic Distribution	Morphologic Features	Host Reaction	Major Differential Diagnoses
Aspergillus species	Worldwide	Septate hyphae of uniform width Regular branching at acute angles	Angioinvasion with ischemic necrosis Acute inflammation	Mucormycosis *Fusarium* Dematiaceous fungi
Mucormycosis	Worldwide, associated with diabetics more than any other mycosis	Pauciseptate hyphae with ribbon-like thin walls. Haphazard branching Optically clear centers	Similar to *Aspergillus*	Similar to *Aspergillus*; *Basidiobolus ranarum*
B ranarum	Southwestern USA; Saudi Arabia, other desert countries	Similar to Mucor; optically clear centers on cross section, "cellophane ball" morphology	Granulomatous reaction with marked eosinophils infiltrate; Splendore-Hoeppli protein	Mucor but not angioinvasive
Candida albicans and similar species	Worldwide	Mixture of budding yeast and pseudohyphae or hyphae;	Usually suppurative, with variable necrosis and ulceration Occasionally	*Aspergillus*

(*continued on next page*)

Table 2
(continued)

Organism	Primary Geographic Distribution	Morphologic Features	Host Reaction	Major Differential Diagnoses
		occasional septate hyphae	granulomatous Rare angioinvasion	
Cryptococcus spp.	Worldwide	Highly pleomorphic (4–7 microns) Uninucleate Narrow based buds Variably mucicarmine positive; Fontana-Masson positive	Usually suppurative; may have extensive necrosis Sometimes granulomatous "Soap bubble" sign	Histoplasmosis
Histoplasma capsulatum var. capsulatum	Worldwide, but endemic in Ohio, Mississippi river basins; parts of Central and South America; St. Lawrence river basin in Canada	Uniform small (2–5 micron), uninucleate ovoid yeast Narrow based buds Intracellular "Halo" effect around organism on H&E	Lymphohistiocytic infiltrate with parasitized histiocytes Occasional granulomas	*Cryptococcus T. marneffei C. glabrata P. carinii* Leishmaniasis
Pneumocystis carinii	Worldwide	Ovoid Cup or crescent shaped if collapsed No buds Internal enhancing detail	Characteristic foamy casts May have suppurative or granulomatous inflammation as well	Histoplasmosis Small parasites *T. marneffei*

acute angles. Because of its affinity for blood vessels, *Aspergillus* may actually occlude vessels in the GI tract and cause ischemia (**Fig. 11**). *Candida* species are often a mixture of budding yeast, hyphae, and pseudohyphae (**Fig. 12**). The dematiaceous, or naturally pigmented, fungi are rarely seen in the GI tract.[31]

Budding yeast encountered in the GI tract include *Histoplasma* spp. and *Cryptococcus* spp. *Histoplasma* are uniformly small and ovoid, with narrow-based buds at the pointed pole.[35,36] There is often a "halo" around the organisms on H&E (**Fig. 13**). *Cryptococcus*[37] also have narrow-based buds but are much more pleomorphic in size and may produce a "soap bubble" effect in tissue due to the dense capsule (**Fig. 14**). *Cryptococcus* species are often mucicarmine positive, but capsule deficient organisms are increasingly common. Fontana-Masson stains are helpful in diagnosing Cryptococcus

when capsule-deficient. *Talaromyces* (formerly *Penicillium) marneffei* is rarely seen in the GI tract, but may occur, especially in endemic areas.[38] Its size is similar to *Histoplasma*, but it does not bud, and large organisms may have a central septation. *Pneumocystis carinii*[39] is similar in size to *Histoplasma*, but it has a cup-shaped morphology and it does not bud. It is also extracellular, with the characteristic foamy-cast tissue reaction (**Fig. 15**).

Ideally, when fungal infection is under consideration, a separate specimen should be submitted for culture. In addition to identification, culture provides the ability to perform antifungal susceptibility testing, which is increasingly important given emerging resistance to antifungal therapy. If fresh tissue is not available, PCR from formalin-fixed, paraffin-embedded tissue can be used for identification, but sensitivity may be limited by formalin fixation.

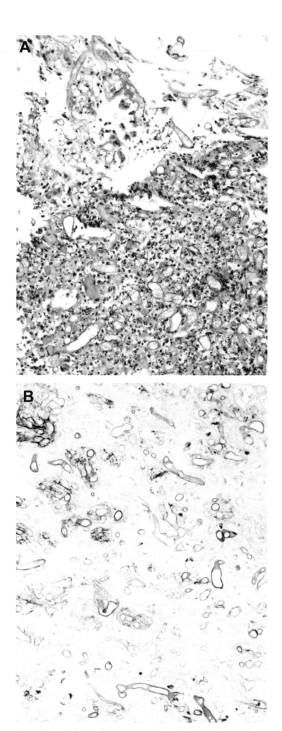

Fig. 9. Exudate from a gastric ulcer shows large, ribbon-like pauciseptate fungi with haphazard branching and optically clear centers on cross-section, typical of Mucor (*A*, H&E, original magnification 80x; *B*, GMS, original magnification 80x).

MEDICALLY IMPORTANT VIRUSES IN THE GASTROINTESTINAL TRACT

Cytomegalovirus (CMV), Herpes simplex virus (HSV), Adenovirus, and Varicella zoster (VSV) are the most commonly encountered viruses in the GI tract, and the pathologic features are summarized in Table 3. Cells infected with CMV show both nuclear and cytoplasmic enlargement. Inclusions are most often seen in endothelial cells, stromal cells, and macrophages, and only rarely in epithelial cells[40,41] (Fig. 16). Inclusions are usually within ulcer bases rather than at the edges of ulcers. Prominent apoptotic epithelial cells are common, and prominent aggregates of macrophages may surround viral inclusions within the inflammatory infiltrate. As noted above, significant endothelial infection can cause vasculitis and ischemia.

The number of inclusions that indicate clinically significant disease remains controversial, and the presence of CMV inclusions in a tissue biopsy does not necessarily correlate with plasma PCR results or viral culture.[42,43] In immunocompromised patients, even isolated CMV inclusions can indicate clinically significant disease, and the lack of plasma PCR positivity does not decrease the significance of rare inclusions. It is also important to note that the more biopsies obtained, the greater the likelihood of finding inclusions. Ultimately, decisions about what constitutes clinically significant CMV infection require the correlation of clinical, histologic, and laboratory information. The need for CMV immunohistochemistry also remains a subject of debate.[44–46] Recent studies have affirmed the use of IHC when no inclusions are found or when suspicious cells are found that require confirmation, but have argued against clinician-initiated or "up-front" ordering.

HSV-1 and HSV-2 infection are indistinguishable morphologically. Histologic findings include neutrophilic inflammation, ulceration, and acantholytic, sloughed epithelial cells.[47] Similar to CMV, prominent aggregates of macrophages may be seen within the inflammatory exudate.[48] The characteristic inclusion is the homogenous "ground glass" inclusion with peripheral chromatin margination. Inclusions may be single or multinucleate and are most often found within squamous epithelium at the edges of ulcers and in sloughed epithelial cells within the exudate (Fig. 17). Occasionally, nclusions may be found deep within ulcers, so-called "deep herpes."[49"] VZV, which rarely infects the gastrointestinal tract,

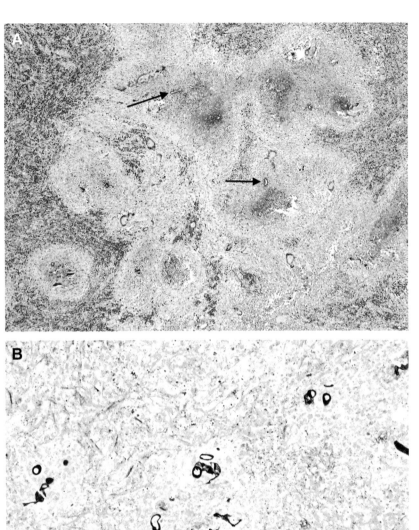

Fig. 10. B. ranarum features an eosinophilic infiltrate, necrosis, granulomas, and Splendore-Hoeppli protein reaction to the organism (arrows; A, H&E, original magnification 8x). The morphology is similar to Mucor, although some have a crinkled "crinkled cellophane ball" appearance (B, GMS, original magnification 40x).

Fig. 11. Occlusion of the underlying blood vessels by *Aspergillus* (*A*, GMS, original magnification 80x) causes ischemia of the gastric mucosa and submucosa (*B*, H&E, original magnification 8x). Note the septate hyphae of uniform width that branch at acute angles, typical of *Aspergillus* and similar species.

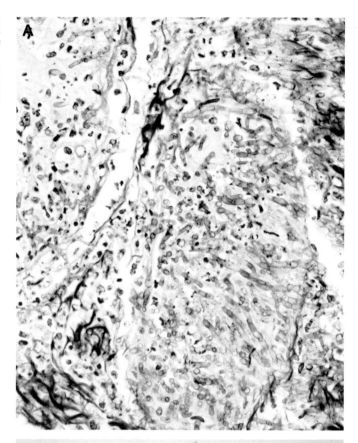

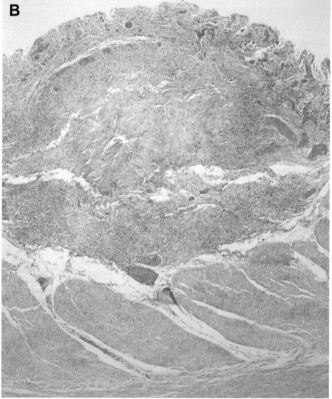

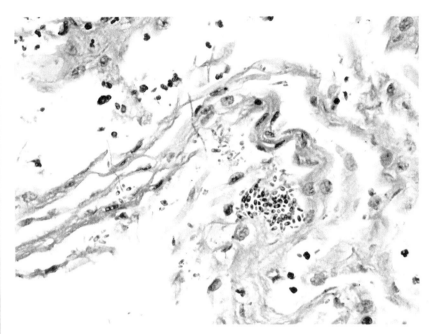

Fig. 12. Candida albicans features a mixture of budding yeast, pseudohyphae, and rare true hyphae, as seen here within the squamous epithelium of the esophagus. The typical inflammatory reaction is comprised of neutrophils (H&E, original magnification 80x).

produces inclusions identical to HSV. There are some notable differences, however, including the likelihood of VZV to involve the stomach and the lack of inflammation in the exudates[50] (Fig. 18).

Adenovirus infection of the GI tract is associated with degenerative changes of the surface epithelium, such as epithelial cell disorder, loss of cell orientation (especially goblet cells), apoptosis, and sloughing of epithelial cells[51,52] Mild villous blunting may be seen in the small bowel. Adenovirus inclusions are known as "smudge cells" due to the enlarged, basophilic nuclei without a clear nuclear membrane. They are exclusively intranuclear and fill the entire nucleus, but the cell itself is not enlarged (unlike CMV). Inclusions are typically within surface epithelial cells, particularly goblet cells, in which they are often crescent-shaped (Fig. 19).

Immunohistochemistry is very useful in distinguishing between these viruses. PCR assays are also available, but cannot necessarily distinguish active disease from viral shedding. Serology has little value in diagnosing HSV or CMV, as assays will be positive in both active and latent disease.

INFECTIONS SUPERIMPOSED ON CHRONIC IDIOPATHIC INFLAMMATORY BOWEL DISEASE

Some pathogens are well known to superinfect patients with CIIBD, often with significant clinical implications. In patients who are experiencing clinical symptom flares, the prevalence of *C. difficile* infection is much higher than patients with inactive CIIBD or patients without CIIBD.[53–56] The use of steroids and immunomodulators are also independently associated with the development of *C difficile* infection, and recurrent *C difficile* infection is common. It is important to note that biopsies may not show the usual findings of pseudomembranous colitis typically seen in patients with non-CIIBD.[56]

The association between CMV and CIIBD has been recognized for decades.[57–59] The clinical significance of rare CMV inclusions on biopsy remains a subject of debate in this patient population, however (see above). CMV infection is associated with steroids and immunomodulators, but not tumor necrosis factor antagonists. *C difficile* is also more common in patients with CIIBD who have CMV infection, and that

Fig. 13. The typical inflammatory reaction to *Histoplasma* is lynphohistiocytic, sometimes with loosely formed granulomas, as seen in this colon biopsy (*A*, H&E, original magnification 8x). The organisms appear to have a "halo" around them on H&E staining (*B*, H&E, original magnification 120x). They are uniformly small (2–5 microns) and have a bud at the more pointed pole (*C*, GMS, original magnification 120x).

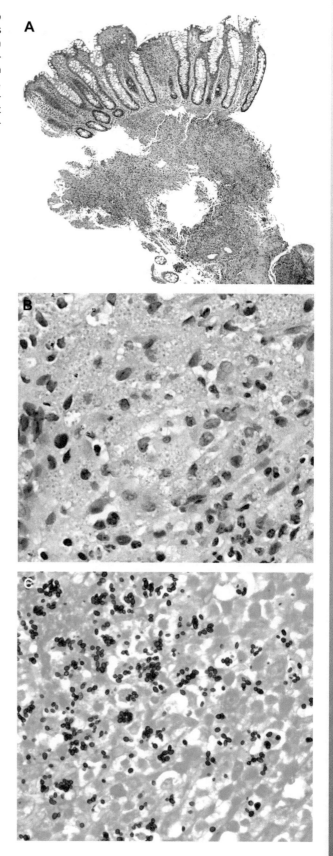

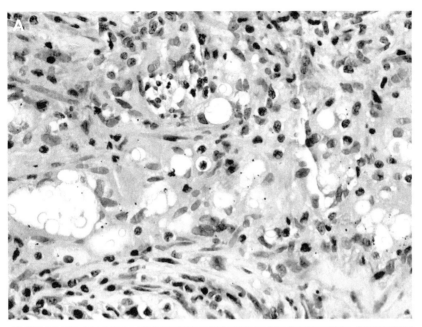

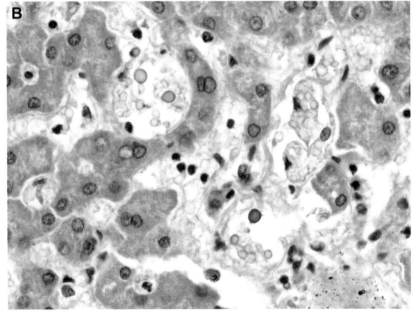

Fig. 14. Cryptococcus has a "soap bubble" appearance in H&E sections due to the capsule (*A*, H&E, original magnification 80x). The typical inflammatory reaction ranges from neutrophilic to granulomatous, and may be mixed. Mucicarmine stain highlights the size pleomorphism; in addition, some organisms are strongly mucicarmine positive whereas others are not, which can happen with capsule-deficient *Cryptococcus* (*B*, mucicarmine, original magnification 120x).

Fig. 15. Pneumocystis car-inii produces the same "foamy cast" tissue reaction in the GI tract that it does in the lung (*A*, H&E, original magnification 20x). It has a distinctive cup-shaped or "ball with the air let out" morphology and it does not bud (*B*, GMS, original magnification 120x).

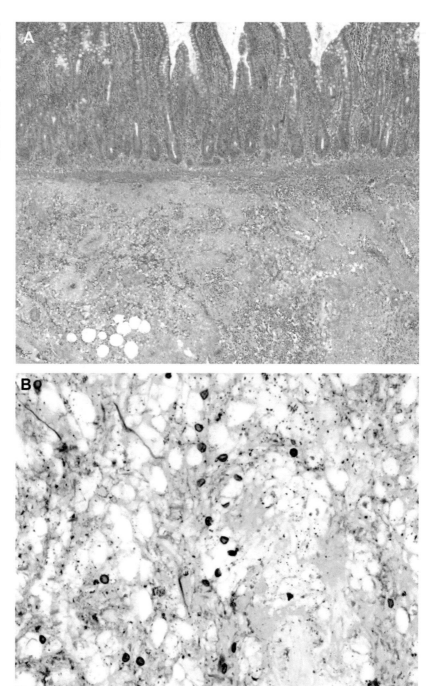

Table 3
Histologic comparison of commonly encountered GI viral infections

	CMV	Adenovirus	HSV/VZV
Location	Stromal and endothelial cells; macrophages; rarely epithelial cells Nuclear and cytoplasmic	Predominantly surface epithelium, especially goblet cells Nuclear	Epithelial cells, usually squamous; rarely deep VZV may involve glandular epithelium Nuclear
Characteristics of inclusion	"Owl's eye" morphology in nucleus; basophilic and granular in cytoplasm	Basophilic "smudge cell" filling entire nucleus; rarely acidophilic inclusions with halo	Homogeneous with "ground glass" appearance or acidophilic with clear halo and peripheral chromatin margination
Associated changes	Cellular enlargement Apoptosis Mixed inflammatory infiltrate Vasculitis	Surface cell disorder; cells not enlarged	Sloughing of epithelial cells, neutrophilic infiltrate; multinucleated cells common

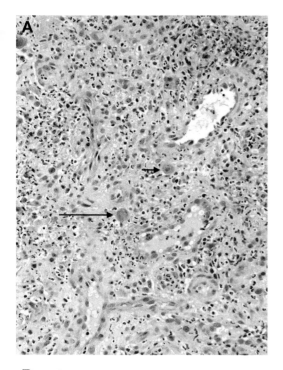

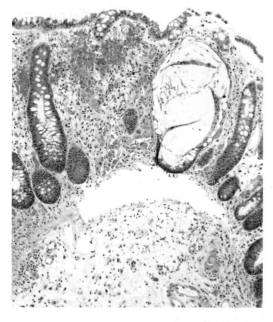

Fig. 16. CMV produces both "owl's eye" nuclear inclusions (*short arrow*) and granular, basophilic cytoplasmic inclusions (*long arrow*) (*A*, H&E, original magnification 80x). The viral inclusions are typically found in endothelial or stromal cells and may be accompanied by inflammation and apototic epithelial cells (*B*, H&E, original magnification 20x). Occasionally inclusions are seen in epithelial cells, especially in the stomach

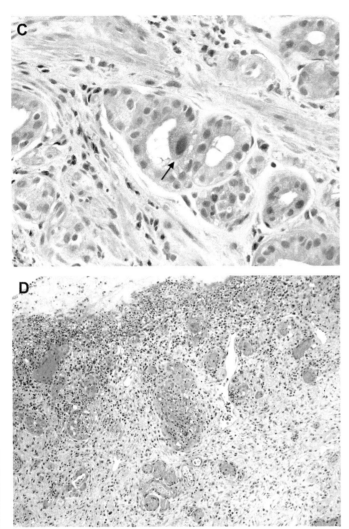

Fig. 16. *(continued)*. (*arrow; C,* H&E, original magnification 80x). This colon biopsy has so many CMV inclusions within endothelial cells that they are occluded and have associated inflammation and fibrinoid necrosis, leading to ischemia (*D,* H&E, original magnification 20x).

combination is associated with poor outcomes (**Fig. 20**).[60]

ANCILLARY STUDIES–OPPORTUNITIES AND CHALLENGES

The ability to use PCR-based assays to detect pathogens in fixed, routinely processed, paraffin-embedded (FFPE) tissue continues to increase, but also poses many challenges. There are no generally accepted recommendations for fixation, processing, and extraction techniques for FFPE tissue. Formalin fixation enhances the degradation of DNA, and causes inhibition of DNA amplification. Some authorities[61] maintain that fixation times of less than 24 hours are optimal, a goal that is rarely achievable with routine specimens. Degradation of DNA also appears to increase if the specimen is fixed at room temperature (which is often the case), and with the length of time of block storage. Fixatives other than formalin (such as mercuric or picric-acid-based fixatives) are thought to limit DNA yield even further. Unfortunately, the lesional tissue in small specimens is often exhausted by the time the specimen is sent for molecular analysis (particularly if many stains were performed), and thus sampling error may cause a negative result even when the patient truly has an infection. Conversely, specimen contamination with

Fig. 17. The "ground glass" inclusions of HSV have basophilic nuclei and peripheral chromatin margination, with associated neutrophils and mucosal acantholysis (*A*, H&E, original magnification 40x; *B*, H&E, original magnification 80x). A prominent mononuclear cell infiltrate that is rich in macrophages may be associated with HSV infection

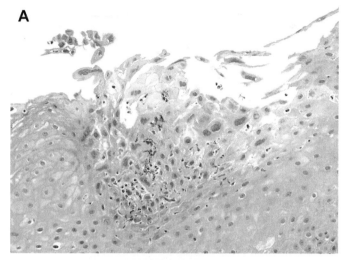

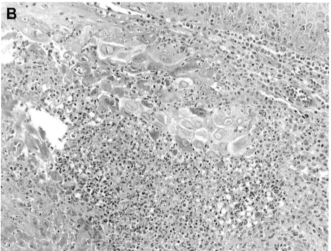

bacteria, yeasts, and molds that exist widely in nature may cause false positive results.

As noted above, stool PCR assays can detect as many as 22 bacteria, viruses, and parasites, often within hours of specimen receipt.[62–65] However, these assays detect pathogens that can differ widely in their epidemiology, virulence, and incidence of co-infection, making the interpretation of positive results challenging. The clinical significance of a positive result is often unclear, and there only a few studies that have correlated biopsy findings with positive stool PCR assays,[66–68] particularly in patients with underlying diseases such as ulcerative colitis.[69]

In summary, the application of molecular testing, while sometimes invaluable, must be done with the understanding (by both pathologists and clinicians) of the limitations of the test. As with

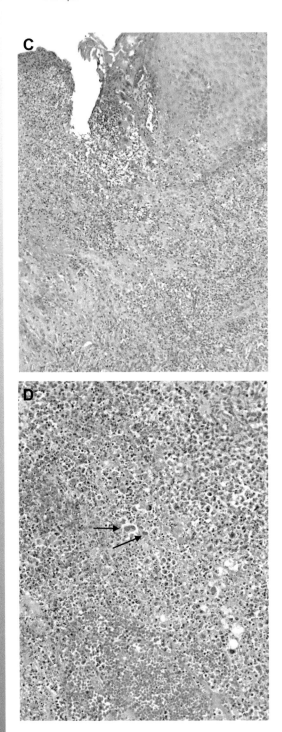

Fig. 17. (*continued*). (*C*, H&E, original magnification 20x). Occasionally HSV inclusions are found deep within ulcers rather than in the squamous epithelium at the edge (*D, arrows*, H&E, original magnification 80x).

Fig. 18. Numerous inclusions similar to HSV are seen at the base of the gastric glands in this case of VZV gastritis with abundant associated apoptotic debris (H&E, original magnification 40x. Courtesy Dr. Rhonda Yantiss).

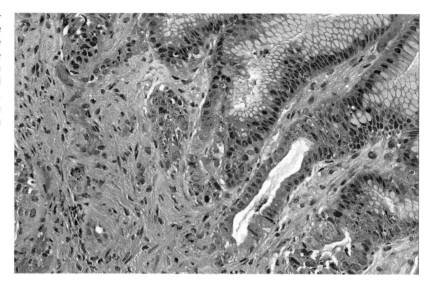

Fig. 19. Adenovirus inclusions are present within the surface epithelium of this duodenal biopsy (*arrows*). The enlarged, basophilic nuclei are known as "smudge cells." There is minimal associated inflammation (H&E, original magnification 80x).

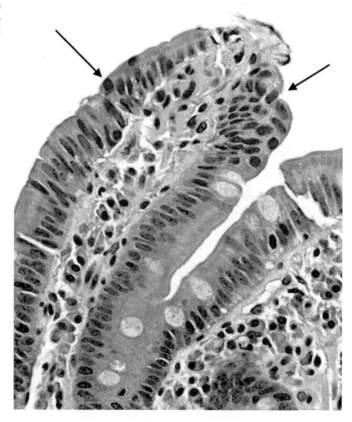

A

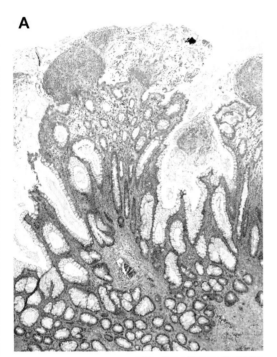

B

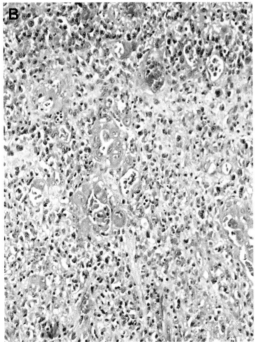

Fig. 20. This patient with an ulcerative colitis flair had both *C. difficile*, featuring typical pseudomembranes (*A*, H&E, original magnification 8x) and CMV, with numerous inclusions at the base of the ulcer (*B*, H&E, original magnification 40x).

all ancillary testing, molecular results must be correlated with the histologic findings, as well as available clinical and laboratory data.

DISCLOSURE

The author has nothing to disclose.

REFERENCES

1. Surawicz CM. The role of rectal biopsy in infectious colitis. Am J Surg Pathol 1988;12(Suppl 1):82–8.
2. Loughrey MB, Shepherd NA. Diagnostic dilemmas in chronic inflammatory bowel disease. Virch Arch 2018;472(1):81–97.
3. Lamps LW. Update on infectious enterocolitides and the diseases that they mimic. Histopathology 2015; 66(1):3–14.
4. Edwards BH. Salmonella and Shigella species. Clin Lab Med 1999;19:469–87.
5. Pegues DA, Hohmann EL, Miller SI. Salmonella including S. typhi. In: Blaser MJ, Smith PD, et al, editors. Infections of the Gastrointestinal tract. New York, NY, USA: Raven Press; 1995. p. 785–809.
6. Dekker JP, Frank KM. Salmonella, Shigella, and Yersinia. Clin Lab Med 2015;35(2):225–46.
7. Kraus MD, Amatya B, Kimula Y. Histopathology of typhoid enteritis: morphologic and immunophenotypic findings. Mod Pathol 1999;12:949–55.
8. McGovern VJ, Slavutin LJ. Pathology of Salmonella colitis. Am J Surg Pathol 1979;3:483–90.
9. Boyd JF. Pathology of the alimentary tract in Salmonella typhimurium food poisoning. Gut 198; 26: 935–944.
10. Speelman P, Kabir I, Islan M. Distribution and spread of colonic lesions in shigellosis: a colonoscopic study. J Infect Dis 1984;150:899–903.
11. Khuroo MS, Mahajan R, Zargar SA, et al. The colon in shigellosis: serial colonoscopic appearances in *Shigella dysenteriae I.* Endoscopy 1990;22:35–8.
12. Mathan MM, Mathan VI. Morphology of rectal mucosa of patients with shigellosis. Rev Infect Dis 1991;13(Supp. 4):S314–8.
13. Islam MM, Azad Ak, Bardhan PK, et al. Pathology of shigellosis and its complications. Histopahtology 1994;24:65–71.
14. Gleason TH, Patterson SD. The pathology of Yersinia enterocolitica ileocolitis. Am J Surg Pathol 1982;6:347–55.
15. El-Maraghi NRH, Mair N. The histopathology of enteric infection with Yersinia pseudotuberculosis. Am J Clin Pathol 1979;71:631–9.
16. Lamps LW, Madhusudhan KT, Greenson JK, et al. The role of *Y. enterocolitica* and *Y. pseudotuberculosis* in granulomatous appendicitis: a histologic and molecular study. Am J Surg Pathol 2001;25: 508–15.

17. Yarze JC. *Aeromonas* as a cause of segmental colitis. Am J Gastroenterol 1998;93:1012–3.

18. Farraye RA, Peppercorn MA, Ciano PS, et al. Segmental colitis associated with *Aeromonas hydrophila*. Am J Gastroenterol 1989;84:436–8.

19. Blaser JM, Parsons RB, Wang WLL. Acute colitis caused by *Campylobacter fetus ss. jejuni*. Gastroenterology 1980;78:448–53.

20. Price AB, Jewkes J, Sanderson PJ. Acute diarrhoea: Campylobacter colitis and the role of rectal biopsy. J Clin Pathol 1979;32:990–7.

21. Arnold CA, Limketkai BN, Illei PB, et al. Syphilitic and lymphogranuloma venereum (LGV) proctocolitis. Am J Surg Pathol 2013;37:38–46.

22. Jawale R, Lai KK, Lamps LW. Sexually transmitted infections of the lower gastrointestinal tract. Virchows Arch 2018;472:149–58.

23. Hoie S, Knudson LS, Gerstoft J. Lymphogranuloma venereum proctitis: a differential diagnosis to inflammatory bowel disease. Scand J Gastroenterol 2011; 46:503–10.

24. Kersh EN, Pillary A, de Voux A, et al. Laboratory processes for confirmation of lymphogranuloma venerium infection during a 2015 investigation of a cluster of cases in the United States. Sex Transm Dis 2017;44:691–4.

25. Griffin PM, Olmstead LC, Petras RE. Escherichia coli 0157:H7- associated colitis: a clinical and histological study of 11 cases. Gastroenterology 1990;99: 142–9.

26. Kelly J, Oryshak A, Wenetsek M, et al. The colonic pathology of E. coli 0157:H7infection. Am J Surg Pathol 1990;14:87–92.

27. Dignan CR, Greenson JK. Can ischemic colitis be differentiated from *C. difficile* colitis in biopsy specimens? Am J Surg Path 1997;21:706–10.

28. Dictar MO, Maiolo E, Alexander B, et al. Mycoses in the transplanted patient. Med Mycol 2000;38(Suppl 1):251–8.

29. Fleming RV, Walsh TJ, Anaissie EJ. Emerging and less common fungal pathogens. Infect Dis Clin N Am 2002;16:915–33.

30. Lamps LW, Lai KK, Milner DA Jr. Fungal infections of the gastrointestinal tract in the immunocompromised host: an update. Adv Anat Pathol 2014;21: 217–27.

31. Pilmis B, Puel A, Lortholary O, et al. New clinical phenotypes of fungal infections in special hosts. Clin Microbiol Infect 2016;22:681–7.

32. Gonzalez CE, Rinaldi MG, Sugar AM. Zygomycosis. Inf Dis Clin N Am 2002;16:895–914.

33. Roden MM, Zaoutis TE, Buchanan WL, et al. Epidemiology and outcome of zygomycosis: a review of 929 reported cases. Clin Infect Dis 2005; 41:634–53.

34. Smilack JD. Gastrointestinal basidiobolomycosis. Clin Infect Dis 1998;27:663–4.

35. Kahi CJ, Wheat LJ, Allen SD, et al. Gastrointestinal histoplasmosis. Am J Gastroenterol 2005;100(1): 220–31.

36. Lamps LW, Molina CP, West AB, et al. The pathologic spectrum of gastrointestinal and hepatic histoplasmosis. Am J Clin Pathol 2000;113(1):64–72.

37. Washington K, Gottfried MR, Wilson ML. Gastrointestinal cryptococcosis. Mod Pathol 1991;4(6): 707–11.

38. Xie Z, Lai J, Peng R, et al. Clinical characteristics of HIV-associated Talaromyces marneffei infection of intestine in Southern China. Int J Infect Dis 2022; 120:48–50.

39. Amin MB, Abrash MP, MEzger E, et al. Systemic dissemination of Pneumocystis carinii in a patient with acquired immunodeficiency syndrome. Henry Ford Hosp Med J 1990;38(1):68–71.

40. Chetty R, Roskell DE. Cytomegalovirus infection in the gastrointestinal tract. J Clin Pathol 1994;47: 968–72.

41. Kraus MD, Feran-Doza M, Garcia-Moliner ML, et al. Cytomegalovirus infection in the colon of bone marrow transplant patients. Mod Pathol 1998;11: 29–36.

42. Durand CM, Marr KA, Arnold CA, et al. Detection of Cytomegalovirus DNA in plasma as an adjunct diagnostic for gastrointestinal tract disease in kidney and liver transplant recipients. Clin Inf Dis 2013;57(11): 1550–9.

43. Yan Z, Wang L, Dennis J, et al. Clinical significance of isolated cytomegalovirus-infected gastrointestinal cells. Int J Surgical Pathol 2014;22:492–8.

44. Juric-Sekhar G, Upton MP, Swanson PE, et al. Cytomegalovirus (CMV) in gastrointestinal mucosal biopsies: should a pathologist perform CMV immunohistochemistry if the clinician requests it? Hum Pathol 2017;60:11–5.

45. McCurdy JD, Enders FT, Jones A, et al. Detection of Cytomegalovirus in patients with inflammatory bowel disease: where to biopsy and how many biopsies? Inflamm Bowel Dis 2015;21:2833–8.

46. Solomon IH, Hornick JL, Laga. AC Immunohistochemistry is rarely justified for the diagnosis of viral infections. Am J Clin Pathol 2017;147:96–104.

47. Goodell SE, Quinn TC, Mkrtichian E, et al. Herpes simplex virus proctitis in homosexual men: clinical, sigmoidoscopic, and histopathological features. New Eng J Med 1983;308:868–71.

48. Greenson JK, Beschorner WE, Boitnott JK, et al. Prominent mononuclear cell infiltrate is characteristic of herpes esophagitis. Hum Pathol 1991;22(6): 541–9.

49. Krystel-Whittemore M, Chan MP, Shalin SC, et al. Deep herpes. Am J Surg Pathol 2021;45(10): 1357–63.

50. Mostyka M, Shia J, Neumann WL, et al. Clinicopathologic features of Varicella Zoster virus infection of

the upper GI tract. Am J Surg Pathol 2021;45(2): 209–14.

51. Qiu Fz, Shen XX, Li GX, et al. Adenovirus associated with acute diarrhea: a case-control study. BMC Infect Dis 2018;18:450.

52. Lion T. Adenovirus Infections in immunocompetent and immunocompromised Patients. Clin Microbiol Rev 2014;27(3):441–62.

53. Garcia PG, Chebli LA, da Rocha Ribeiro TC, et al. Impact of superimposed Clostridium difficile infection in Crohn's or ulcerative colitis flares in the outpatient setting. Int J Colorectal Dis 2018. https://doi.org/10.1007/s00384-018-3105-8.

54. Landsman MJ, Sultan M, Stevens M, et al. Diagnosis and management of common gastrointestinal tract infectious diseases in ulcerative colitis and Crohn's disease patients. Inflamm Bowel Dis 2014;20:2503–10.

55. Maharshak N, Barzilay I, Zinger H, et al. Clostridum difficile infection in hospitalized patients with inflammatory bowel disease: prevalence, risk factors, and prognosis. Medicine (Baltim) 2018;97(5):e9772.

56. Wang T, Matukas L, Streutker CJ. Histologic findings and clinical characteristics in acutely symptomatic ulcerative colitis patients with superimposed Clostridium difficile infection. Am J Clin Pathol 2013;140:831–7.

57. Garrido E, Carrera E, Manzano R, et al. Clinical significance of cytomegalovirus infection in patients with inflammatory bowel disease. World J Gastroenterol 2013;19:17–25.

58. Kambham N, Vij R, Cartwright CA, et al. Cytomegalovirus infection in steroid-refractory ulcerative colitis: a case-control study. Am J Surg Pathol 2004;28:365–73.

59. McCurdy JD, Jones A, Enders FT, et al. A model for identifying cytomegalovirus in patient with inflammatory bowel disease. Clin Gastroenterol Hepatol 2015;13:131–7.

60. McCurdy JD, Enders FT, Khanna S, et al. Increased rates of Clostridium difficile infection and poor outcomes in patients with IBD and cytomegalovirus. Inflamm Bowel Dis 2016;22:2688–93.

61. Turashvili G, Yang W, McKinney S, et al. Nucleic acid quantity and quality from paraffin blocks: defining optimal fixation, processing and DNA/RNA extraction techniques. Exp Mol Pathol 2012;92:33–43.

62. Khare R, Espy MJ, Cebelinski E, et al. Comparative evaluation of two commercial multiplex panels for detection of gastrointestinal pathogens by use of clinical stool specimens. J Clin Microbiol 2014;52(10):3667–73.

63. Buss SN, Leber A, Chapin K, et al. Multicenter evaluation of the BioFire FilmArray gastrointestinal panel for etiologic diagnosis of infectious gastroenteritis. J Clin Microbiol 2015;53(3):915–25.

64. Zhang H, Morrison S, Tang YW. Multiplex PCR tests for detection of pathogens associated with gastroenteritis. Clin Lab Med 2015;35(2):461–86.

65. Leli C, Di Matteo L, Gotta F, et al. Evaluation of a multiplex gastrointestinal PCR panel for the aetiological diagnosis of infection diarrhoea. Infect Dis (London) 2020;52(2):114–20.

66. Axelrad JE, Joelson A, Nobel YR, et al. Enteric infection in relapse of inflammatory bowel disease: the utility of stool microbial PCR testing. Inflamm Bowel Dis 2017;23(6):1034–9.

67. Ihekweazu FD, Ajjarapu A, Kellermayer R. Diagnostic yield of routine enteropathogenic stool tests in pediatric ulcerative colitis. Ann Clin Lab Sci 2015;45(6):639–42.

68. Limsrivilai J, Saleh ZM, Johnson LA, et al. Prevalence and effect of intestinal infections detected by a PCR-based stool test in patients with inflammatory bowel disease. Dig Dis Sci 2020;65(11):3287–96.

69. Hissong E, Mowers J, Zhao L, et al. Histologic and clinical correlates of multiplex stool polymerase chain reaction assay results. Arch Pathol Lab Med 2022;146(12):1479–85.

UNITED STATES POSTAL SERVICE®
Statement of Ownership, Management, and Circulation (All Periodicals Publications Except Requester Publications)

1. Publication Title	2. Publication Number		3. Filing Date
SURGICAL PATHOLOGY CLINICS	025 – 478		9/18/2023

4. Issue Frequency	5. Number of Issues Published Annually	6. Annual Subscription Price
MAR, JUN, SEP, DEC	4	$246.00

7. Complete Mailing Address of Known Office of Publication (Not printer) (Street, city, county, state, and ZIP+4®)

ELSEVIER INC.
230 Park Avenue, Suite 800
New York, NY 10169

Contact Person
Malathi Samayan

Telephone (Include area code)
91-44-4299-4507

8. Complete Mailing Address of Headquarters or General Business Office of Publisher (Not printer)

ELSEVIER INC.
230 Park Avenue, Suite 800
New York, NY 10169

9. Full Names and Complete Mailing Addresses of Publisher, Editor, and Managing Editor (Do not leave blank)

Publisher (Name and complete mailing address)

DOLORES MELONI, ELSEVIER INC.
1600 JOHN F KENNEDY BLVD. SUITE 1800
PHILADELPHIA, PA 19103-2899

Editor (Name and complete mailing address)

TAYLOR HAYES, ELSEVIER INC.
1600 JOHN F KENNEDY BLVD. SUITE 1800
PHILADELPHIA, PA 19103-2899

Managing Editor (Name and complete mailing address)

PATRICK MANLEY, ELSEVIER INC.
1600 JOHN F KENNEDY BLVD. SUITE 1800
PHILADELPHIA, PA 19103-2899

10. Owner (Do not leave blank. If the publication is owned by a corporation, give the name and address of the corporation immediately followed by the names and addresses of all stockholders owning or holding 1 percent or more of the total amount of stock. If not owned by a corporation, give the names and addresses of the individual owners. If owned by a partnership or other unincorporated firm, give its name and address as well as those of each individual owner. If the publication is published by a nonprofit organization, give its name and address.)

Full Name	Complete Mailing Address
WHOLLY OWNED SUBSIDIARY OF REED/ELSEVIER, US HOLDINGS	1600 JOHN F KENNEDY BLVD. SUITE 1800 PHILADELPHIA, PA 19103-2899

11. Known Bondholders, Mortgagees, and Other Security Holders Owning or Holding 1 Percent or More of Total Amount of Bonds, Mortgages, or Other Securities. If none, check box ► ☐ None

Full Name	Complete Mailing Address
N/A	

12. Tax Status (For completion by nonprofit organizations authorized to mail at nonprofit rates) (Check one)
The purpose, function, and nonprofit status of this organization and the exempt status for federal income tax purposes:
☒ Has Not Changed During Preceding 12 Months
☐ Has Changed During Preceding 12 Months (Publisher must submit explanation of change with this statement)

PS Form 3526, July 2014 (Page 1 of 4 (see instructions page 4)) PSN: 7530-01-000-9931 PRIVACY NOTICE: See our privacy policy on www.usps.com.

13. Publication Title	14. Issue Date for Circulation Data Below
SURGICAL PATHOLOGY CLINICS	JULY 2023

15. Extent and Nature of Circulation			Average No. Copies Each Issue During Preceding 12 Months	No. Copies of Single Issue Published Nearest to Filing Date
a. Total Number of Copies (Net press run)			319	306
b. Paid Circulation (By Mail and Outside the Mail)	(1)	Mailed Outside-County Paid Subscriptions Stated on PS Form 3541 (Include paid distribution above nominal rate, advertiser's proof copies, and exchange copies)	228	226
	(2)	Mailed In-County Paid Subscriptions Stated on PS Form 3541 (Include paid distribution above nominal rate, advertiser's proof copies, and exchange copies)	0	0
	(3)	Paid Distribution Outside the Mails Including Sales Through Dealers and Carriers, Street Vendors, Counter Sales, and Other Paid Distribution Outside USPS®	68	67
	(4)	Paid Distribution by Other Classes of Mail Through the USPS (e.g., First-Class Mail®)	0	0
c. Total Paid Distribution (Sum of 15b (1), (2), (3), and (4))		►	296	293
d. Free or Nominal Rate Distribution (By Mail and Outside the Mail)	(1)	Free or Nominal Rate Outside-County Copies included on PS Form 3541	23	13
	(2)	Free or Nominal Rate In-County Copies Included on PS Form 3541	0	0
	(3)	Free or Nominal Rate Copies Mailed at Other Classes Through the USPS (e.g., First-Class Mail)	0	0
	(4)	Free or Nominal Rate Distribution Outside the Mail (Carriers or other means)	0	0
e. Total Free or Nominal Rate Distribution (Sum of 15d (1), (2), (3) and (4))		►	23	13
f. Total Distribution (Sum of 15c and 15e)		►	319	306
g. Copies not Distributed (See Instructions to Publishers #4 (page 83))		►	0	0
h. Total (Sum of 15f and g)		►	319	306
i. Percent Paid (15c divided by 15f times 100)			92.78%	95.75%

* If you are claiming electronic copies, go to line 16 on page 3. If you are not claiming electronic copies, skip to line 17 on page 3.

PS Form 3526, July 2014 (Page 2 of 4)

16. Electronic Copy Circulation		Average No. Copies Each Issue During Preceding 12 Months	No. Copies of Single Issue Published Nearest to Filing Date
a. Paid Electronic Copies	►		
b. Total Paid Print Copies (Line 15c) + Paid Electronic Copies (Line 16a)	►		
c. Total Print Distribution (Line 15f) + Paid Electronic Copies (Line 16a)	►		
d. Percent Paid (Both Print & Electronic Copies) (16b divided by 16c × 100)	►		

☒ I certify that 50% of all my distributed copies (electronic and print) are paid above a nominal price.

17. Publication of Statement of Ownership

☒ If the publication is a general publication, publication of this statement is required. Will be printed in the OCTOBER 2023 issue of this publication. ☐ Publication not required.

18. Signature and Title of Editor, Publisher, Business Manager, or Owner

Malathi Samayan — Distribution Controller   Date 9/18/2023

I certify that all information furnished on this form is true and complete. I understand that anyone who furnishes false or misleading information on this form or who omits material or information requested on the form may be subject to criminal sanctions (including fines and imprisonment) and/or civil sanctions (including civil penalties).

PS Form 3526, July 2014 (Page 3 of 4) PRIVACY NOTICE: See our privacy policy on www.usps.com.

Printed and bound by CPI Group (UK) Ltd, Croydon, CR0 4YY

03/10/2024

01040367-0016